T0296738

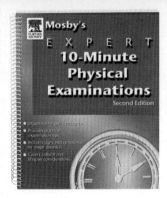

MOSBY'S SUREFIRE DOCUMENTATION

EDITION
2

DOCUMENTATION

How, What, and When
Nurses Need To Document

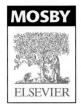

MOSBY

ELSEVIER

11830 Westline Industrial Drive
St. Louis, Missouri 63146

Notice

Previous editions copyrighted 1999

ISBN-13: 978-0-323-03434-0
ISBN-10: 0-323-03434-9

Executive Publisher: Barbara Nelson Cullen
Executive Editor: Cindy Tryniszewski, RN, MSN
Clinical Editor: Colleen Seeber-Combs, RN, MSN
Editorial Consultant: Nancy Priff
Editorial Assistant: Blair Biscardi
Publishing Services Manager: John Rogers
Project Manager: Helen Hudlin
Design Direction: Teresa McBryan

Working together to grow
libraries in developing countries
www.elsevier.com | www.bookaid.org | www.sabre.org

ELSEVIER   BOOK AID International   Sabre Foundation

Printed in the United States of America

Last digit is the print number: 9   8   7   6   5   4   3   2   1

Contents

Contributors and Consultants, vii

Foreword, ix

Overview of Documentation, 1

PART 1   Caring for Patients, 11

    When you perform your initial patient assessment, 15
    When your patient loses a peripheral pulse, 23
    When your patient has chest pain, 28
    When your patient has a myocardial infarction, 34
    When your patient has heart failure, 39
    When your patient is in shock, 46
    When your patient has cardiopulmonary arrest, 52
    When your patient has a new arrhythmia, 57
    When your patient has hypertensive crisis, 63
    When your patient has pneumonia, 68
    When your patient has pneumothorax, 76
    When your patient has an asthma attack, 81
    When your patient has a pulmonary embolism, 86
    When your patient has pulmonary edema, 91
    When your patient has pulmonary tuberculosis, 96
    When your patient has severe pain, 102
    When your patient is confused, 109
    When your patient has a seizure, 114
    When your patient has a cerebrovascular accident, 120
    When your patient is unresponsive, 125
    When your patient aspirates a tube feeding, 130

When your patient has GI hemorrhage, 133

When your patient has hypoglycemia, 140

When your patient has hyperglycemia, 143

When your patient has anaphylaxis, 147

When your patient has a transfusion reaction, 150

When your patient has HIV infection, 154

When your patient has a pressure ulcer, 159

When your patient has an infected wound, 166

When your patient has sepsis, 173

When your patient has an adverse drug reaction, 177

When your patient has I.V. infiltration, 181

When your patient has surgery, 184

When your patient has wound dehiscence or evisceration, 193

PART 2 Dealing with Challenging Patient Situations, 199

When your patient documents her own care, 202

When your patient asks to see his medical record, 204

When your patient's medical record isn't available, 208

When your patient withholds his medical history, 212

When your patient refuses treatment, 215

When your patient is noncompliant, 218

When your patient is in police custody, 220

When your patient leaves against medical advice, 225

When your patient threatens to sue, 228

When your patient makes a sexual advance, 233

When your patient becomes hostile, 236

When your patient threatens to harm someone, 239

When your patient must be restrained, 244

When your patient is anxious, 251

When your patient threatens suicide, 254

When your patient accidentally injures himself, 260

When your patient is caught smoking, 266

When your patient has contraband, 269

When your patient tampers with medical equipment, 272

When your patient hides his drugs, 275

When your patient removes her endotracheal tube, 278

When your patient removes his chest tube, 280

When your patient speaks a different language, 283

When your patient has a hearing impairment, 285

When your patient has a vision impairment, 288

When your patient is obese, 291

When your patient can't give informed consent, 294

When your patient doesn't understand the procedure he's about to undergo, 299

When your patient's equipment fails, 301

When your patient's belongings are missing, 304

When your patient's family questions the quality of care, 306

When you suspect that your patient has been abused, 308

When your patient's visitors won't leave, 311

When your patient is seriously ill, 313

When your patient asks you to witness her last will and testament, 316

When a patient dies, 320

When your patient donates an organ, 323

PART 3 Handling Difficult Professional Problems, 329

When a physician or colleague illegally alters the medical record, 332

When a colleague criticizes your care in the medical record, 335

When you find an inappropriate comment in the medical record, 337

When a physician asks to remove a medical record from the facility, 338

How to handle a physician's questionable order, 342

When you take a telephone or verbal order, 344

When a physician's order is illegible, 347

When a colleague asks you to document her care, 349

When a coworker gives your patient drugs in your absence, 351

When you suspect that a colleague is negligent, 352

How to document care given by unlicensed assistive personnel, 353

When you're asked to countersign a colleague's notes, 356

When you must work on an understaffed unit, 358

When your patient or her family asks you for medical advice, 360

When the physician and family decide to terminate the patient's life support, 363

When the physician writes a "do not resuscitate" order, 366

When you withhold a prescribed drug or other patient care, 369

When someone asks to photograph or videotape your patient, 370

When a member of the media asks for patient information, 372

When your patient is transferred or discharged, 374

How to make a late entry, 377

How to use abbreviations safely, 381

How to complete an incident report, 383

How to avoid the pitfalls of computer documentation, 386

How to protect your patient's privacy when faxing medical records, 389

How to protect patient confidentiality when using the Internet, 392

Index, 395

Contributors
and Consultants

Contributors

Mary Bowen, CRNP, DNS, JD, CNAA
Associate Professor
Vice Chair and Director of Graduate Program
Thomas Jefferson College of Health Professions
Department of Nursing
Philadelphia, Pennsylvania

Ginny W. Guido, RN, MSN, JD, FAAN
Associate Dean and Director of Graduate Studies
University of North Dakota College of Nursing
Grand Forks, North Dakota

Carole Leone, RN, MSN, CIC
Independent Nurse Consultant
Collinsville, Illinois

Reviewers (Consultants)

Cesi E. Ervin, RN, TNS, MICN, PHRN, CEN
President
2nd Opinion Legal Nurse Consultants, Inc.
Mattoon, Illinois

Audrey Dell Maxwell, RN, BS Ed
Director of Education and Program Development
Mary Washington Hospital
Fredericksburg, Virginia

Melisa Bailey, RN, LNC
President
Bailey Consultants
Houston, Texas

Marjorie Jannelle Justice, RN, BSN
Nurse Educator
St. Mary's Health System
Knoxville, Tennessee

Rae W. Langford, RN, EdD
Associate Professor
Texas Women's University
Houston, Texas

Foreword

As a nurse, you have several years of formal education and probably even more years of on-the-job training and continuing education. This combination of knowledge and hands-on experience gives you confidence in your clinical skills and patient care. But are you sure that your expertise is reflected in your documentation? If your care were called into question in court, would your notes reflect your professional competence?

The importance of good documentation can't be overestimated. If you don't document your care, the judge and jury will assume you didn't provide it. If your documentation is incomplete, misleading, or inaccurate, it can raise more legal questions than it can answer. Yet good documentation is your first line of defense in a lawsuit. It also helps protect your professional reputation—and your nursing license.

Perhaps more importantly, solid documentation plays a central role in communicating vital patient information to the rest of the health care team. Concise, thorough, and factual documentation relays critical information about the overall plan of care and it identifies what care has been given and what care remains to be provided. In today's complex, fast-paced, health care environment, it's the essential link that keeps all providers on the same page.

In recent years, handheld computers, bedside electronic documentation systems, and other technological advances have changed how we document. Now computerized medical records can be found in most health care facilities, making documentation faster and easier. But no matter whether you document with a computer keyboard or pen and paper, your notes must be accurate and complete.

Mosby's Surefire Documentation, Second Edition, explains the professional and legal aspects of documentation—and so much more.

This invaluable, up-to-the-minute handbook tells exactly how to document to prevent malpractice charges and how to avoid errors that can throw your documentation off course.

Practical, specific advice sets it apart from other nursing documentation books. *Mosby's Surefire Documentation*, Second Edition, provides expert tips, techniques, and guidance to help you document care for nearly 100 of the most common or challenging situations you face—from caring for a patient with a myocardial infarction to dealing with a colleague who illegally alters a patient's medical record. In clear, concise language thoroughly reviewed by nurse-attorneys, the book explains precisely how to respond in each situation and what to document.

Organization

Mosby's Surefire Documentation, Second Edition, is organized into three parts. The first, "Caring for Patients," tells how to record physical assessment findings and document the clinical care you provide for patients with selected medical conditions. It presents guidelines for recording your assessment findings, interventions, and patient teaching.

The next part, "Dealing with Challenging Patient Situations," explains how to document unusual or complicated situations to show that you've upheld your patient's rights while meeting other professional obligations. For instance, it describes your documentation responsibilities for a patient who can't give informed consent, refuses treatment, leaves against medical advice, asks to see his medical record, becomes hostile, or threatens suicide.

The third part, "Handling Difficult Professional Problems," focuses on safeguarding your legal status when documenting unfamiliar or complicated professional situations. It addresses such topics as altering a patient's medical record, dealing with illegible orders, protecting patient confidentiality, and completing incident reports.

Special Features

As you'll see on the inside covers, special symbols call your attention to important recurring topics throughout the book. For example, *Charting checklist* identifies essential points to record for a particular situation. *Legal brief* explains legal terms or gives practical advice for avoiding legal pitfalls. *Case law closeup* describes a specific court case, explains the court's ruling, and points out the nursing implications. *Tips & advice* helps you solve documentation problems and gives advice on recording data in complex situations. *Did you know?* presents interesting, practical, or little-known points related to the entry.

In every entry, the book embraces diversity. And to maintain a gender-neutral tone while avoiding such awkward terms as "his/her" and "he/she," we've alternated between male and female patients with each entry.

New to this Edition

We've thoroughly revised and improved the second edition to create the most current resource for your documentation needs. Throughout its pages, you'll find:

- Updated content that reflects the latest information related to documentation, including regulations and guidelines from the Health Insurance Portability and Accountability Act (HIPAA) and the Joint Commission on Accreditation of Healthcare Organizations (JCAHO)
- Expanded information about the implications of electronic documentation for nurses
- Additional recurring features to highlight key content in the *Charting checklist*, *Legal brief*, *Case law closeup*, *Tips & advice*, and *Did you know?* formats.

Mosby's Surefire Documentation, Second Edition, is an indispensable resource that you'll to turn to time and again for the most authoritative advice on documentation. Written and reviewed by experienced nurses and nurse attorneys, it will help you hone your documentation skills—and decrease your legal risks.

Mary Bowen, CRNP, DNS, JD, CNAA
Associate Professor
Vice Chair and Director of Graduate Program
Thomas Jefferson College of Health Professions
Department of Nursing
Philadelphia, Pennsylvania

Overview of Documentation

Documenting your patient's care has always been important. But with health care growing increasingly complex, expert documentation skills have become indispensable. Cost constraints, sicker patients, and nurses' growing roles further emphasize the need for a properly documented medical record.

Uses of Documentation

When you document effectively, your patient's medical record reflects your professionalism. It also acts as a continuity-of-care tool, patient protection device, quality management aid, and legal safety net. (See *Meeting basic documentation goals*, page 2.)

Continuity-of-Care Tool. Documentation coordinates health care and improves its quality. Today, the typical patient has several nurses, physicians, pharmacists, therapists, and unlicensed assistive workers. With such a large multidisciplinary team, accurate documentation may be the patient's only protection against fragmented—and possibly dangerous—care.

The patient's medical record must communicate his clinical status, medical treatment plan, nursing plan of care, and responses to interventions. In short, it must tell the entire story of his medical condition and care. All health care providers who read the record should be able to understand the patient's care and needs. (See *Does your documentation stand on its own?*, page 3.)

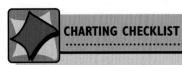
CHARTING CHECKLIST

MEETING BASIC DOCUMENTATION GOALS
When recording your patient's care, use the checklist below to determine if you've met the three basic goals of documentation.

1. Accurately describe the patient's condition and progress
❑ List initial assessment data.
❑ Identify potential and actual problems.
❑ Detail the procedures, treatments, and drugs administered.
❑ Describe the patient's responses to procedures, treatments, and drugs.
❑ Delineate patient teaching, including topics covered and evaluation of patient learning.
❑ List nursing actions.
❑ Name the people you notified of the patient's condition.

2. Communicate clearly, using specific, objective language
❑ Give exact times and dates for assessments, interventions, and other events.
❑ State the facts in a straightforward manner.
❑ Quote the patient directly when appropriate.
❑ Describe only what you've seen, heard, smelled, and touched.
❑ Avoid assumptions and personal opinions.
❑ Use only standard abbreviations and correct spelling.
❑ Make your handwriting neat and legible.

3. Satisfy legal requirements
❑ Write and, if necessary, correct documentation according to facility policy.
❑ Be accurate and truthful.
❑ Allow no omissions, blanks, or unused spaces.
❑ Note all communications with other care providers.
❑ List all assessment findings and nursing actions.
❑ Don't refer to documents that aren't part of the medical record, such as incident reports.
❑ Include your signature and the date.

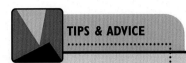

DOES YOUR DOCUMENTATION STAND ON ITS OWN?
A patient's medical record must stand on its own as a complete, accurate picture of his needs and the care he received. To determine whether your documentation meets this objective, review it closely and then ask yourself these questions:

- Did I identify the assessment data I used to formulate the nursing diagnoses and interventions?

- Did I ask key questions during the initial patient interview and later assessments to support or refute the nursing diagnoses?

- Did I base the nursing diagnoses on data obtained from the health history interview, physical examination, and diagnostic test results?

- Did I correlate health history data with physical examination findings and diagnostic test results?

- Did I write realistic expected outcomes?

- Did my nursing interventions relate to the nursing diagnoses and achieve the expected outcomes?

- Did I revise the nursing diagnoses and interventions if patient evaluation data indicated the need for revision?

- Did I communicate patient information to health care team members, as appropriate?

The record must also make sense to others who might review it, such as accreditors, attorneys, educators, researchers, and representatives of insurance companies, peer review organizations, and regulatory bodies.

Patient Protection Device. Documentation creates a record of actions taken to protect the patient from harm. These actions may include notifying appropriate people of changes in his condition and describing events that threaten his well-being.

Quality Management Aid. Medical records provide information about care practices and related problems. By reviewing patient records, quality management staff members can identify trends in care and obtain the data they need to investigate specific quality concerns.

Legal Safety Net. Documentation provides crucial legal protection. Admissible in court, the patient's medical record must be documented in an accurate, complete, systematic, logical, concise, and timely manner. Courts view the medical record as verification of patient care. In the jury's eyes, what isn't documented didn't occur.

By showing that your patient received high-quality care, a well-documented record helps defend you, your colleagues, and your employer against charges of malpractice. Incomplete, inaccurate, falsified, or delayed documentation can have severe legal consequences.

Nurse's Role

Although all health care professionals record patient care, the lion's share of documentation falls on the nurse's shoulders. Every state's nurse practice act addresses documentation.

In 1991, the American Nurses Association (ANA) added data collection to its Standards of Nursing Practice. In 1998, the organization refined and revised its principles for documentation to address issues related to this practice. To meet ANA standards, you must ensure that your documentation is:

- accurate and consistent
- clear, concise, and complete, reflecting your patient's response to nursing care
- timely and sequential

- permanently retrievable
- able to withstand scrutiny during an audit

Documentation Systems

To perform your role expertly, take an organized approach to documentation that promotes accurate, rapid record keeping. Two major systems—source-oriented and problem-oriented documentation—have been used over the years. Others include the traditional narrative notes system, which now usually is combined with another format, and newer systems, including focus charting, problem-intervention-evaluation charting, and charting by exception.

Source-Oriented Documentation. In source-oriented documentation, each professional discipline keeps separate records. For instance, nurses record nurses' notes and physicians write progress notes. This means you must consult several sources to get a complete, accurate picture of the patient's condition and care. If your facility uses a source-oriented system exclusively, you'll need to take extra steps to communicate patient information to other health care team members.

Problem-Oriented Documentation. Introduced in the late 1960s, problem-oriented documentation aids communication among team members. Based on assessment findings, team members create a problem list, formulate an initial plan of care for each problem, use multidisciplinary notes, and write a discharge summary that tells whether each problem was resolved. Typically, they record routine assessment and care on flow sheets.

Problem-oriented progress notes may be organized by the acronym SOAP:

- **S**ubjective data—what the patient says
- **O**bjective data—information gathered through physical examination
- **A**ssessment—analysis based on subjective and objective data
- **P**lan—actions to be implemented

Some facilities add more elements. The SOAPIE format includes **I**mplementation of interventions and treatments and **E**valuation of patient responses. The SOAPIER format includes **R**evision as needed, based on evaluation.

Newer versions eliminate subjective and objective data and start with assessment—a combination of subjective and objective data. Thus, the new acronym is AP, APIE, or APIER.

Narrative Notes. When writing narrative notes, you record assessment data, interventions, and patient responses in a straightforward, chronological form. Many nurses fall back on narrative notes in emergencies or unexpected situations because the system is easy to learn and flexible enough for virtually any care setting. When used as the primary documentation system, narrative notes have major disadvantages:

- They reflect the author's subjective viewpoint.
- They don't allow easy tracking of problems and trends.
- They complicate information retrieval.
- They may make care appear disorganized.
- They can be repetitive and time-consuming.
- They don't always reflect the nursing process.

Focus Charting. Introduced in the early 1980s, focus charting identifies patient-centered concerns, or foci. A focus may be a nursing diagnosis, a sign or symptom, a patient behavior, a special need, or an acute change in the patient's condition. Caregivers organize notes according to the DAR framework. **D** stands for patient assessment data, **A** for actions or interventions taken, and **R** for the patient's response.

Focus charting highlights patient concerns, incorporates aspects of the nursing process, and can be adapted to any clinical setting. Writing accurate, logical notes using this system can be challenging.

PIE Documentation. Another innovation of the early 1980s, PIE documentation groups information into three categories: Problem, Intervention, and Evaluation. Besides keeping a running list of nursing diagnoses and a daily patient assessment flow sheet, caregivers write structured progress notes that consist of:

- the problem, labeled **P,** written as a nursing diagnosis
- interventions, labeled **I,** describing the nursing actions taken
- evaluation of interventions, labeled **E**

By integrating the plan of care into the nurses' notes, PIE documentation eliminates the need for a separate plan of care. It may be time-consuming and repetitious and doesn't allow for documentation of expected outcomes. Also, it's not suited for long-term-care patients.

Charting by Exception. When you use charting by exception (CBE), you document only abnormal or significant findings or deviations from established norms. This system eliminates lengthy, repetitive notes and makes trends or changes in the patient's condition more obvious.

Effective use of CBE depends on written standards of practice that identify nurses' basic patient responsibilities and intervention protocols. Facilities using CBE must have critical pathways or interdisciplinary plans of care that address every possible patient problem.

Easy to use at the bedside, CBE reduces documentation time and gives all health care team members immediate access to patient data. But it raises legal concerns. For example, it doesn't give a complete picture of the patient's evolving condition because it requires qualitative observations only for important clinical changes. Also, it doesn't provide a written record of communication among health care team members. In *Lama v. Borras*, nurses couldn't prove that they met the needs of their patient, who showed signs of severe infection after surgery for a herniated disk. They also couldn't prove that they reported signs of infection to the surgeon. The court concluded that "intermittent charting failed to provide the sort of continuous danger signals that would be most likely to spur early intervention by health care providers." (*Lama v. Borras*, 16F.3d 473 1st Cir.[PR] 1994.)

Computerized Documentation

No matter which system is used, most health care facilities rely on computerized documentation to some degree. Typically, a large centralized computer is linked to smaller terminals in each work area or at each bedside. To gain access to a patient's medical record, you type in your password and enter the patient's code number. The computer screen then displays the patient's record.

Entering patient data by computer and storing it in one easily accessible location can make documentation more precise, accurate, legible, and timely. It also promotes multidisciplinary networking. Computers can enhance patient care by providing standardized protocols and teaching guidelines to health care team members. They can facilitate data management and communication. They also reduce the time spent filing, searching for, and retrieving patient information. This frees caregivers to spend more time meeting patients' needs.

But computers are expensive to install and maintain. During times of peak computer use, processing may slow. During routine servicing or unexpected computer failure, patient information may be unavailable. Also, critics fear that computers may dehumanize the workplace, reduce caregiver–patient interactions, and provoke fears about the confidentiality of medical records.

Nursing Information Systems. Developed to supplement existing hospital information systems, computerized nursing information systems link nursing resources to educational applications. Besides helping to manage standardized patient information, they promote documentation of all nursing process steps. Some programs signal the nurse if part of the nursing process is omitted when documenting patient care. Newer programs also prevent the nurse from ending a documentation session if the record is incomplete.

Documentation in Your Facility

Whether your facility uses traditional narrative notes or a more modern documentation system on computer, you need to document your actions expertly. To help you do this, *Surefire Documentation* presents detailed guidance in three areas.

Part 1 shows you how to document all aspects of routine care for patients with a wide range of acute and chronic conditions. Part 2 describes how to deal with challenging situations related to your patients, such as noncompliance, inability to give informed consent, and organ donation. Part 3 highlights your role in documenting difficult professional problems, such as those related to your health care team and facility. For example, its entries cover taking verbal and phone orders, faxing medical records, and dealing with colleagues who alter medical records.

● ● ●

So no matter which documentation system your facility uses, you can apply the information in this book. By doing this, you can create documentation that reduces your legal risks and provides the best possible patient care.

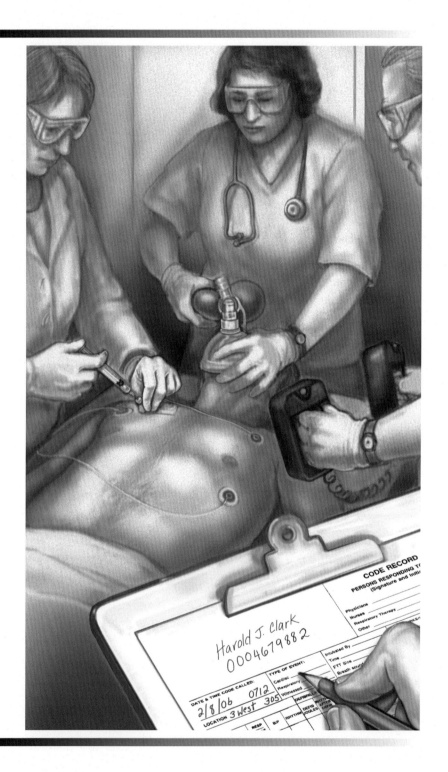

PART 1

Caring for Patients

How crucial is nursing documentation? As an information-sharing tool and a link between disciplines in a health care facility, good documentation may be the best way to promote continuity of care. Thorough, accurate documentation of the patient's physical, mental, and emotional condition is a fundamental nursing responsibility. Every time you document an assessment finding, intervention, or topic you've taught, you're helping to ensure the most effective treatment for your patient.

From a legal standpoint, documentation is the best protection the patient, health care team, and health care facility have. If you fail to record your assessment, interventions, and teaching, you're not just depriving other team members of information they need to treat patients effectively. You're also putting yourself, your colleagues, and your employer in legal jeopardy. Remember—jurors rely heavily on medical records to determine whether care was provided. Many malpractice cases that involve nurses arise from suspected failure to monitor a patient's condition or report changes in his clinical status—situations that wouldn't have arisen if the nurse had documented the patient's care properly.

Documentation and Quality-of-Care Evaluation

Patient outcomes are more important than ever in evaluating the quality of care provided—a fact that casts nursing documentation in an even brighter spotlight. Your documentation in the patient's medical record should clearly reflect your evaluation of the patient's response to nursing care measures.

Organizing Your Data

You no doubt recognize the importance of thorough documentation. But it's not always easy to make documentation a priority.

Time constraints may make other patient care activities seem more important, especially during a crisis. When you consider the amount of information you must record, you may be tempted to push documentation to the bottom of your must-do list.

You can make documentation less burdensome by organizing the information into these logical categories:

- What the patient tells you: information you obtain directly from the patient (or from indirect sources, if the patient is incapacitated)
- What you assess: information you collect from physical assessment (vital sign measurement, inspection, palpation, percussion, and auscultation)
- What you do: interventions you perform in response to assessment findings
- What you teach: instruction you give to the patient and family.

These categories serve as the framework for the entries in Part One. Each one covers documentation for a specific clinical situation.

Document What the Patient Tells You

During the health history interview, gather information about the patient's current symptoms, past health status, previous medical treatments, and responses to those treatments. All these facts help the health care team identify successful treatments to incorporate into the management plan.

Information you collect during the interview also serves as the basis of your teaching plan. By determining the patient's knowledge of his disorder, drugs, and health promotion measures, you can identify and prioritize appropriate teaching topics.

Identify the Best Information Sources. Ideally, you should obtain information directly from the patient. In some situations—for instance, if your patient is unconscious—you'll need to interview family members, refer to the patient's medical records, and consult other health care team members to find out what you need to know. If you can't obtain information from the patient or his family, explain why. For example, you could write, "Patient is unconscious; no family is present." Be sure to document as many details as you can, leaving no gaps or uncertainties that a retrospective review might reveal.

Quote the Patient Directly. Record the patient's exact words, placing quotes around them. This helps others clearly differentiate his words from yours.

If your patient has allergies, document his description of the allergic responses he has experienced. (What a patient reports as an allergy may be an expected or adverse effect of a drug.) Record information about his allergies in as many places as possible. At the very least, it should appear on the initial assessment form, the medication administration record, the nursing plan of care, the front of the patient's chart, and the patient's identification band.

Document What You Assess

Next, document your findings from vital sign measurement, inspection, palpation, percussion, and auscultation. Describe abnormal findings in detail, paying special attention to those that relate to the patient's current condition. Also document findings related to symptoms the patient has denied. These pertinent negatives can be as useful as other data in determining the underlying problem.

Be Objective and Specific. Use objective language and avoid making judgments when documenting assessment data. For instance, if you write, "The patient's heart rate was only 60," this suggests that you think his heart rate is low.

Whenever possible, quantify your findings by citing specific numbers or ranges. Instead of "Mr. Jones says he gets up a lot during the night to urinate," for example, write, "Mr. Jones states he gets up 7 or 8 times during the night to urinate." Avoid phrases like "a little" and "a lot"—they're open to wide interpretation.

Be Concrete. Describe only what you see, hear, feel, and smell during your assessment. Don't document your interpretation of the patient's behavior. Instead of "Mary Smith was crying because of her depression," for example, write, "Mary Smith was crying during the assessment."

Document What You Do

Your documentation should show that you took appropriate actions based on your assessment of the patient's condition. Record interventions as you perform them or soon afterward. Otherwise, you may forget to record important information. Note the time of each intervention to avoid the appearance that you took too long to intervene after assessing a significant finding.

Document the Patient's Response. Just because you've documented an intervention doesn't mean that your patient benefited from it. To indicate the effectiveness of an intervention, describe the patient's response—whether positive or negative. Be sure to evaluate his emotional response as well as his physical response.

Record Referrals. Document the details of discharge planning. Your documentation should indicate whether additional resources, such as home care, are needed and any referrals you make to secure those resources. Also record your meetings with staff members from other disciplines who are involved in the patient's care.

Document What You Teach

A patient's progress during your care and after discharge may depend on how well he understands his condition, treatment plan, and home care. When you document your teaching, clearly indicate the patient's understanding of the instructions you've provided. Also note any family members or support people who were present during patient teaching and the extent of their involvement in discharge planning. If family members or support people plan to take a key role in patient care after discharge, document their understanding of your teaching as well. If you think that the patient or a member of his support system needs additional instructions, note this so that other health care team members can cover that topic in their teaching.

How Documentation Helps You Evaluate the Plan of Care

All the information you obtain from the health history interview, physical assessment, nursing interventions, and the patient's response to interventions contributes to the plan of care. Thorough documentation helps you evaluate the plan and revise it as needed.

WHEN YOU PERFORM YOUR INITIAL PATIENT ASSESSMENT

As you conduct and document the initial patient assessment, keep in mind that the entire health care team will use this information throughout the patient's stay. If your patient's care is challenged in court, the thoroughness, accuracy, and legibility of your documentation can prove crucial.

Begin your assessment with the health history interview, focusing on the patient's chief complaint. Document everything she tells you. If necessary, obtain data from other sources too—family members, friends, and medical records.

Next, perform a complete physical examination, recording all findings. Be sure to include pertinent negatives—absence of a significant finding, such as "no abdominal tenderness" in a patient with abdominal distention.

Then, depending on your findings, perform and document rapid interventions needed to address urgent medical problems you've uncovered. Finally, document that you taught the patient about all topics relevant to her care and condition.

Document What the Patient Tells You

During the health history interview, use simple terms and avoid complex medical language. Record the patient's chief complaint exactly as she relates it, placing quotation marks around her words. Then begin a detailed health history, which can include the areas described below.

Current Health Status. Document the signs, symptoms, or changes in health status that led the patient to seek medical care.

Find out which prescription drugs she takes. Record their names, dosages, and administration times and routes, as well as the time she took the last dose. Ask whether she's taking nonprescription drugs; record the name of each one along with her reason for taking it. Document allergies to drugs, foods, or other substances.

Next, list factors the patient mentions that could increase her risk for infection, including steroid use, chemotherapy, recent organ transplantation, recent exposure to infectious diseases, and high-risk behaviors (such as IV drug use and unprotected sex).

Document complaints of burning or discomfort during urination, urinary frequency, incontinence, and difficulty starting the urine stream. For a male patient, document a history of prostate enlargement.

Record reports of diarrhea or constipation, and document laxative or stool softener use. Document the patient's usual bowel patterns.

Past Health Status. Ask the patient to describe her medical history, including previous hospitalizations, diagnostic tests, surgeries and other treatments, chronic conditions, and acute illnesses. Also record falls, trauma, and accidents she has experienced. Note the date for each item she reports, along with the treatment administered. Then list immunizations she has received and childhood diseases she has had.

Family Health Status. Ask the patient about the general health of her immediate family members. Find out the cause of death for deceased members. Thoroughly document her answers.

Occupation. Record the patient's occupation. Be sure to note potentially harmful occupational hazards or exposures she reports.

Developmental Considerations. Document the patient's age, growth, physical abilities and limitations, and cognitive abilities. To help determine her growth and developmental needs, evaluate and document her activities of daily living and physical capacity to perform them. (See *Documenting growth and developmental information: What JCAHO requires.*)

Personal Habits. Explore the patient's personal habits and lifestyle, and carefully record what she tells you. Include her use of alcohol, over-the-counter and "street" drugs, caffeine, and tobacco. State the number of years she has used the substance she reports using.

Then find out about the patient's sexual behavior. Ask whether she is sexually active. Document a history of high-risk sexual behavior or sexual difficulties. Be sensitive when asking questions about sexuality—many patients are embarrassed or feel threatened when discussing this topic.

If your patient is of child-bearing age, ask if she uses contraception. Also ask if she has ever been pregnant and, if so, how many live births she has had. Document menstrual irregularities, fertility problems, and menopausal symptoms.

Religious and Cultural Influences. Ask the patient to describe her religious and cultural background. Both may have a bearing on health practices and beliefs, so be sure to document her answers completely.

Health Promotion Patterns. Document measures the patient regularly takes to stay healthy. Evaluate her dietary pattern by recording her average daily food intake. Ask about food preferences, and find out whether she has a nutritional disorder. Then evaluate and document her compliance with dietary restrictions. Also record problems related to nutrition, such as nausea, vomiting, abdominal pain, and difficulty chewing or swallowing.

Next, find out whether and how often the patient exercises, and record this information. Document her usual sleep patterns. Record the name and phone number of her primary health care provider.

Educational Level. Assess and record the patient's educational level. Then determine her ability to read and understand the information presented to her.

DID YOU KNOW?

DOCUMENTING GROWTH AND DEVELOPMENTAL INFORMATION: WHAT JCAHO REQUIRES

The Joint Commission on Accreditation of Healthcare Organizations (JCAHO) requires health care professionals to assess each hospitalized patient's physical, psychological, and social status. Guidelines published in 1998 *Hospital Accreditation Standards* require assessment of the patient's growth and development and provision of age-appropriate care.

In most cases, you'll document growth and developmental needs as part of the admission assessment. The following examples show how you might document such needs for patients of various ages:
- *Male, age 70.* Mr. Harris talks about the recent loss of two close friends.
- *Female, age 58, who suffered a hip fracture.* Ms. Robinson is concerned about her elderly uncle. She is the sole caregiver for the 88-year-old man and does not know how she will care for him now that her injury prevents her from taking care of herself.
- *Male, age 17, who has paraplegia.* Billy describes his frustration with being dependent on his mother. He wants to attend a school on the West Coast and live in a dormitory.
- *Male, age 2, with respiratory syncytial virus infection.* Ryan cries for his mother and refuses to drink liquids.

Communication Barriers. Note obvious communication barriers. For instance, if the patient has a foreign accent, document how well she speaks and understands English. If her English is poor, arrange for an interpreter. Also check for and document speech or comprehension problems and hearing or vision deficits.

Home Environment. Document information about the patient's home environment, including details that may indicate abuse. If you suspect abuse, follow your facility's policy and state's laws for reporting the situation, and document your actions.

Help the patient identify home safety hazards. Document them along with related teaching you provide.

Advance Directive. Ask the patient whether she has an advance directive. If she does, attach a copy of the document to her medical record. If she doesn't, ask if she would like relevant information. Arrange for the social services department to assist her.

Document What You Assess

After completing the health history interview, perform a physical examination, recording the information you gather in as much detail as possible. Start by taking the patient's vital signs and measuring her height and weight. Then move on to inspection, palpation, percussion, and auscultation. Record normal and abnormal findings. Be sure to note physical responses you elicit, such as tenderness on palpation.

Vital Signs, Height, and Weight. Obtain and record the patient's heart rate, respiratory rate, temperature, and blood pressure. Measure her height and weight, noting the type of scale used, time of day, and clothing the patient is wearing. Record any recent weight gain or loss the patient reports.

Head and Neck. When assessing the patient's head and neck, check for and document asymmetry, unusual hair distribution, and other abnormal findings, such as lesions, lumps, edema, and erythema. Then look for jugular vein distention.

Palpate the carotid pulses one at a time, and document their rate and intensity and any abnormal findings. Then auscultate and document bruits you hear over the carotid arteries.

Next, note the location, size, and mobility of palpable lymph nodes. Then record the results of cranial nerve testing.

Eyes, Ears, Nose, and Throat. Evaluate and document the patient's visual acuity. Note whether she wears eyeglasses or uses other vision correction devices. Assess and document eye movement, tearing, color recognition, scleral characteristics, and pupillary reaction to light.

If appropriate, evaluate the patient's hearing, documenting the results and noting whether she uses a hearing aid. Include your observations of the external ear, auricle, and tympanic membrane.

Next, note nasal flaring or obstruction. Document the color and consistency of secretions, and note abnormalities.

Document dental or gum abnormalities you detect as well as the use of dentures. Record your observation of the patient's mouth and throat and her swallowing ability. Then assess and document movement of the facial muscles and joints and integrity of the gag reflex.

Nervous System. Evaluate and document the patient's coordination, motor and sensory functions, reflexes, nerve functions, level of consciousness, memory, cognitive ability, judgment, speech, and mental and emotional status. Also document complaints of headache, blurred vision, vertigo, and lightheadedness.

During this assessment, evaluate and document the patient's orientation to person, place, time, and situation. Also determine whether she exhibits knowledge of current events. If you detect confusion or memory loss, record specific examples. Also document your assessment of the patient's speech and thought processes and ability to understand what she is told. Note whether she can communicate her needs and perform activities of daily living. Describe her attention span, and note signs of anxiety, agitation, and irritability.

Respiratory System. Evaluate and document the patient's respiratory rate and rhythm, use of accessory breathing muscles, chest expansion, and skin and nail bed color. Record chest auscultation findings and document tracheal position. Then percuss the chest and assess for fremitus. Also evaluate for dyspnea and chest pain, and note cough and sputum production.

Cardiovascular System. Document your patient's pulse rate, rhythm, and intensity. Record orthostatic blood pressure changes.

Then auscultate and document heart sounds, and record reports of chest pain and shortness of breath.

Next, evaluate the arms and legs for edema, capillary refill, temperature, and color; record your findings. If electrocardiography is performed, document the rhythm, rate, and any abnormalities of the heart that it shows.

Gastrointestinal System. Inspect the patient's abdomen, and document whether it is flat, round, symmetrical, distended, or concave. Then record your findings as you auscultate bowel sounds and percuss the abdomen and liver. Describe the location of the liver border, and note any ascites. Document areas of abdominal tenderness or guarding. Palpate the spleen and kidneys, and record your findings. If you detect an abnormality, describe its location, such as the right upper abdominal quadrant.

Elimination. Note the color, clarity, amount, and odor of the patient's urine. Record the stool color and consistency, and check it for blood. Document your assessment of the perianal area for skin abnormalities, hemorrhoids, and loss of sphincter tone.

Reproductive System. Document abnormalities you see when inspecting the genitalia. Also note scars in this area and abnormal vaginal or penile drainage. For a female patient, inspect and palpate the breasts as well, and document your findings.

Musculoskeletal System. Evaluate and document the patient's range of motion, gait, posture, symmetry, body alignment, muscle strength, and joint movement. Note deformities and edema around joints. If she reports musculoskeletal pain, record whether the pain worsens with movement. Describe the use of assistive devices, such as a cane, walker, wheelchair, prosthesis, or orthotic device.

Skin. Assess the color, tone, texture, moistness, hygiene, and turgor of the patient's skin. Also note hair distribution, and inspect for lesions; record your findings. Evaluate the condition of her nails and hair. Document areas with obvious skin breakdown. Pay special attention to skin problems reported during the interview, such as rashes and itching.

Psychosocial Status. Document noteworthy nonverbal behavior, such as lack of eye contact. Also record stressors in the patient's life, and describe the mechanisms she uses to cope with them.

Document What You Do

Take actions to resolve immediate or acute problems your assessment has uncovered, and document these actions as soon as possible. Suppose, for example, a newly admitted patient with diabetes has not eaten all day after taking her full insulin dose in the morning. Appropriate nursing actions include notifying the physician, checking the patient's blood glucose level, and giving her a snack, as appropriate.

Patient Identification. Provide your patient with proper identification, including allergies and special precautions. Make sure that the patient's unique identifying information, such as her name and medical record number, is consistent and correct in all paperwork and electronic or computer-based systems. Verify with her that the information on the identification form and jewelry inventory is correct, and document that you did this.

Orientation. Orient your patient to her surroundings, and explain your facility's policies on smoking, visiting hours, and other relevant matters. Record your actions.

Safety and Security. Document specific measures you take to ensure your patient's safety and protect her privacy and confidentiality. If she has a history of falls, take safety measures and follow your facility's fall prevention policy. Then document the steps you took. Make an itemized inventory of her belongings, indicating whether they will stay with her, be sent home, or be turned over to the security department. Encourage the patient to send valuables home or have them locked up; document your actions and her response. If her belongings are sent to the security department, document the location of the security receipt and the name of the person who signed it.

Document What You Teach

Detailed, reliable documentation is essential for discharge planning, which begins as soon as the patient is admitted. Information you obtain from your initial assessment will help you determine your patient's readiness to learn and identify areas in which she requires instruction. At the time of admission, focus on introducing pertinent subjects, including the following:

- hospital environment
- patient rights, including the right to privacy (See *Complying with HIPAA*.)
- disease process
- prescribed drugs, including their names, dosages, administration times and routes, adverse effects, and storage

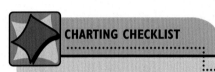

CHARTING CHECKLIST

COMPLYING WITH HIPAA

The Health Insurance Portability and Accountability Act (HIPAA) helps protect the patient's privacy by safeguarding health care information, such as medical records, medical data collected by or communicated to health care providers by oral, electronic, or paper routes, as well as any information that relates to the patient's health, health care, or payment history. HIPAA gives patients better control over their personal health records and gives health care providers uniform standards of practice related to the disclosure of health care information.

Here's how you can comply with HIPAA standards when documenting assessment findings or other medical information:

❑ When admitting a patient, provide a copy of her privacy rights.

❑ When taking a health history or providing care, keep your voice low and ask others to leave the room, if possible.

❑ Keep medical records in a secure location. If charts are held at the nurse's station, shield the names from the view of people who pass by.

❑ When documenting electronically, make sure the computer screen isn't visible to visitors and others.

❑ Distribute a patient's private information on a need-to-know basis. This rule applies to information given in writing, by phone or fax, and in electronic form. Check your facility's policies and procedures or consult an administrator to determine whether you need patient authorization before sharing information. Also, when you need a patient's private information, remember to request only the data relevant to her care.

❑ Remove any patient identifiers, such as her name and social security number, from documents that you transmit by fax or e-mail. If needed, you may add a cover sheet that tells why you're sending the documents.

- scheduled tests and procedures
- safety measures, including the use of side rails and call buttons
- ambulation privileges
- nutritional needs, supplements, or restrictions
- signs and symptoms to report
- community resources
- home care

To provide a baseline for later teaching sessions, thoroughly document your assessment of the patient's understanding of every topic you teach. Use measurable concepts, such as "Patient is able to verbalize symptoms, demonstrate use of the call button, and correctly answer questions." Finally, document areas in which she requires further teaching.

WHEN YOUR PATIENT LOSES A PERIPHERAL PULSE

Loss of a peripheral pulse may signal interruption of circulation—a potentially life-threatening event. If your assessment reveals this finding, you'll need to act rapidly. Besides reviewing your patient's medical history, you must quickly evaluate his current health status. You'll also need to record your findings accurately to ensure prompt, effective treatment.

Document What the Patient Tells You

Record an abbreviated version of the patient's medical history, especially noting a previous diagnosis of peripheral vascular disease, diabetes mellitus, heart disease, arterial occlusive disease, or other disorders that may predispose the patient to an arterial occlusion. If he reports chronic skin ulcers, injury, trauma, surgery, or wounds in the affected area, record that information. Pinpoint the exact location of the affected area, and detail treatments the patient received for the condition.

Next, document reports of pain, weakness, numbness, tingling, and decreased sensation in the arm or leg that has lost the pulse.

Determine whether the patient's symptoms are relieved by rest, and note this in the medical record. Also document other symptoms, even if they seem unrelated to the absent pulse. Because decreased circulation in an arm or leg may reflect a systemic problem, you'll need to check for and document signs and symptoms of reduced cardiac output, such as hypotension, decreased level of consciousness, and chest pain.

Document What You Assess

Although signs and symptoms vary with the cause of the absent peripheral pulse, you can expect these abnormal findings in the affected arm or leg:

- weakness
- pain
- numbness
- tingling
- discolored nail beds or skin
- edema
- sluggish capillary refill
- cool skin

Make sure you describe the affected arm or leg in detail, including its circumference, skin temperature and appearance, nail bed color, briskness of capillary refill, and the patient's ability to move the arm or leg.

Next, compare the affected arm or leg with the opposite one, and record your findings to help determine the circulatory status of the pulseless arm or leg. Measure the circumference of both arms or legs at two or more places. (See *Documenting your measurements.*)

Then, using a Doppler device if possible, auscultate for a pulse in the arm or leg. Record the presence or absence of a bruit. If you see an open area or a break in the skin, document its location, size, and color and carefully describe the lesion's edges. Also document the amount, color, and odor of drainage.

Next, record information that might help determine the cause of the pulse loss. To do this, measure the apical pulse and determine whether a pulse deficit exists; assess level of consciousness; measure blood pressure; evaluate urine output; and note dyspnea,

TIPS & ADVICE

DOCUMENTING YOUR MEASUREMENTS

If your patient loses his peripheral pulse, the circumference of the involved arm or leg may change. This may indicate whether his underlying condition is improving or worsening. To ensure accurate assessment over time, always measure the arm or leg at exactly the same location each time and thoroughly document the location you're using.

When possible, mark the patient's skin at the top and bottom edges of the measuring tape. If you're using such skin markings as a guide, note this in your documentation. For instance, you might write, "Right leg circumference: 30″ midthigh, 20″ midcalf, measured using skin markings."

If you can't mark the patient's skin, refer to an easy-to-find landmark to indicate where you took the measurement. For a thigh measurement, you might use the bend of the knee, as the following example shows: "Placed bottom edge of measuring tape on right anterior thigh 6″ above bend of knee."

You can also use a preprinted diagram to document measurement sites or to indicate skin abnormalities. To record a wound's location, for example, you can indicate its color and size in the margin. If the patient has multiple areas of skin breakdown, assign a number or letter to each area, and then reference the areas in the narrative section of your note. For instance, you may write, "Cultures taken from right leg wound A." You can also indicate changes in skin color or temperature on the human outline.

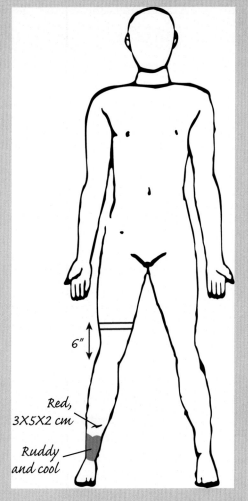

6″

Red,
3X5X2 cm

Ruddy
and cool

chest or back pain, abdominal pain or distention, and nausea or vomiting. These assessments help identify the cause of the lost pulse, such as shock, hemorrhage, or aneurysm.

Document What You Do

As you intervene during the patient's acute illness and his recovery, use the information below to guide your documentation and tailor the written plan of care to the patient's needs.

Frequent Monitoring. Document your assessment of the affected arm or leg and the patient's overall condition every 1 to 2 hours, or as indicated. Include vital signs; skin condition, temperature, and color; capillary refill; edema; presence or absence of pain; and presence or absence of blood flow by Doppler device. Compare these assessment findings with earlier findings.

Removal of Constricting Items. If compartment syndrome has caused the loss of your patient's pulse, assist with removal of the constricting item; document your actions. For example, if the syndrome is resulted from a tight bandage or cast, record its immediate removal, which should occur before other interventions.

Drugs and IV Therapy. If the physician prescribes drugs, such as vasodilators, to improve your patient's circulation, document the drug name, dosage, and administration time and route. Always measure and record your patient's blood pressure before giving a vasodilator. Also, keep in mind that vasodilators commonly cause orthostatic hypotension, so you'll need to take—and document—precautions to avoid patient injury.

If the physician prescribes anticoagulant therapy, document the patient's activated partial thromboplastin time (APTT), prothrombin time (PT), and international normalized ratio (INR) of prothrombin time before initiating therapy and every 6 to 24 hours thereafter, as ordered. Before anticoagulant therapy starts, record evidence that your patient may be at risk for bleeding, such as a history of heme-positive stools, GI bleeding, or ulcers. If his APTT, PT, and INR are abnormal, document that you notified the physician of the results and record the physician's response.

If the physician orders IV fluids or blood transfusions, such as to treat underlying hypovolemia or bleeding, document all agents you administer. Include the time and date you initiated the infusion, the type of catheter and dressing used, and your assessment of the IV site, dressing, delivery device, and patency of the IV line. During the infusion, monitor and record the patient's hemodynamic status to evaluate his response to IV therapy.

If the patient will be receiving a blood transfusion, place a signed transfusion consent form in his medical record before the transfusion begins, and document that the blood identification has been checked against the patient's identification band and verified by two nurses. During the transfusion, record his vital signs as directed by facility policy. Record signs and symptoms of a transfusion reaction and your interventions, such as stopping the transfusion. Also document the patient's response to the transfusion and changes in his vital signs and hemodynamic values.

Pain Management. If your patient reports pain in the pulseless arm or leg, document the measures you take to decrease the pain, such as using special positioning of the arm or leg or giving analgesics. Note the patient's response to pain-relief interventions. For example, you may note, "Patient rates his pain as a 2 on a 0-to-10 scale, with 0 indicating no pain and 10 indicating the worst pain imaginable, 1 hour after receiving the analgesic."

Proper Positioning. If tests show an arterial obstruction, which contraindicates elevating the affected arm or leg, document that you're keeping the patient lying flat.

Pressure Relief. Record your interventions to relieve pressure on the affected arm or leg—essential for preserving its skin and tissue integrity. For a leg, record the type of mattress the patient has; use of a heel protector, foot cradle, or footboard; and frequency of repositioning.

Activity. If you assist your patient with active or passive range-of-motion exercises, document the type of exercise performed, its duration, and the patient's tolerance. Note movement limitations or weaknesses he exhibits. Also document the safety precautions you take and the use of antiembolism stockings, if ordered.

Document What You Teach

Your documentation must include the teaching you provide to help your patient prevent the underlying condition from recurring. Evaluate and note in the record whether the patient and family understand your teaching. As appropriate, include the following topics in your teaching and documentation:

- disease process
- diagnostic tests, such as Doppler ultrasonography, ventilation-perfusion scan, and x-rays
- recommended procedures, such as angioplasty
- prescribed drugs, such as heparin, warfarin, vasodilators, and thrombolytics, including their names, dosages, administration times and routes, adverse effects, and storage
- necessary precautions and follow-up tests if the patient must take an anticoagulant
- use of antiembolism stockings, if ordered
- recommended activity and exercise levels
- proper positioning of the arm or leg
- avoidance of constrictive clothing, leg crossing, and staying in one position for prolonged periods
- smoking cessation
- proper nutrition
- signs and symptoms to report
- wound and skin care
- scheduled follow-up visits

WHEN YOUR PATIENT HAS CHEST PAIN

Because chest pain may indicate a myocardial infarction (MI) or another potentially fatal condition, always take this symptom seriously. Act quickly to perform a focused assessment and intervene promptly as indicated. Remember—documentation of your assessment findings must convey the essential information the health care team needs to guide treatment, especially when your patient's life is in danger.

Document What the Patient Tells You

When documenting your patient's chest pain, record her exact description of this symptom, placing quotes around her words.

Ask her to rate pain severity on a scale of 0 to 10, with 0 indicating no pain and 10 indicating the worst pain imaginable.

Then have your patient point to the exact pain location; document her response. Ask whether the pain radiates to other parts of her body, such as her jaws, shoulders, arms, or back. Document accompanying symptoms the patient reports, such as shortness of breath and nausea. Whenever possible, record her own words, not your interpretation of them.

Next, document the pain's duration. Ask when the pain started and whether it is steady or intermittent. Determine whether the patient has had chest pain before. If she has, ask her to compare her current pain with that in previous episodes; carefully document her response.

Ask whether any factor (such as activity) triggered the chest pain. Find out whether anything makes it better (such as rest or nitroglycerin) or worse (such as breathing deeply). Assess and document her emotional status, noting, for instance, if she is anxious or reports a feeling of impending doom.

Health History. Document pertinent health history information, such as a history of heart disease, hypertension, or hypercholesterolemia. Note other risk factors for heart disease, such as a family history of it, advanced age, history of smoking, diabetes mellitus, obesity, and a sedentary or stressful lifestyle. Document the use of estrogen or oral contraceptives. Also record chronic diseases, hospitalizations, procedures, and surgeries the patient reports.

Obtain a drug history, recording the names, dosages, and administration times and routes for all drugs the patient uses. Record the time of her last dose of each. Document drug and other allergies the patient reports.

Document What You Assess

Measure the patient's vital signs, especially noting tachycardia or bradycardia, an increased respiratory rate, and abnormally high or low blood pressure. Record your auscultation of heart sounds, including their strength and clarity. If you hear abnormal sounds, note the stethoscope location. Document whether the patient's heart rate is regular or irregular.

Then document patient actions (such as guarding and holding the chest) and behaviors (such as anxiety and restlessness) that suggest she's in pain. Note changes in her mental status too, such as decreased level of consciousness, disorientation, and confusion.

Next, evaluate the patient's respiratory rate and pattern. Record dyspnea, use of accessory breathing muscles, and jugular vein distention. Obtain and document the patient's pulse oximetry reading. Then assess her skin, recording such abnormalities as coolness, clamminess, pallor, and cyanosis.

Arrange for your patient to undergo a baseline 12-lead electrocardiogram (ECG). Then review it with the physician to detect abnormal rhythms and other changes. If permitted by facility policy, place a copy of the tracing at the bedside for quick comparison during future ECG evaluations.

Document What You Do

As you intervene during the patient's acute illness and recovery, expect to implement and document the following general interventions. Because many interventions for a patient with chest pain depend on the underlying condition—for instance, if diagnostic tests reveal that your patient has had an MI—she may require additional interventions. As always, document your interventions and the patient's responses.

Frequent Monitoring. Record your patient's vital sign measurements every few minutes until her chest pain subsides and then every hour or as ordered. As required by your facility, use a flow sheet with columns to record the patient's heart rate and rhythm, respiratory rate, and blood pressure. If the flow sheet includes several blank columns, you can label one "Pain" and document the patient's 0-to-10 pain rating next to her vital signs. In the other blank columns, record her signs and symptoms, as well as the treatments administered.

Document the times you obtain laboratory samples, such as blood samples for cardiac isoenzymes or troponin. Record the results and your communication of the results to the physician.

Record the patient's fluid intake and output every 4 to 8 hours. Notify the physician of a significant imbalance or urine output below 30 ml/hour. Document the time of notification, the physician's response, and your actions.

Oxygen Therapy. Record your patient's initial pulse oximetry reading, respiratory assessment findings, and arterial blood gas (ABG) analysis results. If the physician prescribes oxygen, document the time oxygen therapy began, the oxygen flow rate, and the delivery device used, such as a nasal cannula or face mask. Document vital sign measurements and pulse oximetry readings frequently until these findings return to a normal range and every 4 hours thereafter. Document the oxygen flow rate together with the pulse oximetry reading and ABG levels.

Continuous Cardiac Monitoring. Document the time the patient was first placed on a cardiac monitor and your teaching about the reason for monitor use. Also record which lead is being displayed.

Obtain a rhythm strip, and label it with the patient's name, time and date, and lead displayed. Place a rhythm strip in your patient's medical record as often as your facility requires, any time her condition changes, and whenever you note ectopic beats or an arrhythmia on the ECG tracing. For each strip, note the heart rate and rhythm, PR-interval and QRS-complex duration, and, if present, ST-segment elevation or depression. If you detect a significant change in the patient's rhythm strip, document the change. Then notify the physician and record the time of notification, the physician's response, and your actions.

Drug and IV Therapy. Document the names, dosages, and administration times and routes of drugs you administer. Before and after giving a drug such as nitroglycerin or morphine, measure and document the patient's vital signs. If vital sign measurements cause you to question whether or not to give the drug, document that you communicated your concern to the physician, along with the physician's name and the time and method of notification—for instance, by pager, cell phone, or answering service or in person. (See *Should you honor orders from a physician's assistant?*, page 32.) Record the physician's response and your subsequent interventions. To help gauge the patient's response to drugs, assess and document chest pain severity on a 0-to-10 pain rating scale each time you administer a dose.

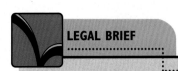

LEGAL BRIEF

SHOULD YOU HONOR ORDERS FROM A PHYSICIAN'S ASSISTANT?
What should you do if a physician's assistant orders nitroglycerin and morphine
to relieve your patient's chest pain? Should you administer them—or request
an order directly from the physician? You won't find an across-the-board
answer. Although several authorities and agencies have issued opinions on the
subject, no definitive ruling exists. Consult with your state board of nursing for
guidance and direction. And document the actions you take, such as trying to
verify the drug dosage with the physician. Also try to work with your facility's
administrators to establish policies and procedures for handling such situations or to develop standing orders, if appropriate.

What the Authorities Say
Washington State Nurses Association v. Board of Medical Examiners (605, P.2d 1269)
states that "the actions of the physician's assistants should be considered
as the actions of the supervising physician." Iowa Attorney General Opinion
(No. 78-12-41, 12/30/78) held that "the nurse was legally obligated to carry out
the orders of a physician's assistant, if those orders were carrying out the
intent of the supervising physician."

Michigan Attorney General Opinion (No. 5220, 1997) stated that "the
nurse was legally obligated to carry out the orders of a physician's assistant,"
if those orders were carrying out the intent of the supervising physician. It also
held that "the nurse had the same legal duty to question the order of the
physician's assistant as she did an order of a physician."

The Joint Commission on Accreditation of Healthcare Organizations
recognizes physician's assistants as "part of the hospital's medical staff."

If your patient is receiving IV drugs, document your assessment of the IV site, the date and time the IV line was inserted
and by whom, catheter size, dressing type and condition, and IV
line patency. If the patient is receiving drugs such as IV nitroglycerin, document the date and time the IV bag was hung, infusion
rate, delivery device, and patient's response.

Activity. If appropriate, record that the patient is on bed rest
to minimize cardiac workload. Document your instructions to
her about activity limitations. If exertion could worsen her
condition, document the frequency and necessity of your assistance to meet such needs as nourishment and elimination.

Communication. Document your communications with other health care team members. For example, record the physician's name, the time you first notified him of the patient's chest pain, and the orders he gave. Continue to document the times of all communications throughout your care.

Emotional Support. If your patient has had an MI, provide emotional support to help her cope with the physical and psychosocial implications of her condition. Document the measures you take to relieve her anxiety, such as encouraging her to express her feelings and administering an antianxiety drug.

Transfer to ICU. If the patient must be transferred to the intensive care unit (ICU) for hemodynamic monitoring, document the aspects of her condition that indicate the need for such monitoring. Also document your report to the ICU nurse, and make a written record of the patient's belongings. Note the name of the person who accompanied her on the transfer and which monitoring devices were in place. Finally, document how well she tolerated the transfer.

Document What You Teach

Tailor the teaching plan to your patient's condition and treatment. For instance, if she has chronic heart disease, focus on teaching her how to manage her condition for the rest of her life. Document your teaching and her understanding—not just for legal purposes but also to help health care team members coordinate their teaching. As appropriate, teach the following topics and document that you did so:

- heart anatomy and physiology
- disease process
- diagnostic tests, such as ECG stress testing and cardiac catheterization
- treatments, such as heart surgery and coronary angioplasty
- signs and symptoms of an MI
- signs and symptoms to report
- actions to take when chest pain occurs
- prescribed drugs, including their names, dosages, administration times and routes, adverse effects, and storage
- ways to reduce cardiac risk factors, such as by stopping smoking

- nutrition, including dietary restrictions
- activity and rest recommendations
- resources for further information and support

WHEN YOUR PATIENT HAS
A MYOCARDIAL INFARCTION

When caring for a patient who's experiencing a myocardial infarction (MI), accurate documentation can be as critical as rapid response. Your documentation can help ensure effective emergency treatment and tailor the plan of care to your patient's specific needs.

Document What the Patient Tells You

In this emergency, you probably won't have time to gather and document a complete health history. Once the crisis passes, be sure to question the patient or a family member or check medical records to obtain pertinent information.

To begin, document recent reports of crushing, substernal chest pain that radiates to the left arm, jaw, neck, or shoulder blades. Ask the patient to rate the pain's severity on a scale of 0 to 10, with 0 indicating no pain and 10 indicating the worst pain imaginable. Document his response, along with the time the pain started and factors that seem to improve or worsen it.

Next, determine whether the patient has a history of atherosclerosis, coronary artery disease, or hyperlipoproteinemia. If he does, record the date the condition was diagnosed and its treatment, including drugs, activity guidelines, and dietary restrictions. If he smokes cigarettes or did so in the past, record the number of packs he smoked per day and the number of years he smoked.

If he reports a history of hypertension and knows his most recent systolic and diastolic readings, document these readings to provide a baseline for comparison with current values. Record whether he complies with his hypertension treatment plan.

Find out whether the patient has a history of diabetes mellitus. If so, record the date of diagnosis and the details of his treatment plan, including the type and dosage of the oral antidiabetic drug or insulin he takes. To help determine the effectiveness of diabetes treatment, document how often he monitor his blood glucose level at home, which methods he uses, and his most recent blood glucose level.

Then record the patient's reported activity level, including the types of activity and exercise he performs and the number of days per week he exercises. If he describes a sedentary lifestyle, record this. If he's obese, document his weight and recent history of weight loss or gain.

If the patient has a family history of heart disease, note which family members are affected. You may want to use a genogram to record this information. (See *Constructing a genogram,* page 36.)

If the patient reports a previous MI, record the date and any complications. To aid your assessment of previous MI treatments and the patient's response, review the past medical record and document pertinent findings.

Ask whether the patient has recently had symptoms that typically precede or accompany an MI: indigestion or heartburn, more frequent angina attacks, feelings of impending doom, increased fatigue, and episodes of nausea, vomiting, or shortness of breath. Document his response fully. Discuss with the physician significant information you gather during the health history interview.

Document What You Assess

Although signs and symptoms of MI vary among patients, you should assess for and document the following expected abnormal findings:
- anxiety
- restlessness
- dyspnea
- tachypnea
- diaphoresis
- jugular vein distention
- cool, mottled skin
- diminished peripheral pulses

- S_4 or S_3 (abnormal heart sounds)
- paradoxical splitting of S_2
- systolic murmur
- pericardial friction rub
- low-grade fever
- tachycardia and hypertension (with an anterior MI)
- bradycardia and hypertension (with an inferior MI)

TIPS & ADVICE

CONSTRUCTING A GENOGRAM

A genogram, such as the one shown here, reveals family relationships and health history patterns. It may indicate a family history of heart disease and other familial diseases and disorders. To construct your patient's genogram, fill in the ages of all living family members, the ages at which deceased family members died, and the causes of death. Note whether the family history includes diseases with a known or suspected familial or genetic tendency.

Be sure to include a key that identifies all important people and details in the patient's life. The key should explain the symbols you used to denote male, female, living, and deceased.

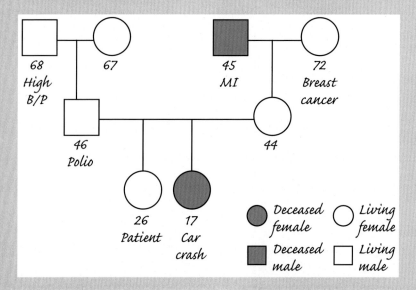

Document What You Do

As you intervene during the patient's acute illness and recovery, use the following guidelines to ensure accurate documentation and to refine your plan of care.

Vital Sign Checks and Pain Assessments. Document your patient's heart and respiratory rates, temperature, blood pressure, and pain level every 1 to 2 hours during the acute phase of the MI and every 4 hours thereafter, or according to facility policy. If he experiences chest pain or develops complications, check his vital signs more frequently. Compare the results of each vital sign measurement with previous findings.

ECG Tracking and Continuous Cardiac Monitoring. Obtain a baseline tracing from a 12-lead electrocardiogram (ECG) and place it in the patient's chart. Then obtain one ECG tracing daily, or as ordered, to document return of the ST segment to baseline as well as Q-wave formation in the affected leads.

Document the time you start and stop continuous cardiac monitoring. To show that you're monitoring the patient appropriately, indicate which lead is displayed. For instance, note that you're displaying modified chest lead 1 (MCL_1) to show that you've chosen the best lead to detect arrhythmias and ischemic changes.

Obtain a rhythm strip and place it in the patient's medical record as often as required by your facility. (Some facilities require nurses to obtain a rhythm strip at the beginning and end of each shift.) Also post a rhythm strip when your patient develops chest pain or an arrhythmia or when an ECG change occurs. On the strip, write the patient's name, the time and date the strip was recorded, the lead used, the patient's heart rate and rhythm, PR-interval and QRS-complex duration, and, if present, ST-segment elevation or depression.

Hemodynamic Monitoring. Because an MI impairs the heart's ability to meet the body's oxygen demands, be sure to closely monitor and document your patient's hemodynamic status. If he has a pulmonary artery catheter in place, document all readings— especially pulmonary artery pressure and pulmonary artery wedge pressure. For an accurate record of the patient's progress, evaluate and document his cardiac output, cardiac index, and systemic vascular resistance every 2 hours or more frequently, as indicated.

Drug and IV Therapy. Document the names, dosages, and administration times and routes for all drugs you give. Before administering a drug that reduces myocardial oxygen demand and improves cardiac output (for instance, a nitrate, beta blocker, or calcium channel blocker), obtain and record the patient's blood pressure and pulse rate. Throughout drug therapy, stay alert for adverse effects on his blood pressure and pulse rate.

For each IV site used, document the location, catheter type and size, IV solution administered, infusion rate, and appearance of the site, dressing type and condition, and delivery device. Keep in mind that different sites may be used for thrombolytic therapy, other infusions, or blood sampling.

Oxygen Therapy. Document the time you start and stop oxygen therapy, the oxygen flow rate, and the delivery device, such as a nasal cannula or face mask. Also record the patient's pulse oximetry readings and arterial blood gas values, as appropriate.

Nutrition. Document the diet ordered, such as a 2-g/day sodium, low-fat, low-cholesterol diet. Evaluate and record your patient's compliance with dietary restrictions, and note your actions to promote compliance. For instance, if you contact the dietitian to review the diet with the patient, record the time of this contact and the dietitian's name. Also document your patient's response to interventions and his compliance.

Document What You Teach

As you implement and document the teaching plan for your patient, be sure to cover these essential topics:
- normal heart anatomy and physiology
- pathophysiology of coronary artery disease and MI
- diagnostic tests, including ECG and cardiac isoenzyme tests
- cardiac catheterization
- treatments, such as percutaneous transluminal coronary angioplasty, coronary atherectomy, coronary artery stent placement, and coronary artery bypass grafting
- prescribed drugs, including their names, dosages, administration times and routes, adverse effects, and storage
- signs and symptoms to report
- activity and exercise recommendations

- proper nutrition, including dietary restrictions
- sexual activity
- smoking cessation
- cardiac rehabilitation after discharge
- support groups and other resources for support and information, such as the American Heart Association

WHEN YOUR PATIENT HAS HEART FAILURE

S uccessful drug therapy for heart failure focuses on reducing fluid volume, decreasing peripheral vascular resistance, and preventing or limiting ventricular remodeling. To help your patient manage her disease at home, you'll help her modify her lifestyle, for example, by restricting her sodium and fluid intake and recognizing warning signs of complications. Your thorough documentation helps the health care team determine effective interventions and create a long-range treatment plan for your patient.

Document What the Patient Tells You

When obtaining your patient's health history, assess for and document signs, symptoms, and risk factors that could contribute to heart failure. If the patient has a history of heart failure, collect information about past treatments she has received, noting their effectiveness.

Ask the patient to relate her medical history, especially heart or circulatory diseases she has had. Along with this information, record the date of each diagnosis and treatment she received.

Document past or present signs and symptoms of heart failure she describes, and note whether she has new or worsening symptoms. In particular, ask about shortness of breath, edema, cough, tachycardia, chest pain, orthopnea, and fatigue. Record her responses in detail.

As necessary, ask the patient to elaborate on her symptoms. For example, if she says she gets tired from walking shorter and shorter distances, ask her exactly how far she can walk now before tiring compared with how far she could walk previously. Your documentation might read, "Patient states she previously could walk up to one block before feeling slightly short of breath. One week ago, she noted that she became short of breath after walking approximately 10 feet." If appropriate, use the New York Heart Association (NYHA) classification system to further characterize the patient's functional ability. (See *Using the NYHA classification system to document the effects of heart failure.*)

Next, elicit and record information about the patient's diet and recent dietary changes. Document your assessment of her sodium, fat, and cholesterol intake and her understanding of how an

TIPS & ADVICE

USING THE NYHA CLASSIFICATION SYSTEM TO DOCUMENT THE EFFECTS OF HEART FAILURE

For your patient with heart failure, get a general idea of her condition by asking specifically which activities she can—and can't—perform. Then in your notes, record your patient's functional ability in relation to the New York Heart Association (NYHA) classification system, as described below.

Class	Patient Symptoms
Class I	No activity limitation. Patient has no undue fatigue, palpitations, or dyspnea with ordinary physical activity that requires 7 metabolic equivalents of a task (METs) or more, such as walking briskly uphill.
Class II	Slight activity limitation by symptoms. Patient is comfortable at rest, but experiences fatigue, palpitations, or dyspnea with ordinary physical activity of 5 to 7 METs, such as yard work and housecleaning.
Class III	Activity limitation by symptoms. Patient is comfortable at rest but experiences fatigue, palpitations, or dyspnea with ordinary physical activity of 2 to 5 METs, such as walking slowly and cooking.
Class IV	Inability to perform physical activity. Patient displays symptoms with ordinary physical activity of 1 to 3 METs, such as bathing or dressing, and may even have symptoms at rest.

improper diet can contribute to heart disease. Note whether she has gained or lost weight recently and whether she weighs herself at the same time each day.

Ask about urination patterns, and document recent changes in urine output and frequency of urination. Also inquire about her daily fluid intake, and document her answer.

If the patient reports a history of hypertension, document this along with her most recent blood pressure reading, if known. Record the names and dosages of drugs she is using and her perception of the reason for using each one. Also document whether she complies with the prescribed drug regimen. Using her own words, record exactly how she uses her drugs. Finally, document recent changes in the amount of her daily activity, and determine whether she's been under new or unusual stress.

Document What You Assess

Perform and document a thorough patient assessment to establish a baseline. As treatment progresses, your documentation will help the health care team track the patient's condition.

Vital Signs Checks, Weight Measurements, and Pain Assessments. Record the patient's pulse and respiratory rates and blood pressure every 4 hours—more often if they're unstable. Document whom you notified and how you intervened for abnormal values and changes, especially tachycardia, tachypnea, and hypotension.

When measuring vital signs, also document daily weights—a valuable indicator of fluid gain or loss for a patient with heart failure. If your patient has pain, especially chest pain, record her rating of it on a 0-to-10 scale.

Respiratory System. Auscultate the patient's lungs every 1 to 2 hours or more frequently if needed. Document adventitious breath sounds and changes from the previous assessment-especially increased congestion and decreased air movement. Notify the physician of changes, and document that you did so.

Then evaluate for and record the use of accessory breathing muscles and signs and symptoms of decreased perfusion and hypoxia. Document the time dyspnea occurs and precipitating factors. Ask the patient if anything has improved the dyspnea in the past, and record her answer.

Cardiovascular System. Check for jugular vein distention. When documenting this finding, include the degree of distention. Document your assessment of heart sounds every 1 to 2 hours. Be sure to record abnormal sounds, especially S_3 or a prominent systolic murmur, which may indicate fluid overload.

Tissue Perfusion. Record indicators of decreased tissue perfusion, especially pallor, diaphoresis, and cool, clammy skin. Also note confusion and decreased level of consciousness, which may signal decreased cardiac output.

Fluid Balance. Assess for and document signs and symptoms of fluid overload. If your patient has edema, note its location and whether it's pitting or nonpitting. Record the degree of pitting, if present. Document changes from the previous assessment.

Document What You Do

As you intervene to manage your patient's heart failure, document exactly what you did, when you did it, and the patient's response. This will help you identify effective interventions and refine your plan of care as needed.

Fluid Balance. Eliminating excess fluid is one of the treatment goals for a patient with heart failure. Document a complete record of the patient's fluid intake and output. Include as intake IV fluids or drugs the patient is receiving as well as such foods as gelatin dessert and ice cream.

You'll probably record intake and output on a flow sheet or special I&O record. If you document fluid balance in narrative notes, clearly indicate the time you detected a fluid gain or loss. For example, you might write, "The patient is minus 1,500 ml from 0700 until 1500."

If urine output drops below 30 ml/hour or a fluid imbalance occurs, notify the physician. Document that you did so, along with the physician's orders and your interventions.

Drug and IV Therapy. Document the names, dosages, and administration times and routes for drugs you give. Measure and record the patient's vital signs before and after giving a drug that could alter hemodynamic status—for instance, digoxin, a beta blocker, a nitrate, or an angiotensin—converting enzyme inhibitor.

Before giving a diuretic, obtain and record the patient's fluid balance, most recent serum potassium level, and blood pressure. As with any drug you administer, document the patient's response.

If your patient is receiving IV therapy, document the location of the IV site, date and time of IV line placement, delivery device, cannula size, dressing type and condition, and assessment findings at the site. For a patient with an intermittent indwelling catheter, note the presence of blood return and the use of saline or heparin flushes to keep the line patent.

Oxygen Therapy. Before giving supplemental oxygen, document the patient's initial pulse oximetry reading, vital sign measurements, respiratory assessment findings, and arterial blood gas (ABG) analysis results. Note whether she has a history of chronic obstructive pulmonary disease, which influences the amount of supplemental oxygen she can receive. When indicated, document that you notified the physician of significant laboratory results. (See *Reporting critical laboratory results,* page 44.)

Be sure to document the time oxygen therapy was started, the oxygen flow rate, and the delivery device, such as a nasal cannula or face mask. Record the patient's vital sign measurements and pulse oximetry readings every 1 to 2 hours until the findings fall within normal limits and then every 4 hours or according to your facility's policy. Record ABG levels, noting the time the blood sample was drawn and the oxygen level the patient was receiving at the time.

Close Monitoring. To track your patient's condition, frequently assess and document her vital signs, heart rhythm, respiratory status, and weight. Record her vital sign measurements every 4 hours and whenever her condition changes—more often if her vital signs are unstable. Weigh her daily before breakfast and after she voids; note the time you obtained the weight and whether this measurement reflects a significant change. To ensure that all caregivers weigh her on the same scale, document which scale you used.

Next, record the time you initiated cardiac monitoring and the lead you're using. Document that you explained the reason for the monitor. Obtain a rhythm strip, and label it with the date and

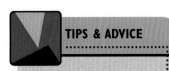

TIPS & ADVICE

REPORTING CRITICAL LABORATORY RESULTS
Always record critical laboratory results clearly and accurately. Identify the physician you notified of the result, the time of notification, and the orders you received. Include the following in your notes:
- full name of the physician you notified
- date and time of notification
- specific information you reported to the physician
- orders the physician gave, or a statement that no orders were received

Documenting Pertinent Negatives
Always document pertinent negatives about a physician's orders. For instance, if the physician doesn't change the treatment plan after you tell him that your patient with heart failure has a serum potassium level of 3.3 mEq/L, ask directly whether he wants to change the treatment. If he says he doesn't, document this to show you're aware of the usual and customary treatment of hypokalemia.

By recording this pertinent negative, your documentation clearly indicates that the deviation in standard practice didn't result from lack of knowledge or foresight on your part. If you think the deviation will harm the patient, discuss this with the physician. If he still doesn't alter the treatment plan, notify your immediate supervisor or follow your facility's policy.

time, your patient's name, her heart rate and rhythm, PR–interval and QRS–complex duration, and, if present, ST–segment elevation or depression. Place a new rhythm strip in the medical record as often as your facility requires, whenever the patient's condition changes, and any time an ectopic beat or arrhythmia appears. Document significant changes in the rhythm strip, and notify the physician. Then record your notification, the physician's response, and your actions.

If your patient has a pulmonary artery catheter inserted, record the date and time it was inserted, the name of the physician who inserted it, and how well the patient tolerated the procedure. Frequently record your observation of the site. Also document catheter readings—especially pulmonary artery pressure, pulmonary artery wedge pressure, and cardiac output—as often as ordered.

Document and notify the physician if these values change or if the patient's condition worsens. Record your notification, the physician's response, and your interventions.

Energy Conservation. Document instructions you give your patient about energy conservation. Also describe specific patient activities that take place. For instance, you may write, "Patient transferred from bed to commode with assistance of one nurse. Patient denies shortness of breath or weakness when moving from bed to commode."

Nutrition. Document the diet the physician ordered, such as a low-sodium, low-fat, low-cholesterol diet. Note your patient's dietary compliance, and record the percentage of each meal she eats. Also document your instructions about the prescribed diet. If appropriate, document a referral to the dietitian.

If the patient has a fluid restriction, meticulously record how much fluid she drinks with and between meals. Document the instructions you provide about fluid rationing, and note her compliance.

Document What You Teach

To help your patient manage heart failure after discharge, provide comprehensive teaching about the disease and treatment plan. Document all teaching you provide, along with measurable indicators of her understanding. Be sure your teaching and documentation include the following topics:
- heart anatomy and physiology
- disease process
- nutrition, including dietary or fluid restrictions and referral to a dietitian
- daily weights
- drugs, including their names, dosages, administration times and routes, adverse effects, and storage
- signs and symptoms to report
- activity limitations and energy conservation
- cardiac rehabilitation activities or physical therapy
- diagnostic tests
- home monitoring, such as blood pressure measurement and Holter monitoring

WHEN YOUR PATIENT IS IN SHOCK

C areful documentation of health history and physical examination findings can help identify the type of shock your patient is experiencing—cardiogenic, hypovolemic, or distributive (which includes septic, neurogenic, and anaphylactic shock). If the patient can't answer questions, gather key information from medical records and family members.

Document What the Patient Tells You and What You Assess

Document your findings often for a patient in shock. Record all assessment information you obtain, even if it seems irrelevant. For faster documentation, consider recording vital sign measurements, hemodynamic parameters, and IV fluids and drugs on a flow sheet. Keep in mind that using a flow sheet doesn't mean that you can neglect your narrative notes. (See *Recognizing the drawbacks of flow sheets.*)

When collecting health history information, especially note factors that might have predisposed your patient to shock. As appropriate, focus on:

- conditions that increase the risk for *hypovolemic* shock, such as hemorrhage, blood or fluid loss, trauma, a coagulation disorder, surgery, diuresis, and excessive vomiting or diarrhea
- conditions that pose a danger of *cardiogenic* shock, such as myocardial infarction, heart failure, arrhythmias, and valvular disease
- conditions that contribute to *distributive* shock, such as immunosuppressive therapy, steroid therapy, chronic illness, invasive devices, surgery, and malnutrition

Vital Signs. Assess and document your patient's vital signs frequently. Vital sign changes can be the earliest indicators of shock. Measure and document his pulse rate, noting threadiness, weakness, and irregularity. Because hypotension commonly accompanies shock, measure and document your patient's blood pressure often, noting significant changes from previous values.

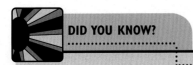

RECOGNIZING THE DRAWBACKS OF FLOW SHEETS
Flow sheets offer several advantages to the busy nurse—for example, they're quick and easy to use. They also have drawbacks. For instance, they typically don't provide much space to record information. Also, using them may mean duplicating your documentation if you also record a narrative note for the information you enter on the flow sheet.

Coping with Space Constraints
On most flow sheets, you must squeeze a lot of information into a small space. You'll need to write as neatly and legibly as possible so others can understand your data. If possible, ask your facility's flow sheet designer to allot more space to entries and to leave some columns blank to allow tracking of nonstandard parameters, such as bed position.

Avoiding Duplication
Some nurses write a narrative note for the information they enter on a flow sheet. Besides doubling the work, this practice increases the risk that your documentation will be inconsistent, creating a potential legal quagmire.

When Should You Write a Narrative Note? At times, you should write a narrative note—not to duplicate flow sheet information but to clarify it and show that you took appropriate action. Suppose you indicate on the flow sheet that your patient's blood pressure is 89/50 mm Hg. Then you should write a narrative note documenting your action in response to this abnormally low reading. Your narrative note might read, "Dr. Jonason was notified of low blood pressure at 1215. Normal saline solution 500 ml administered IV over 30 minutes, as prescribed. BP 106/62 at 1300."

Fluid Balance. Depending on your patient's condition, you may need to weigh him daily to gauge his hydration and response to treatment. Documenting daily weights also helps determine proper drug dosages.

Tissue Perfusion. Document the quality of peripheral pulses, noting whether they're weak, diminished, or absent. (Keep in mind that in shock, perfusion in the arms and legs decreases.) Also assess and document the patient's skin color and temperature, noting mottling, coolness, and clamminess.

Record urine output hourly; falling output signals shock progression. Check for and document jugular vein distention (which occurs in cardiogenic shock) or flatness (which may accompany hypovolemic or distributive shock). Next, evaluate skin turgor and capillary refill, and document your findings.

Then evaluate and record changes in the patient's level of consciousness, staying alert for disorientation, restlessness, anxiety, and confusion. Such changes could signal decreased cardiac output and impaired oxygenation. Finally, auscultate and document bowel sounds, which may diminish in late stages of shock.

Respiratory System. Document your findings as you auscultate breath sounds. Record the respiratory rate, rhythm, and depth, and describe crackles and other abnormalities. Frequently document pulse oximetry readings, and record arterial blood gas (ABG) levels each time you obtain them. When documenting ABG levels, note how much supplemental oxygen the patient is receiving and describe changes in his condition. Remember—documenting ABG levels frequently is crucial to detecting the acid–base imbalances that commonly occur in shock, such as respiratory alkalosis and metabolic acidosis. Notify the physician of significant findings; document this action, the time of notification, and your interventions.

Laboratory Test Results. Expect to send samples and specimens for laboratory testing frequently. Document all results, including complete blood count, blood urea nitrogen, serum electrolytes, serum lactate, serum creatinine, blood culture, prothrombin time, partial activated thromboplastin time, erythrocyte sedimentation rate, serum and urine osmolality, urine specific gravity, and urine sodium. Notify the physician of abnormal findings; record the time of notification, the physician's response, and your actions.

Document What You Do

To help prevent your patient from deteriorating, act rapidly—and document each intervention promptly. Monitor his response to interventions continuously, and record all findings.

Airway, Breathing, and Circulation. Document that you've assessed and ensured the patient's airway, breathing, and circulation (ABCs). Make sure your notes reflect that ensuring ABCs was your priority and that it preceded other interventions.

Until your patient is stabilized, record his pulse and respiratory rates and blood pressure every 15 minutes—or more frequently if indicated. Record his temperature every 1 to 2 hours. Also document pulse oximetry readings, respiratory assessment findings, and ABG levels. If you're administering oxygen, document the time oxygen therapy was begun, the flow rate, and the delivery device used (such as nasal cannula or face mask).

Once the patient is stabilized and these values fall within normal limits, document them every 4 hours or when the patient's clinical condition changes. After oxygen therapy begins, record serial ABG levels, noting the oxygen flow rate.

Endotracheal Intubation and Mechanical Ventilation. If the patient's respiratory status and ABG levels don't improve, he may require mechanical ventilation. Document the time of intubation, the physician or person who performed it, and the size of the endotracheal tube. Also record that the patient was hyperventilated with 100% oxygen before the procedure to ensure adequate oxygenation. Such documentation could prove crucial if a lawsuit arises from complications of mechanical ventilation.

After tube placement, clearly mark the tube's exit point from the mouth or nose with a marking pen or tape, and record how far it was inserted. Document that the tube is intact and properly taped. Record that you auscultated for breath sounds and that a chest x-ray was done to confirm tube position. Then document chest x-ray results, adding that you communicated them to the physician. If required by facility policy, also document that tube placement was confirmed by carbon dioxide detector. Record the time mechanical ventilation began, the ventilation mode, fraction of inspired oxygen, and other ventilator settings.

Drug Therapy. The powerful drugs used to treat shock require close monitoring to evaluate the patient's response. Also monitor his hemodynamic status frequently and record the results carefully.

For instance, if your patient is receiving dopamine, an adrenergic drug, record his vital sign measurements and hemodynamic readings to evaluate the drug's effects and help determine the proper dosage. Also measure and record his urine output because dopamine up to 5 mg/kg/minute increases renal blood flow. And record his baseline peripheral vascular status because high doses of dopamine may adversely affect the systemic vascular response.

When documenting vasoactive drug administration, indicate the patient's dosage in commonly ordered units, such as micrograms per kilogram per minute or micrograms per minute. This is more precise than simply documenting that the drug is infusing at a particular rate per hour because the amount administered per hour may depend on the concentration of the IV mixture.

Volume Replacement. Document your administration of IV fluids, volume expanders, and blood transfusions. Include the time and date you initiated the infusion, assessment findings at the IV site, catheter type, dressing type, and patency of the IV line. During the infusion, record hemodynamic status, urine output, and respiratory status.

If the physician prescribes a blood transfusion, place a signed transfusion consent form in the patient's record before beginning the transfusion. Also document that the blood identification has been checked and verified against the patient's identification band by two nurses. During the transfusion, document the patient's vital signs as often as your facility requires. Note signs or symptoms of a transfusion reaction and record your actions, such as stopping the infusion. Record the patient's response to the transfusion, changes in vital sign measurements and hemodynamic status, and physician notification of significant changes.

Hemodynamic Monitoring. If your patient has a pulmonary artery catheter in place, document readings, especially pulmonary artery pressure and pulmonary artery wedge pressure, as often as ordered. Record cardiac output every 4 hours or as appropriate. Because the patient's position in bed may alter readings, document for each reading whether he's in a position other than supine with the head of the bed flat.

If the pulmonary artery catheter is inserted or changed during your shift, record the date and time of its insertion or change, the physician who inserted or changed it, assessment findings from the site, and how the patient tolerated the procedure. Note any changes in readings and the patient's condition and your interventions to manage the changes. Record hemodynamic status frequently during drug administration and after changing drug dosages.

ABG Analysis. If your facility's policy allows you to draw arterial blood samples for ABG analysis, document site preparation, Allen's test results, and the equipment and artery used. After the blood sample has been drawn, record that pressure has been applied to the site, note the site's appearance, and document your assessment of distal circulation.

Record ABG levels, along with the time the sample was drawn, amount of oxygen the patient was receiving, and changes in his condition. Also document that you notified the physician of the levels, and record the time of notification and related interventions.

Intraaortic Balloon Pump. If an intraaortic balloon pump (IABP) is used to augment the heart's pumping action, record the frequency of counterpulsation and the assisted systolic and diastolic pressures. Also document your assessment of the insertion site and dressing changes or other care you perform.

Throughout IABP use, record hourly assessments of circulation to the involved leg or arm, including its pulse and skin color and temperature. Include your comparison of the involved arm or leg with the opposite arm or leg.

Fluid Intake and Output. Document the patient's fluid intake and output every hour. If you detect an imbalance, if urine output drops below 30 ml/hour, or if output does not change appropriately in response to therapy, document these findings and notify the physician. Document your notification, the physician's orders, and your actions.

Document What You Teach

Typically, a patient in shock can't respond to—and may not understand—your instructions. Although you won't be able to teach him directly, you can instruct his family members. Besides documenting the patient's cognitive status, record the teaching you provide to family members and their understanding of it. Essential topics to cover in your teaching and documentation include the following:

- disease process
- procedures and treatments

- activity limitations
- safety measures
- prescribed drugs, including their names, dosages, administration times and routes, adverse effects, and storage
- signs and symptoms the patient may experience
- hygiene and infection prevention

WHEN YOUR PATIENT HAS CARDIOPULMONARY ARREST

In the controlled chaos of lifesaving interventions during cardiopulmonary arrest, documentation may seem like a low priority. But in this crisis, as well as in others, recording the details of the patient's condition and documenting the quick, appropriate response of the health care team are crucial.

In such a situation, one nurse usually acts as the recorder, documenting the health care team's interventions. If you're the designated recorder, keep in mind that documentation of the arrest and interventions should follow advanced cardiac life support guidelines.

After the crisis ends, the lead physician and nurse-recorder should review and sign the nurse-recorder's documentation, indicating that they agree with its content. (See *Which data go where?*)

Document What the Patient Tells You

If you witnessed your patient's cardiopulmonary arrest, record what she said before she became unresponsive, such as a report of chest pain. Gather other health history data, including drug therapies and allergies, from the medical record to help determine the cause of the arrest.

Document What You Assess and What You Do

In this emergency, assessment and intervention almost occur simultaneously. If you're the designated recorder, record the time

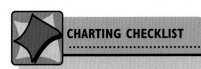

CHARTING CHECKLIST

WHICH DATA GO WHERE?
For your patient in cardiopulmonary arrest, deciding which data to record on the code sheet and which to document in standard nursing documentation can be tricky. Remember that the code sheet is streamlined for quick, accurate documentation during fast-paced activity. And recall that a code officially begins when the code call goes out; it ends when the physician in charge declares that it's over. Here's a list of data to record in each type of record.

Code Sheet
Enter the following information on the code sheet:
❑ Patient's name
❑ Date and time the code began
❑ Time of physician notification
❑ Names of participating team members
❑ Name of the attending physician
❑ Time when each resuscitation measure began
❑ Chronological list of assessment findings (including heart rhythm, pulse rate, and laboratory test results), treatments (including cardiopulmonary resuscitation and defibrillation or cardioversion), drugs (including their names, dosages, and administration times and routes), and procedures (including central venous line insertion, intubation, and pacing)
❑ Time of family notification
❑ Patient's status and disposition at the end of the code
❑ Time when the code ended

The lead physician and nurse-recorder must sign the code sheet. The nurse-recorder signs her name and writes "recorder" after it to show that she documented the information but didn't perform the interventions.

Standard Nursing Documentation
Record the following information in standard nursing documentation:
❑ Events leading to the initial call that triggered the code
❑ Assessment findings that led the health care giver to call the code
❑ Name of the person who initiated the code call
❑ Treatment being administered, if any, when the code call was made

End the standard nursing documentation with the statement "See code sheet." After the code ends, document a complete assessment of the patient's condition and your ongoing interventions.

the patient was found unresponsive and general observations, such as her specific position in bed or that she was found clutching her chest. If another staff member witnessed a noteworthy event just before the arrest, such as a fall or an abnormal rhythm on the cardiac monitor, document this information. Also record the time of the initial call for help by the first health care giver on the scene.

Then record all assessment findings and actions. Indicate in your notes that the patient's airway has been opened and her breathing assessed. If no breaths are felt and no chest movements are seen, record these facts. Then document the start of resuscitation. Indicate that the patient received two slow breaths and was checked for a carotid pulse. Record pertinent negatives too, such as absence of breathing and a pulse.

Indicate the time chest compressions and rescue breathing began. Document whether one- or two-person cardiopulmonary resuscitation (CPR) was performed. Note the times when CPR was interrupted for a pulse check. If the patient wasn't already on a cardiac monitor, document that cardiac monitoring was initiated, and describe the heart rhythm that appears. Also document the administration of high-flow oxygen and CPR continuation.

Endotracheal Intubation. If the patient required intubation, record the time of intubation, the physician who performed the procedure, and the endotracheal tube size. Document that the patient was hyperventilated with 100% oxygen before the procedure. If the physician had difficulty intubating the patient, record the frequency of oxygen administration during the procedure.

After tube placement, mark the tube's exit point, and record how far the tube was inserted. Also document that the endotracheal cuff was checked for leaks and that a chest x-ray was done to confirm proper tube placement. Then record the results of the x-ray. Note that the tube was secured with tape or an endotracheal stabilizing device. Record the amount of air in the cuff, and note that cuff pressure is less than 20 mm Hg. Document breath sounds, including their equality and adventitious sounds. Your documentation helps verify that the tube was placed correctly— or that ventilation problems occurred.

IV Therapy. Document that IV access was established. Record the site's location and appearance, catheter size, dressing's appearance, and IV line patency. If more than one IV line was started, note the location and appearance of each. If a central venous line was inserted, record the name of the physician who inserted it, its location, site preparation, and blood return. Record changes in the patient's condition during central venous line insertion as well as bilateral assessment of breath sounds to rule out pneumothorax. Document the results of the postprocedure chest x-ray to verify catheter placement.

Interventions for Ventricular Fibrillation or Tachycardia. If the cardiac monitor shows ventricular fibrillation or ventricular tachycardia, prepare for defibrillation or cardioversion. Record the time of defibrillation or cardioversion, paddle placement, use of protective gel pads or conductive paste, and the number of joules delivered. Be sure to document each episode of defibrillation or cardioversion and its effects on the patient's condition and heart rhythm.

Interventions for Asystole. If the cardiac monitor shows asystole, document confirmation of that finding in more than one electrocardiographic lead. If the physician initiates transcutaneous (external) pacing, document the duration of asystole before initiation of cardiac pacing. Record electrode positioning and pacer settings. If electrical capture appears, note the heart rate and include a rhythm strip in the patient's medical record. Also document signs of mechanical capture, such as palpation of a carotid pulse. If drugs such as epinephrine or atropine are given, record the dosages, administration times and routes, and effect on the patient's condition.

Interventions for Pulseless Electrical Activity. If the patient experiences pulseless electrical activity, document that the absence of blood flow was verified by Doppler device. Document administration of ordered drugs, such as epinephrine, and apparent effects on the patient's condition.

Other Interventions. Record the names, dosages, and administration times and routes of all drugs given, such as lidocaine, bretylium, magnesium sulfate, and procainamide. If blood is drawn, document which tests were ordered and at what time. Then record the results and related interventions.

Terminating Resuscitation. If interventions prove unsuccessful and the physician terminates resuscitation, document the physician's name, the time, and specifics of the patient's condition. Be sure to note pertinent negatives, such as no pulse and no respiratory activity.

Return to Spontaneous Rhythm. If resuscitation succeeds and the patient regains a spontaneous heart rhythm, record the time the rhythm returns, the specific rhythm present, and the patient's vital sign measurements. Make sure your documentation reflects that her airway, breathing, and circulation are supported. Document your patient's response to interventions and the results of continuous monitoring.

Document What You Teach

During the crisis, when the patient is unresponsive, direct your teaching to family members. Document your explanations of procedures and the patient's condition to the family, along with the emotional support offered. Record that you showed family members to a waiting area and updated them frequently on the patient's condition. Note that they were prepared for changes in the patient's appearance and condition before being allowed to visit her after resuscitation Also document whether family members remained present during the code (if permitted by your facility) and the name of the person designated to provide support and answer their questions. Be sure your teaching and documentation include:

- disease process
- procedures and treatments, such as x-rays
- activity limitations
- safety measures
- prescribed drugs, including their names, dosages, administration times and routes, adverse effects, and storage
- signs and symptoms to report
- nutrition, including dietary restrictions
- explanation of equipment, such as a cardiac monitor and mechanical ventilator
- communication techniques use by the patient and family

WHEN YOUR PATIENT HAS A NEW ARRHYTHMIA

Although some arrhythmias, such as atrial fibrillation, can be chronic and stable, every new arrhythmia deserves close inspection. Because you're on the front line of patient care, you must be ready to detect new arrhythmias quickly, provide appropriate treatments, and evaluate the patient's response accurately. These actions help ensure a good outcome. So does your documentation of them. And a key part of that documentation is the patient's electrocardiogram (ECG) tracings.

An ECG tracing provides a graphic representation of the heart's electrical activity. Each ECG lead displays activity from a different view of the heart's left ventricle. A multichannel recorder, such as a 12-lead ECG, supplies multiple views, usually at one point in time. In contrast, a continuous cardiac monitor typically provides one or two views all the time, which allows uninterrupted monitoring for arrhythmias.

If your patient is recovering from cardiac surgery or is otherwise at risk for arrhythmias, expect to place him on a continuous cardiac monitor while he's hospitalized. Your careful documentation of his baseline cardiac rhythm and any new arrhythmias can help guide his care and prevent complications.

Document What the Patient Tells You

Meticulously record your patient's health history. This information can help you and the physician determine the patient's need for cardiac monitoring and help you identify arrhythmias that may develop. For example, suppose a wide complex tachycardia of unknown origin occurs. If the patient's medical record shows a history of Wolff-Parkinson-White (WPW) syndrome, you'll know that he's at risk for a reentrant arrhythmia related to WPW syndrome and you can provide the appropriate treatment. Other history data that can help identify arrhythmias include cardiac and pulmonary diseases and therapy with such drugs as digoxin or theophylline.

Also document symptoms that may herald an arrhythmia, such as palpitations, skipped heartbeats, weakness, lightheadedness, faintness, dyspnea, nausea, or chest pain. Record whether symptoms are constant or intermittent. Also chart other symptoms that suggest a complication of an arrhythmia, such as unilateral weakness or slurred speech.

Document What You Assess

When your patient has a new arrhythmia, act quickly to assess it. If the arrhythmia is paroxysmal or intermittent, try to obtain a rhythm strip of the arrhythmia's onset and termination. If the arrhythmia is continuous, activate the continuous recording function on the cardiac monitor, which also documents the results of interventions, such as carotid sinus massage and drug therapy. Remember—the cardiac monitor is a diagnostic tool that also provides an important piece of documentation for the medical record. By providing a clear tracing of an arrhythmia (including its onset, duration, and termination), the record gives the health care team important clues for future care. For the clearest view of an arrhythmia, make sure you select the best lead for its type. (See *Lead placement counts when recording an arrhythmia.*)

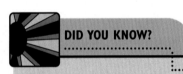

DID YOU KNOW?

LEAD PLACEMENT COUNTS WHEN RECORDING AN ARRHYTHMIA
Your choice of lead for monitoring an arrhythmia can critically affect the quality of the resulting ECG tracing. Your patient's health history or baseline ECG tracing can help you select the most appropriate lead, as shown below.

History Data or Baseline ECG Tracing	Best Leads to Use
Atrial arrhythmias	II or III
Bundle branch block	V_1 or V_6 (or MCL_1 or MCL_6)
History of wide-complex tachycardias	
Unknown history of arrhythmias	V_1 (or MCL_1)

Rapidly assess the patient for signs of circulatory compromise, such as hypotension, weakness, or a decreased level of consciousness. Also perform a focused head-to-toe assessment; record all assessment findings.

Arrhythmia. Place a recording of the arrhythmia in the patient's chart, according to facility protocol. Make sure it contains at least 6 seconds of the ECG tracing to make measurement easier. Document the lead—such as lead II or MCL_1—and your measurement of key intervals, such as the PR interval, QRS duration, and QT interval. Also measure and chart the heart rate and your interpretation of the arrhythmia. If the patient has a pacemaker, record any failure to sense or capture. If the patient has an implantable defibrillator, note whether it fired during the arrhythmia and whether it successfully terminated the arrhythmia. Also document the recovery rhythm, such as sinus bradycardia. If the monitor doesn't mark the strip with identifying information, label the strip with the patient's name and room number, as well as the date and time.

Vital Signs. Record your patient's heart rate, blood pressure, and respiratory rate as soon as you detect an arrhythmia. Then continue to document these vital signs at least every 4 hours or more frequently, depending on the arrhythmia.

When documenting the heart rate, use the patient's heart sounds instead of palpating a pulse. That's because the arrhythmia can affect pulse amplitude—and you might not correctly count the number of beats.

When recording the blood pressure, consider the arrhythmia's likely effects. An arrhythmia that begins suddenly (such as atrial fibrillation) or produces an abnormally slow or fast heart rate can cause a precipitous drop in blood pressure. Sustained ventricular tachycardia or fibrillation can produce a low or absent blood pressure.

Heart Sounds. Auscultate the heart sounds, particularly noting irregular or extra sounds, such as S_3 or S_4, which may signal heart failure or ischemia; document unusual heart sounds. Be aware that a patient with atrial fibrillation can't produce S_4 because this extra heart sound requires atrial contraction, which is missing in atrial fibrillation.

Breath Sounds. If the arrhythmia produces heart failure, listen for and record adventitious breath sounds, such as crackles, which could indicate pulmonary congestion. Also check the medical record for a history of pulmonary disease, which can produce sonorous or sibilant wheezes and may trigger an arrhythmia, such as multifocal atrial tachycardia.

Vascular System. Document your jugular vein findings, which may include an absent a-wave in a patient with atrial fibrillation. Also record peripheral pulse characteristics; pulses may be weak or vary in amplitude in a patient with an arrhythmia because not every heartbeat moves blood to the periphery. If the patient has ventricular fibrillation, expect to document pulselessness, but expect to find a pulse in a patient with ventricular tachycardia. Also assess for and document an apical-radial pulse deficit caused by reduced peripheral perfusion from ectopic beats. For a patient with atrial fibrillation, record signs of acute vascular complications. For example, thromboembolism may arise, causing dyspnea if the embolus lodges in a pulmonary vessel; cerebrovascular accident may occur, possibly producing hemiparesis.

Diagnostic Test Results. At least initially, your patient is likely to have a continuous cardiac monitor to assess his arrhythmia and detect new ones. Document the use of the monitor and, if possible, place a baseline rhythm strip in the patient's chart. Also place a 12-lead ECG tracing in the chart to help confirm the arrhythmia and monitor for ischemia.

Note the results of baseline laboratory tests that are ordered, which may include coagulation studies, serum electrolyte levels, and blood levels of drugs, such as digoxin. If you suspect hypoxemia, also record the results of arterial blood gas analysis.

Document What You Do

Some arrhythmias don't require treatment, such as those that don't produce cardiac compromise. But many arrhythmias demand treatment of their cause, such as fluid overload, digitalis toxicity, electrolyte imbalance, or hypoxemia. Your documentation should reflect your treatment of the arrhythmia or its cause, as well as the patient's response to the treatment.

Airway, Breathing, and Circulation. Document that you've assessed and ensured the patient's airway, breathing, and circulation (ABCs). Make sure that your notes reflect that ensuring ABCs was your priority and that it preceded other interventions.

For a patient with a life-threatening arrhythmia, such as ventricular tachycardia or ventricular fibrillation, perform advanced life support. In the chart, note the initial call for assistance, and assign a recorder to document the events that follow. The chart should indicate that you opened the patient's airway and provided positive-pressure ventilations and chest compressions, while another health care team member retrieved the defibrillator. It also should include the number of defibrillation attempts and the amount of energy used for each one. In addition, it should note the patient's cardiac rhythm, whether it changes or not. If the physician orders cardioversion for a patient who is breathing and has a pulse, the chart should show that you provided IV sedation before the procedure.

Drug and IV Therapy. If a large-bore IV catheter isn't in place already, insert one in the antecubital or similar vein. Document that you've confirmed correct catheter placement in the vein before administering drugs and IV solutions. Record the name, dosage, administration times, and routes of all drugs given. For drugs given as part of the code, put their information on the code sheet. For drugs given to treat a non–life-threatening arrhythmia, such as atrial fibrillation, record their information in the medication administration record and your notes. If anticoagulants are prescribed before the arrhythmia is corrected (as in atrial fibrillation), document the plan of care in the notes. Also note whether an IV drug will be given later in oral form. No matter which antiarrhythmic you give, keep in mind that it may worsen an existing arrhythmia or cause a new one. So throughout therapy, continue to monitor your patient's rhythm strip, especially for prolonged QT intervals; document this action.

Additional Diagnostic Tests and Treatments. Record blood test results, such as abnormal levels of digoxin or other drugs. If the physician orders monitoring of therapeutic levels of drugs, such as procainamide, note the time of blood sample collection in relation to drug administration, such as for a trough level.

If an external pacemaker is ordered to treat severe bradycardia or advanced heart block, document that you've applied it. Record patch placement on the chest and back, including skin preparation. (Be sure to clip—not shave—chest and back hair, and avoid areas with nitroglycerin paste or ointment or over bony prominences.) Also record settings for heart rate parameters, mode, and energy output. Verify that the energy output setting is sufficient to produce adequate capture on the ECG display without undue patient discomfort. Note that you've explained the procedure to the patient and warned him that the pacemaker discharge may cause a shocking sensation. Document the administration of sedatives or anxiolytics, if prescribed.

If the physician performs electrophysiology studies (EPS), document that you prepared the patient by describing the test and explaining that he may lose consciousness if an arrhythmia is induced. Record whether you administered or withheld antiarrhythmics beforehand, as ordered. On your facility's preprocedure checklist, record routine preparations, such as removing dentures and ensuring that the patient receives nothing by mouth. After the EPS, check the patient's venous access site (usually in the femoral vein) for bleeding or hematoma; document your actions. Monitor his vital signs and cardiac rhythm as often as required by facility policy. Also note if a treatment was performed during EPS, such as ectopic focus ablation or permanent pacemaker insertion.

Document What You Teach

A patient with an arrhythmia may have a long, complicated hospital stay while the health care team works to determine the arrhythmia's cause and its most effective treatment. Documentation of your teaching is vital because it helps communicate to colleagues what teaching has already taken place and what still needs to be done. Whether you document teaching in your narrative notes, in the nursing care plan, or on a patient-teaching form, be sure to include these important areas:

- disease process
- procedures and treatments
- home diagnostic tests, such as 24-hour Holter monitoring

- activity limitations
- signs and symptoms to report
- prescribed drugs, including their names, dosages, administration times and routes, adverse effects, and storage
- pacemaker or defibrillator care, if indicated
- incision care, including self-assessment for signs of infection
- diet
- follow-up appointments with the physician
- emergency access information, such as calling 911
- support group information

WHEN YOUR PATIENT HAS HYPERTENSIVE CRISIS

If your patient's diastolic blood pressure suddenly rises above 120 mm Hg and if she has renal failure or other signs of organ damage, suspect hypertensive crisis. This medical emergency requires prompt attention and treatment to avoid complications that can produce lasting effects, such as brain damage. When hypertensive crisis strikes, prepare to record events not only in your nurse's notes, but also on a flow sheet. That's because you need to measure your patient's blood pressure often—if not continuously—and to record those measurements frequently.

Document What the Patient Tells You

When your patient develops hypertensive crisis, documentation of a thorough health history can help pinpoint the cause. Be sure to ask about a history of chronic, uncontrolled hypertension; subarachnoid or cerebrovascular hemorrhage; cerebral infarction; pheochromocytoma; renal failure; and pregnancy complicated by eclampsia or preeclampsia. Also inquire about the sudden withdrawal of antihypertensive drugs, the use of monoamine oxidase (MAO) inhibitors with tyramine-rich food (such as aged cheese), and the use of recreational drugs, such as cocaine or crack.

If the patient reports that she suddenly stopped taking a prescribed antihypertensive, carefully document her reasons for this, including lack of understanding of the drug regimen, unpleasant adverse reactions, inconvenient scheduling, lack of affordability, or simple forgetfulness. Avoid being judgmental, especially in your documentation.

Also record the patient's reported signs and symptoms, such as blurred vision, diplopia, dizziness, tinnitus, vertigo, nosebleeds, muscle twitching, chest pain, palpitations, nausea, vomiting, behavior changes, and decreased level of consciousness. If the patient has a headache, determine its location (frontal headaches are common in hypertensive crisis), severity, and aggravating and alleviating factors.

Document What You Assess

The first several blood pressure measurements you record are likely to be manual ones taken with a sphygmomanometer. For these measurements, record the systolic and diastolic blood pressure. However, as you deflate the cuff, listen for Korotkoff sounds to become muffled and then disappear. If a gap of 10 mm Hg or more exists between their muffling and disappearance, record the blood pressure as three numbers: the systolic pressure, the point where the sounds become muffled, and the point where they disappear. For example, you might record 180/100/82.

Then use an automatic blood pressure cuff until an arterial line is established. Set the cuff to record measurements every 5 minutes or more frequently, as ordered. Document each blood pressure measurement on a vital sign flow sheet.

In hypertensive crisis, your patient is likely to need an arterial line for continuous blood pressure monitoring. Be sure to explain arterial line insertion to the patient and record your care before and after the procedure. (See *Documentation reminders for arterial line insertion*.) In addition to recording systolic and diastolic blood pressure readings, note the patient's mean arterial pressure (MAP).

Also document other vital signs, such as the patient's heart and respiratory rates and temperature. Measure and record her fluid intake and output, particularly noting decreased urinary output.

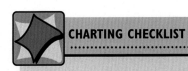

DOCUMENTATION REMINDERS FOR ARTERIAL LINE INSERTION

To monitor your patient's blood pressure continuously during hypertensive crisis, the physician usually inserts an arterial line in a radial artery. Before the procedure, review the patient's records for a history of radial artery removal (such as with coronary artery bypass grafting) or vascular grafting in the affected extremity. Then take and document the following steps to help ensure a good outcome:

Before the Procedure

❑ Explain the procedure to the patient and her family members.

❑ Make sure that a signed informed consent is in the patient's chart.

❑ Assess the circulation in her affected extremity by checking the skin color and temperature, capillary refill in the nail beds, and the presence and amplitude of the distal pulses. If the Allen test is performed to assess radial and ulnar artery patency, document the results.

❑ Prepare a flush bag of heparinized saline, as ordered. Check to make sure that heparin isn't contraindicated for the patient. Place the flush bag in a pressure bag and attach it to the pressure tubing system at the bedside. Purge air from the system.

❑ If a transducer isn't part of the tubing system, attach one and flush it; cap all stopcocks.

❑ Inflate the pressure bag to 300 mm Hg.

❑ Immobilize the patient's arm as the physician inserts the catheter. Then help suture it in place. Apply a sterile dressing over the insertion site.

After the Procedure

❑ Connect the tubing to the arterial catheter. Immobilize the patient's arm with an arm board, if needed.

❑ Level and zero the transducer according to facility policy and procedure. Observe the waveform on the cardiac monitor. Run a strip of the baseline tracing and place it in the patient's chart.

❑ Record blood pressure measurements, especially the mean arterial pressure, on a vital sign or critical care flow sheet.

❑ Frequently assess circulation in the extremity until the catheter is removed.

Then perform a head-to-toe assessment to detect complications of hypertensive crisis; document your findings.

Eyes. If you're skilled in using an ophthalmoscope, inspect the patient's retina. Check for and document papilledema (enlarged optic disc) and retinal hemorrhage or exudates.

Neurologic System. Assess for and record decreased level of consciousness, irritability, or confusion. Examine the patient for signs of cerebrovascular accident (CVA), noting such findings as hemiparesis, weakness, and slurred speech in the chart. Also document signs of hypertensive encephalopathy, such as seizures, and of focal deficits, such as cortical blindness or sensory impairment.

Cardiovascular System. During auscultation, listen for extra heart sounds, such as S_3 and S_4. Be sure to note these sounds in the chart because they often occur in hypertension and heart failure, which is a complication of hypertension. Based on your vascular assessment findings, record jugular vein distention or peripheral edema.

Diagnostic Test Results. Although some diagnostic tests may be postponed until hypertensive crisis has been resolved, review the results of initial tests to help determine the cause of the crisis and detect its complications. Place a copy of the test results in the appropriate area of the patient chart. Then in your nurse's notes, record that you read the abnormal results and reported them to the physician.

Review the patient's 12-lead electrocardiogram (ECG) tracing and document tachycardia, arrhythmias, or T-wave or ST-segment changes that suggest myocardial ischemia or infarction. Also record your observation of increased height or voltage in the QRS complexes from precordial leads—possible signs of left ventricular hypertrophy.

Make note of abnormal urinalysis results, such as proteinuria and low specific gravity, which can point to renal impairment. Also document red blood cells, granular casts, or blood in the urine, which may signal renal-induced hypertension. From other urine tests, record an abnormal protein level and creatinine clearance, which suggest renal impairment, and elevated levels of catecholamine (epinephrine and norepinephrine), which may indicate pheochromocytoma. If test results from a 24-hour urine collection confirm a decreased creatinine level, make a note of that also.

Renal ultrasonography can help pinpoint renal disease, and renal arteriography can help diagnose renal artery stenosis; record the results of these tests, too.

Document abnormal blood test results, such as elevated blood urea nitrogen or creatinine levels. Also record the results of tests that reveal left ventricular hypertrophy or heart enlargement, such as echocardiography and chest x-rays.

Document What You Do

To treat hypertensive crisis, plan to lower the MAP by 25% and the diastolic pressure to 100 to 110 mm Hg over several hours. Don't try to reduce the blood pressure more rapidly, because that can cause complications, such as cerebral edema. When treating the patient, closely monitor her for complications and frequently record her blood pressure and MAP measurements on a critical care flow sheet.

Close Monitoring. To track your patient's condition, frequently monitor her vital signs and connect her to a continuous cardiac monitor. Place a baseline rhythm strip in her medical record and add one or more strips per shift, as directed by facility policy. If the patient has an arrhythmia, also place a strip in her chart. Then in your nurse's notes document that you recognized the arrhythmia, notified the physician, and intervened promptly. As ordered, begin continuous pulse oximetry and record the patient's oxygen saturation. Provide supplemental oxygen if her oxygen saturation falls below 92%. Also monitor and record her fluid intake and output at least every 4 hours.

Drug and IV Therapy. Insert at least one IV catheter for IV antihypertensive therapy, keeping in mind that some drugs must be given in a separate IV infusion. In the patient's medication administration record and your nurse's notes, document administration of the prescribed antihypertensive. If the physician orders nitroprusside sodium, be sure to record the precautions you take to administer it safely:

- Always use an infusion pump to deliver nitroprusside sodium accurately. Use a dedicated IV line or port to infuse the drug.

- Wrap the drug container in a light-filtering cover, which is usually provided by the manufacturer.
- Inspect the solution for discoloration before administration.
- Titrate the drug as prescribed to lower the blood pressure safely. If hypotension occurs, decrease the infusion rate or stop the infusion.
- Watch for signs of thiocyanate and cyanide toxicity, such as nausea, vomiting, and muscle spasms.
- Monitor blood test results for signs of thiocyanate or cyanide toxicity. Record elevated cyanide and thiocyanate levels as well as signs of metabolic acidosis, such as an elevated anion gap.

When the target blood pressure is reached, discontinue IV drugs and begin oral antihypertensive therapy, as prescribed.

Document What You Teach

During hypertensive crisis, document your teaching, which should focus on the patient's immediate needs during hospitalization. Once the crisis has passed, target your teaching toward discharge planning. Be sure your teaching and documentation include:
- disease process
- procedures and treatments, such as arterial line insertion
- signs and symptoms to report
- prescribed drugs, including their names, dosages, administration times and routes, adverse effects, and storage
- importance of adhering to the prescribed drug, activity, and diet regimen
- dietary changes, including a low-sodium, low-fat diet
- follow-up appointments with the physician
- follow-up diagnostic tests

WHEN YOUR PATIENT HAS PNEUMONIA

Documentation for a patient with pneumonia can help avoid complications, promote his progress toward self-care, and prevent recurrences. During the health history interview and physical examination, stay alert for risk factors or other conditions that make your patient vulnerable to the disease.

Document What Your Patient Tells You

After documenting a complete health history, ask your patient to describe his symptoms. Then document them using his own words. Record the time of symptom onset, noting whether it was sudden or gradual. Ask about and record associated symptoms, such as fever, chills, cough, sputum production, weakness, fatigue, pain, and anorexia.

Risk Factors. To further identify risk factors for pneumonia, note the patient's age and ask about a history of recent hospitalizations or surgery, chronic conditions, cardiopulmonary disease, immunosuppressive therapy, decreased level of consciousness, and past bouts of pneumonia. Record complaints of difficulty eating, chewing, or swallowing, which predispose the patient to developing aspiration pneumonia. Document whether he has received a pneumococcal vaccine. If he did, note the administration date.

Finally, record his report of allergies to drugs, foods, chemicals, and environmental elements, such as dust, pollen, and pets.

Pain. Document chest pain, headache, or other pain your patient reports. Using his own words, record the pain's characteristics, including intensity and duration. Note factors that he says make the pain better (such as splinting the chest while coughing and applying heat) or worse (such as coughing and breathing deeply).

Document What You Assess

Assess and record the patient's vital sign measurements every 4 hours or more often if he's unstable. If you detect a fever, tachycardia, tachypnea, or hypotension, document this finding, notify the physician, and document your notification. When measuring vital signs, also reassess the patient's pain and record its intensity and other characteristics. Record all laboratory test results you obtain, such as arterial blood gas (ABG) levels.

Respiratory Status. Record the respiratory rate and rhythm. Then auscultate for breath sounds and document abnormalities, such as diminished breath sounds or crackles. Next, record percussion findings, such as areas of dullness, which may indicate consolidation. Also record other findings, including dyspnea, nasal flaring, use of accessory breathing muscles, and abnormal breathing patterns.

If the patient has a cough, document its frequency and its effectiveness in clearing secretions. If the cough is productive, describe the amount of sputum produced, frequency of sputum production, and sputum color, odor, and other characteristics.

Oxygenation. Record physical findings that reflect the patient's oxygenation, such as nail bed color and respiratory effort. Record pulse oximetry readings at the time of your initial assessment. Then obtain and document oximetry readings whenever the patient's condition changes or as required by the physician or facility policy. If the patient is receiving supplemental oxygen, note the amount of oxygen being administered at the time of the oximetry reading, along with the oxygen flow rate and delivery device. Do the same when recording ABG levels. Always record and report significant levels or important changes from previous ABG levels.

Next, document the patient's skin color, turgor, and temperature as well as capillary refill. Particularly note diaphoresis, pallor, and cyanosis, which may signal decreased oxygenation.

Finally, document your patient's level of consciousness. Stay especially alert for confusion or disorientation—a sign of hypoxia or hypercapnia—and report this immediately.

Document What You Do

Record your interventions as you initiate them. This helps show that you provided timely and appropriate care and can prove legally significant if the patient's care becomes an issue for litigation. (See *The court's lesson on failure to monitor patients,* pages 71-72.)

Frequent Monitoring. Record your patient's vital sign measurements every 4 hours or more often if he's unstable. Carefully document changes in temperature, heart and respiratory rates, and blood pressure.

Record respiratory findings often to help show whether the patient's condition is improving or deteriorating. Document breath

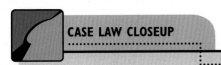

CASE LAW CLOSEUP

THE COURT'S LESSON ON FAILURE TO MONITOR PATIENTS
Anywhere, at any time, a patient with a condition such as pneumonia can suddenly worsen. That's why it's so important to monitor for and treat any significant changes. As far as the court is concerned, it's equally as important to document those efforts.

Understanding the Case
Nowhere is that concept more apparent than in *Brandon HMA, Inc. v. Bradshaw*[1], a case in which Mrs. Bradshaw's pneumonia rapidly took a turn for the worse. Upon admission to an acute care setting, she was stabilized, had a chest tube inserted on the left side, and received orders for Tylenol Extra Strength and Lorcet Plus every 6 hours for pain and Ativan as needed for anxiety. Then she was transferred to a general medical unit.

During the evening shift, nurse's notes indicated that Mrs. Bradshaw was checked periodically. The notes showed that her vital signs remained stable, she was medicated as needed for pain and anxiety, and she experienced no distress. This information was given to the night shift staff via an audiotaped nursing report.

At midnight, night shift staff members began to enter the patient's room. The charge nurse started a new bag of intravenous (IV) solution. However, no vital signs were taken, and no notes were made in the patient's record.

A short time later, the licensed practical nurse (LPN) took Mrs. Bradshaw's vital signs and recorded a slightly elevated temperature. He also recorded that she was having pain in her left side. At 2:00 A.M., the LPN gave Mrs. Bradshaw Tylenol Extra Strength tablets for continuing pain. The LPN didn't take vital signs but, after consulting the charge nurse, administered Ativan for agitation.

At 2:40 A.M., Mrs. Bradshaw was in high-Fowler's position and reported that worsening pain. The LPN noted that her respirations were "short and rapid" and repeated the dose of Lorcet Plus, believing that she needed more pain medication. At 3:00 A.M., the charge nurse entered the room to hang another IV bag.

When the LPN returned at 3:30 A.M., Mrs. Bradshaw was in severe respiratory distress and had nausea, disorientation, and diaphoresis. He took her vital signs again and then consulted the charge nurse but didn't indicate that this was an emergency. At 3:40 A.M., they both came to the room, found the patient cyanotic, and called a code. Mrs. Bradshaw was revived, but sustained severe hypoxic brain damage. The patient's family sued for negligence.

---

[1]*Brandon HMA, Inc. v. Bradshaw, 809 So. 2d 611 (Mississippi, 2001).*

Continued

CASE LAW CLOSEUP

THE COURT'S LESSON ON FAILURE TO MONITOR PATIENTS—cont'd
How the Court Ruled
The Supreme Court of Mississippi upheld a $9,000,000 award to Mrs. Bradshaw for several reasons. First, nothing in the chart validated the charge nurse's claim that it was her habit to inspect the patient whenever she would hang a new bag of IV fluid. If she had inspected Mrs. Bradshaw at 3:00 A.M. when she brought in the second IV bag, she would have noticed greatly altered respirations. That would have been her first clue to the patient's changing condition.

Second, the court faulted the LPN for giving the patient another Lorcet Plus dose at 2:40 A.M. without considering the narcotic's ability to depress her already compromised respirations, for failing to retake her vital signs before giving the narcotic, and for failing to check them afterward.

Finally, there was no code sheet to validate what happened during the code that successfully resuscitated Mrs. Bradshaw. The court noted that, although it wasn't certain what the code sheet would show, the staff's failure to complete the required form showed a lack of professionalism at the facility and prevented the patient's attorney from presenting the full facts of the case.

The Lesson Learned
This case highlights the need to properly monitor and care for patients—and to thoroughly document assessment findings and related care. Of course, even with the best care, a patient's health can suddenly worsen, especially if she has respiratory compromise and a chest tube. However, it's unpardonable to allow a patient's overall condition to worsen this much without noticing it or recognizing critical signs and symptoms.

Accurate documentation may not have made much difference to this case's outcome. Yet such documentation would have helped the court verify that the patient received appropriate nursing care. And it would have prevented the court from holding that the care given to this patient was unprofessional.

sounds, sputum production and characteristics, pulse oximetry readings, cough, ability to clear secretions, dyspnea, breathing patterns, and other significant findings.

Next, document your patient's initial pulse oximetry reading, along with vital sign measurements and ABG levels. If the physician prescribes oxygen, document the time you initiated oxygen therapy, the oxygen flow rate, and the delivery device used (such as a nasal cannula or face mask). Monitor vital signs and pulse oximetry values at least every 4 hours until they fall within normal limits, and then check every 4 to 8 hours, as ordered.

To document fluid balance—an important indicator in pneumonia—record intake and output every 4 hours. Document a significant fluid imbalance, your notification to the physician, and your interventions.

Drug and IV Therapy. Record the times of specimen collection for sputum and blood cultures, which usually precede antibiotic therapy. Also document the time antibiotic therapy began, along with the drug names, dosages, and administration times and routes. As appropriate, record drug administration in the medication administration record. (See *Using a medication administration record,* page 75.)

After giving the first IV dose of an antibiotic the patient has never received before, record pertinent negatives, such as "no signs or symptoms of an allergic reaction." If a reaction occurs, document it in detail, along with the name of the drug, administration time, and name of the physician you notified. If you receive orders for treating the allergic reaction, document this fact and the time you implemented them.

If the physician prescribes hydration, document the type of IV fluid given, date and time you initiated the infusion, infusion rate, and infusion device used. Then record the location and appearance of the IV site, the date and time the IV line was inserted, cannula size, type and condition of dressing, patency of the line, and the patient's tolerance for the infusion.

Secretion Clearance. Document any difficulty your patient has clearing secretions. Also record measures you take to promote clearance, such as elevating the head of the bed, encouraging frequent coughing and deep breathing, performing chest physiotherapy, and suctioning. Record the patient's response to these interventions and resulting changes in his status.

Sample and Specimen Collection. If your facility's policy permits you to draw arterial blood samples for ABG analysis, document site preparation, Allen's test results, equipment and artery used, and pressure application after blood withdrawal. After sample collection, record your observation of the site, pulse palpation, and assessment of adequate distal circulation. Record all ABG levels, noting the time the sample was drawn, amount of oxygen the patient was receiving at the time, and changes in his condition.

Also document the time other blood samples or sputum specimens were collected, collection method used (for instance, "Blood was obtained from patient's central venous access device"), and the time you reported results to the physician. Explain the specimen collection process to the patient, and document this teaching.

Nutrition. Record your assessment of the patient's diet and appetite, including the percentage of meals he eats. Note that you're helping him choose foods high in nutritional value that he can easily eat. If he's too weak or fatigued to eat without help, note assistance you give at meals. If he requires aspiration precautions, document that you've instituted and maintained those precautions. Also record referrals you make to the dietitian, noting the time the dietitian consults with the patient.

Activity. Record your patient's activity level, noting changes from his usual activity level at home. During activity, assess and document dyspnea if it occurs. If he's bedridden or sedentary, document that you encouraged him and provided assistance to increase his activity level, if appropriate.

Document What You Teach

Your teaching and the patient's accurate understanding can promote a quick, uneventful recovery and help prevent recurrences of pneumonia. By documenting your teaching and the patient's understanding, you confirm that your patient has the information he needs to maintain optimal health. Include these topics in your teaching and documentation:

- disease process
- drugs, including their names, dosages, administration times and routes, adverse effects, and storage
- coughing and deep-breathing exercises
- hygiene

- infection prevention
- signs and symptoms to report
- recommended preventive vaccines
- hydration
- nutrition
- activity and rest
- resources for further information and support

CHARTING CHECKLIST

USING A MEDICATION ADMINISTRATION RECORD

Most health care facilities require nurses to document drug administration in the medication administration record (MAR). When making entries in the MAR, follow these guidelines:

❑ Use two lines when transcribing orders, unless your facility has a different policy. On the first line, indicate the drug's name and prescribed dosage. Then on the second, note the administration route and frequency and other pertinent information, such as a stop date.

❑ When transcribing a medication dosage, use a leading zero, as in "0.2 mg." Avoid a trailing zeros, as in "2.0 mg."

❑ To record the time, use a 24-hour clock. For example, write "1400 hours" instead of "2 P.M."

❑ Record pertinent information, such as vital sign measurements, where indicated on the MAR. For example, before administering digoxin, note the patient's heart rate in the appropriate box.

❑ Use only standard abbreviations approved by your facility.

❑ After recording the patient's first dose, sign your full name and licensure status, and place your initials in the appropriate space.

❑ Indicate the site used, if you're giving a drug by intramuscular or subcutaneous injection.

❑ Enter information in the MAR as soon as possible after giving the drug so that other health care providers have access to the most recent drug information.

❑ Above all, learn—and follow—your facility's policies and procedures for drug documentation.

WHEN YOUR PATIENT HAS PNEUMOTHORAX

P neumothorax occurs when air accumulates between the visceral and parietal pleurae, which commonly causes the adjacent lung to collapse. In *open pneumothorax,* traumatic injury or another event causes a chest wall opening, which allows air to enter and accumulate. In *closed pneumothorax,* a disease such as emphysema weakens the surface of the visceral pleura, allowing air accumulation. Other causes of pneumothorax include procedures and treatments, such as central catheter insertion or mechanical ventilation that causes barotrauma.

Sometimes, air accumulates gradually and may not lead to complete collapse of the lung. A small pneumothorax may even resolve spontaneously. Other times, air accumulates rapidly, entering the pleural space on inhalation, but not escaping on exhalation. This happens in *tension pneumothorax,* which results in lung collapse and mediastinal shift and requires immediate intervention.

For a patient with pneumothorax, your timely documentation of assessment findings, interventions, and responses to treatments can make her hospital stay run more smoothly. That's because proper documentation clearly communicates all pertinent information to the health care team, resulting in better care.

Document What the Patient Tells You

When your patient develops pneumothorax, record everything she says about her symptoms. If her breathing is so impaired that she can't speak, ask a family member about what she has been experiencing. If she can speak, expect her to describe labored, possibly painful breathing. She may report sudden, sharp, pleuritic pain over the affected area. She may also feel restless and hungry for air and may have a sense of impending doom. Document each symptom in detail, noting its onset, duration, severity, quality, and location, as well as factors that aggravate or alleviate it.

If time allows, record a focused health history and review it for risk factors of pneumothorax. Be sure to ask about a history of pulmonary disease, such as emphysema; injury, such as chest trauma; and recent medical procedures, such as central line insertion.

Document What You Assess

If you suspect that your patient has pneumothorax, quickly assess her for signs of the disorder and its complications, such as hypoxemia and respiratory distress. Document your findings—and your communication with the physician—in your nurse's notes.

General Appearance. Assess your patient's general appearance. Check the color of her skin and mucous membranes, particularly noting ashen skin or cyanosis. Observe for anxiety, diaphoresis, and gasping for air. Look for signs of respiratory distress, such as sternocleidomastoid contractions, intercostal and suprasternal retractions, nasal flaring, and chest hyperexpansion. Document all pertinent findings.

Vital Signs. Record the patient's vital signs and stay alert for tachypnea, tachycardia, and hypertension—all signs of respiratory impairment.

Neck Structures. When examining the patient's neck, assess for and record jugular vein distention and tracheal deviation toward the side opposite the affected lung. These signs suggest that tension pneumothorax has caused a mediastinal shift. Document your immediate notification of the physician about these findings.

Chest and Back. As you assess the patient's chest and back, look for and record asymmetrical chest movement—a sign of lung collapse. Also document any hyperresonance on percussion and decreased or absent breath sounds on the affected side. In the chart, note whether you detect subcutaneous emphysema or crepitus during chest wall palpation. These findings suggest that air has escaped into the surrounding subcutaneous tissue.

Diagnostic Test Results. If a pulse oximeter is available, record the patient's oxygen saturation; note a reading below 92%, which signals hypoxemia. Also check her oxygen saturation via arterial blood gas analysis.

Prepare the patient for a chest x-ray to confirm the presence, location, and size of her pneumothorax. In the chart, record whether the x-ray is performed in the radiology department or

at the bedside. If the patient must go to the radiology department, document the name and title of the nurse who escorted
her, the availability of emergency equipment while she's off your
unit, the time the patient left and returned to the unit, and how
well she tolerated the procedure. Also note if the patient was
placed on portable oxygen or a cardiac monitor before, during,
and after her trip to the radiology department.

Document What You Do

If your patient's pneumothorax is small, she may simply require
close observation while the trapped air resorbs and the pneumothorax resolves on its own. But if pneumothorax causes lung
collapse and impaired ventilation, she may need rapid interventions, such as chest tube insertion. Before, during, and after any
interventions, carefully record your actions and the patient's
response to them.

   Interventions for Open Pneumothorax. If a chest wall
opening produces tension pneumothorax (as with chest trauma
or inadvertent chest tube removal), act quickly and record your
interventions. Document that you covered the puncture site with
an occlusive dressing, such as petroleum gauze, and securely
taped it in place. Then record that you helped the patient into a
high-Fowler's position to improve chest expansion and aid ventilation. Document that you provided supplemental oxygen as
ordered, noting the amount, the delivery system (nasal cannula or
face mask), and the patient's response. If a chest tube isn't available immediately, document that you helped insert a large-bore
needle to release trapped air and improve ventilation. When a
chest tube becomes available, record the steps you took to assist
with insertion. (See *What to document about chest tube insertion,*
pages 79-80.)

   Interventions for Closed Pneumothorax. Treatment for
closed pneumothorax may require chest tube insertion. If the
patient also has hemothorax or other fluid accumulation, she
may need a second chest tube inserted at the base of her lungs.
If pneumothorax is not resolved with one or more chest tubes,
the patient may undergo pleurodesis. This procedure uses instillation

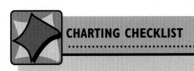

WHAT TO DOCUMENT ABOUT CHEST TUBE INSERTION
For pneumothorax, the most effective treatment is insertion of a chest tube, which is usually connected to a drainage system that flows by gravity or suction. Your patient care related to chest tube insertion is critical. So is meticulous documentation of your actions before and after the procedure, especially if complications arise.

Before the Procedure
❏ Explain the procedure to the patient and her family members.

❏ Assemble the equipment using sterile technique.

❏ Help the patient into the proper position—usually in the side-lying position with the affected side up.

❏ Assist with local anesthetic injection and antiseptic application before chest tube insertion. For pneumothorax, expect to prepare a site near the apex of the lungs in the second intercostal space.

After the Procedure
❏ Once the chest tube is inserted, attach it to a drainage system and placing the draining device lower than the patient's chest. Reinforce all connections with tape.

❏ Help suture the chest tube in place.

❏ Apply an occlusive dressing. Regularly check the dressing for drainage and the surrounding tissue for signs of infection or subcutaneous emphysema.

❏ Attach the drainage system to wall suction, if prescribed.

❏ Record the results of a STAT chest x-ray that confirms tube placement. Note the results of daily chest x-rays to evaluate the resolution of pneumothorax.

❏ Auscultate the patient's breath sounds bilaterally to help assess for lung reinflation. Check her vital signs frequently.

❏ Maintain tube patency by keeping them free of kinks and tangles.

❏ Avoid routinely milking or stripping the tubes. If you notice a clot, gently milk the tubing, as ordered.

❏ If pleural fluid drains into the collection chamber, mark the chamber with the date and time at the end of each shift. In your notes or on a flow sheet, record the amount of drainage per shift, as well as the total amount.

Continued

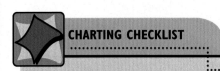

WHAT TO DOCUMENT ABOUT CHEST TUBE INSERTION—cont'd

❑ Check for intermittent bubbling in the water-seal chamber and tidaling (rising of the level with inspiration and falling with expiration), which should be present. Note that continuous bubbling can signal a leak.

❑ Encourage the patient to cough and take deep breaths to help reexpand her lung.

❑ Provide analgesics, as prescribed, to promote comfort and improved range of motion on the affected side.

of an irritant, such as tetracycline, to sclerose the pleural membranes, causing them to adhere and seal the air leak. For a patient receiving pleurodesis, document that you explained it to her and that you provided analgesia, as prescribed.

Resolution of Pneumothorax. When the patient's chest x-ray shows that pneumothorax has resolved and that the lung has reexpanded, prepare her for chest tube removal. In your notes, record other signs of pneumothorax resolution, such as clear breath sounds on the affected side and a lack of bubbling in the water-seal chamber. Document that you clamped the chest tube several hours before its removal as ordered and that the patient experienced no respiratory distress.

After chest tube removal, note that you immediately covered the site with an occlusive dressing, such as petroleum gauze, and taped it in place. Then document that you assessed for signs of respiratory distress, auscultated breath sounds, and checked vital signs frequently. Record that you encouraged the patient to take deep breaths, cough, and use an incentive spirometer to help maintain lung expansion.

Document What You Teach

Patient teaching and support should occur throughout your patient's hospital stay. Because pneumothorax and its treatment, such as chest tube insertion, can cause pain and anxiety, don't forget to record your comfort measures and emotional support. Also be sure that your teaching and documentation include:

- disease process
- procedures and treatments, such as chest tube insertion
- passive and active range-of-motion exercises on the affected side
- importance of coughing and deep breathing
- use of an incentive spirometer
- signs and symptoms to report
- prescribed drugs, including their names, dosages, administration times and routes, adverse effects, and storage
- home care for chest tube insertion site, including self-assessment for signs of infection
- diet
- follow-up appointments with the physician

WHEN YOUR PATIENT HAS AN ASTHMA ATTACK

Potentially life-threatening, an acute asthma attack calls for prompt, accurate assessment and expert intervention—and complete documentation of those actions. To avoid future asthma attacks and help maintain an optimal activity level, the patient also needs effective teaching. Thorough documentation of your assessment, interventions, and teaching directs his plan of care during the acute episode. It can also help safeguard his long-term health.

Document What the Patient Tells You

Even after stabilizing a patient with an acute asthma attack, difficulty breathing and speaking may prevent him from supplying information. If he can nod or shake his head, ask essential yes-or-no questions and record his responses. If he's accompanied by a family member or friend, obtain information from that person.

Then check the patient's medical record for data about a history of asthma or other respiratory problems, current drug use, and allergies. Be sure to note whether he uses oxygen, a nebulizer, or an inhaler at home, and document whether he's taking a steroid to treat asthma. If he is, record the dosage and the date he started taking it. Also find out whether he takes peak–flow measurements at home. Ask about and document his best measurement.

Next, record data about the current asthma attack, including its onset, duration, and accompanying symptoms. Ask the patient or his companion how often he experiences asthma attacks and whether the current episode differs from previous attacks. Carefully document the answers. Then identify and record recent exposure to irritants, such as smoke, allergens, and chemicals. Ask about symptoms of recent respiratory tract infections, such as fever and productive cough. Also document the treatments that have helped terminate previous asthma attacks. In addition, ask about and record a history of any related disorders, such as gastroesophageal reflux disease, which often accompanies asthma.

Document What You Assess

Record your findings from a rapid assessment. Include the following expected abnormal findings, if present, and any others you detect:
- wheezing and dyspnea
- diminished or absent breath sounds
- difficulty speaking or performing activities (from dyspnea)
- tachypnea
- use of accessory breathing muscles
- productive cough
- tachycardia
- hypotension
- anxiety and diaphoresis
- signs of decreased oxygenation, such as cyanosis
- change in level of consciousness

If diagnostic test results are available, record pulse oximetry readings, arterial blood gas (ABG) levels, and peak–flow measurements.

Document What You Do

To prevent the asthma attack from progressing, intervene rapidly and record your actions as you take them. Expect to implement and document some or all of the interventions described below.

Oxygen Administration. If the physician prescribes oxygen, document the time you initiated oxygen therapy, the flow rate, and the delivery device (such as a nasal cannula or face mask). Monitor and document vital sign measurements and pulse oximetry readings every 1 to 2 hours as appropriate until these values fall within normal limits. Then monitor and document them every 4 hours. Record ABG levels from samples drawn after oxygen therapy begins, noting the oxygen flow rate.

Nebulizer or Inhaler Administration. Document each time your patient receives a nebulizer or inhaler treatment. Record the dosage, administration technique (including whether the patient self-administered it), and his response to the treatment. Before and after each treatment, record peak-flow measurements to evaluate the effectiveness. Note, too, if the patient reports that his symptoms are subsiding or worsening.

Drug and IV Therapy. Document the names, dosages, and administration times and routes of drugs you administer, along with teaching you provide about the drugs. Record the patient's response to each drug and adverse reactions that occur. If he's receiving theophylline, record blood theophylline levels and document signs of toxicity. If he's receiving a corticosteroid, document your teaching about adverse reactions and the need to taper the dosage rather than stopping the drug abruptly.

If you're administering IV drugs or fluids, record the infusion rate, IV site appearance, and line patency. Also document each time you hang a new IV bag and change the tubing. Note the delivery device used (such as an IV pump or controller), and record changes you make in the flow rate. Be sure to evaluate and document the patient's response to IV therapy.

Sample and Specimen Collection. If your facility's policy permits you to draw arterial blood samples for ABG analysis, document site preparation, Allen's test results, equipment and artery used, and pressure application after blood withdrawal. After drawing samples, document your observation of the site, pulse palpation, and assessment of distal circulation. Record ABG levels each time a sample is drawn, noting the amount of oxygen the patient was receiving and changes in his condition.

For other blood samples obtained for laboratory tests, note the time of withdrawal, the site used, and the patient's response. Document test results when they become available, along with your notification to the physician, his orders, and your interventions.

If ordered, obtain a sputum specimen for culture and sensitivity testing. Document the time the specimen was obtained, noting its color and other characteristics.

Oxygenation. Record interventions you take to improve oxygenation, such as positioning the patient upright, teaching about proper breathing and relaxation techniques, and pacing his activities.

Emotional Support. Provide emotional support during your patient's acute asthma attack. Document indicators of his emotional state, your interventions to ease anxiety, and his response.

Document What You Teach

To help your patient lead a normal, active life, provide comprehensive teaching about asthma and its treatment. Document each topic you cover, the method used to teach it, and the patient's understanding. Based on your established teaching outcomes, use measurable terms to evaluate his understanding, such as, "Patient demonstrated correct use of inhaler in three of four attempts." (See *Documenting teaching outcomes*.)

Be sure to include the following topics in your teaching and documentation:

- respiratory system anatomy and physiology
- disease process
- significance of peak-flow measurements
- what to do if peak-flow measurements worsen or if an acute asthma attack occurs
- prescribed drugs, including their names, dosages, administration times and routes, adverse effects, and storage
- corticosteroid use, if applicable
- use of a prescribed inhaler or nebulizer
- care of an inhaler and other respiratory equipment used at home
- signs and symptoms to report
- hygiene and infection prevention
- breathing techniques

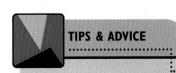

DOCUMENTING TEACHING OUTCOMES

Teaching outcomes fall into three categories. *Cognitive outcomes* measure the patient's understanding of the information taught, such as symptoms to report to the physician. *Psychomotor outcomes* reflect his ability to perform a task, such as obtaining a peak-flow measurement. *Affective outcomes* measure changes in the patient's behavior, such as adhering to dietary restrictions.

To be effective, teaching outcomes should be clear and measurable so that other health care team members can easily evaluate what the patient has learned. When writing outcomes, include the topic taught, desired patient behavior, and criteria for evaluating each outcome. For best results, start each outcome with an action verb and restrict the outcome to a single concept, action, or behavior. For examples of well-written and poorly written outcomes, review the chart below.

Well-Written Outcomes	Poorly Written Outcomes
The patient with asthma will demonstrate the ability to:	The patient with asthma will demonstrate the ability to:
Cognitive Outcomes	
• state when to take each prescribed drug	• know his drug schedule
• describe symptoms leading to an asthma attack	• know when he is in danger of having an asthma attack
• name asthma triggers to avoid	• understand what asthma triggers to avoid
Psychomotor Outcomes	
• measure his peak flow rate accurately	• take his peak flow rate
• use an inhaler and a spacer correctly	• use an inhaler
• clean his spacer properly	• care for his spacer
Affective Outcomes	
• maintain a twice-daily record of his peak-flow measurements	• understand the relationship between peak-flow measurements and asthma
• verbalize his concerns about the need to make changes in his environment	• adjust to limitations imposed by asthma
• keep scheduled physician appointments	• realize the importance of seeing his physician

- identifying and avoiding precipitating factors
- pacing activities with rest
- dietary and fluid recommendations
- stress management and relaxation techniques
- additional sources of information and support

WHEN YOUR PATIENT HAS A PULMONARY EMBOLISM

Without prompt assessment and treatment, pulmonary embolism can lead to serious complications and, possibly, death. If you suspect a pulmonary embolism, notify the physician at once and take emergency steps to safeguard the patient's life. Then, as soon as possible, document the findings that led you to suspect pulmonary embolism.

When the patient's condition allows, review her history for factors that predispose her to this disorder. Then perform a thorough physical examination, focusing on her respiratory status and oxygenation. To show efficient nursing care and ensure clear communication with the rest of the health care team, document your interventions as you initiate them, along with the patient's response.

Document What the Patient Tells You

Record predisposing factors that the patient reports, such as a history of recent surgery, myocardial infarction, heart failure, atrial fibrillation, venous insufficiency, thrombophlebitis, polycythemia vera, chronic illness, trauma, and immobilization after a fracture. Add other risk factors that you note, such as smoking, advanced age, and obesity. Note recent pregnancy, childbirth, oral contraceptive use, and estrogen replacement therapy.

If your patient reports chest pain, ask her to describe it in detail, and record her answer in her own words. Include its precise location and time of onset. Record her rating of pain severity on a scale of 0 to 10, with 0 indicating no pain and 10 indicating the worst pain imaginable. Ask about and record factors that she says make the pain worse (such as breathing deeply and coughing) or better (such as lying still and splinting the chest while coughing). If she reports shortness of breath, document when she first noted this symptom. Also assess and record her anxiety level and note whether she reports a sense of impending doom.

Document What You Assess

Focus your assessment and documentation on the patient's respiratory status and oxygenation. If you suspect that a blood disorder has contributed to the pulmonary embolism, check her most recent hemoglobin, erythrocyte, and thrombocyte values. Document that you notified the physician of abnormal values, along with the notification time and the physician's orders. Also, if you suspect that deep vein thrombosis has led to pulmonary embolism, check the patient's calves for erythema and edema and assess for Homans' sign; document your findings.

Respiratory System. Document your assessment of the patient's respiratory status every 1 to 2 hours or as appropriate. Include the respiratory rate and rhythm, chest expansion characteristics (such as asymmetry), and any tachypnea, dyspnea, shallow breathing, or accessory muscle use.

Record the time of breath sound auscultation, noting such abnormalities as diminished breath sounds, wheezes, crackles, and friction rub. Document whether the patient has a cough. If the cough is productive, describe the amount of sputum produced and its characteristics.

Oxygenation. To document the patient's oxygenation, record your assessment of her skin for circumoral cyanosis, pallor, coolness, clamminess, and diaphoresis. Also document pertinent negatives, such as absence of pallor. If the patient was admitted for thrombophlebitis, record your assessment of the affected leg, including its temperature and any edema, redness, or tenderness. Because impaired oxygenation can decrease the patient's level of consciousness, check for and record disorientation, confusion, and stupor.

Document the patient's pulse oximetry reading each time her condition changes. Write down the oxygen concentration she's receiving at the time of the reading. If she's not receiving oxygen, note that she's on room air. Record arterial blood gas (ABG) levels each time a sample is drawn, and note the amount of oxygen she was receiving and any changes in her condition.

Document What You Do

Act quickly to help your patient with a pulmonary embolism maintain adequate oxygenation and gas exchange. Try to document each intervention as you perform it, and then record the patient's response. (See *Documenting by "AIR."*)

TIPS & ADVICE

DOCUMENTING BY "AIR"
Designed to avoid repetition of previously documented information, the AIR (Assessment, Intervention, Response) format promotes clear, concise recording of the patient's condition and nursing interventions—especially when used with flow sheets and the nursing plan of care. Using "AIR" allows you to document continual care. This can prove especially useful when the patient response you document doesn't reflect a final outcome. Here's an explanation of AIR documentation, followed by a sample.

A: Assessment
Summarize your assessment findings, including trends (worsening or improvement) and your impressions of the patient's problem. Organize the data into appropriate sections, using headings such as "Admission note" and "Discharge teaching."

I: Intervention
Describe your actions and those of other caregivers in response to assessment findings. Group information under the same headings you used in the "Assessment" section. You may want to include plans for additional monitoring or care.

R: Response
Document your patient's response to interventions, using the same headings you used for the other sections. Be aware that if the patient's response isn't expected for several hours or days after the intervention, another nurse may document it.

Oxygen Therapy. If the physician prescribes oxygen, document the time you initiated oxygen therapy, the flow rate, and the delivery device (such as a nasal cannula or face mask). Record your patient's tolerance of and compliance with oxygen therapy.

Monitor and document vital sign measurements and pulse oximetry readings at least every hour until these values fall within normal limits. Then monitor and document values every 4 hours or with any change in the patient's condition. Also record ABG levels obtained after oxygen therapy begins, and note the oxygen flow rate at the time the blood sample was drawn.

A: At 1240, patient had labored respirations of 24 breaths/minute. Breath sounds diminished in Ⓡ base. Skin cool and clammy. Fingernails cyanotic. _____ A. Casey, RN

I: At 1300, Dr. Williams notified of change in patient's clinical status and physical findings. Dr. Williams' verbal orders at that time included STAT ABGs and O_2 therapy to begin at 4 liters/minute. ABG sample obtained by respiratory therapist. Patient placed in semi-Fowler's position and nasal O_2 started at 4 liters/minute as prescribed. ____ A. Casey, RN

R: At 1330, patient's respiratory rate 20 breaths/minute. Skin cool but no longer clammy. Nail beds show no cyanosis. Patient states he feels "much better." He appears comfortable while supine. ____ A Casey, RN

Anticoagulant Therapy. If the physician prescribes an anticoagulant, document the patient's baseline prothrombin time (PT), activated partial thromboplastin time (APTT), and international normalized ratio (INR) of prothrombin time before giving the first dose. Also document the date and time the IV line was inserted, catheter size, IV site location and appearance, and type and condition of dressing.

Before beginning a heparin infusion, check the patient's medical record for her most recent height and weight to help determine the correct dosage. If the record doesn't indicate her recent height and weight, weigh her if she's stable enough or ask family members if they know her height. Be sure to document this crucial information. Then record the time and date the infusion began, the infusion rate, delivery device (such as IV pump), and bolus doses given. Document follow-up APTT 6 hours after heparin therapy starts or after the infusion rate changes.

If the physician changes the order from heparin to warfarin, document the prescribed warfarin dosage and administration time and route. Record the patient's INR daily or as ordered, and record the time you notified the physician of significant results. Throughout anticoagulant therapy, check for and record signs and symptoms of bleeding, including epistaxis and bloody urine or stools, and document that you notified the physician if any were found.

Oxygenation. Document interventions used to promote oxygenation, such as positioning the patient, encouraging frequent rest periods, and assisting with activities of daily living to prevent fatigue. If you give a prescribed analgesic to control pain and ease breathing, record the dosage, administration time and route, and the patient's response.

As appropriate, implement and document comfort measures, such as assisting with relaxation techniques. Remember—breathing difficulties commonly cause anxiety, which can further compromise oxygenation.

Document What You Teach

Depending on the cause of pulmonary embolism, your patient may require extensive teaching to prevent a recurrence. Thoroughly document your teaching plan, your assessment of the patient's readiness to learn, and her understanding of the material taught. Include these topics:

- respiratory system anatomy and physiology
- disease process
- signs and symptoms of respiratory insufficiency
- dietary restrictions
- prescribed anticoagulant therapy
- other prescribed drugs, including their names, dosages, administration times and routes, adverse effects, and storage
- bleeding precautions
- signs and symptoms to report
- required follow-up tests, such as PT, APTT, and INR
- ways to prevent future episodes, such as by using antiembolism stockings if ordered

WHEN YOUR PATIENT HAS PULMONARY EDEMA

Accurate documentation helps identify the cause of pulmonary edema and guides the health care team toward the most effective treatment. Pulmonary edema can rapidly progress to respiratory failure. By focusing your documentation on the key points described below, you can help your patient avert this acute emergency.

Document What the Patient Tells You

As necessary, gather information from the patient, family members, and existing medical records. In particular, document reports of chest pain. Using the patient's own words, record the pain's exact location, time of onset, duration, severity (on a scale of 0 to 10), exacerbating factors (such as taking a deep breath), and alleviating factors (such as sitting upright).

Also check for and record preexisting cardiac or respiratory conditions that can precipitate pulmonary edema, past episodes of heart failure or acute respiratory distress syndrome, and a history of other predisposing factors, such as kidney or liver disease. Then record the names of drugs the patient reports taking and allergies he describes.

Document What You Assess

During the acute crisis, record the patient's vital sign measurements frequently and obtain his weight daily. Also thoroughly document the crucial findings described below.

Respiratory System and Oxygenation. Document your frequent auscultation of the patient's breath sounds, including adventitious sounds (such as crackles and wheezes). Note dyspnea, labored breathing, and use of accessory breathing muscles. Also document whether the patient has a cough. If he does, check for sputum production and describe the amount, color, and odor of the sputum, as well as other characteristics.

Then record significant skin findings, such as diaphoresis, abnormal temperature, clamminess, and cyanosis. Look for and document signs and symptoms of hypoxia, such as anxiety and restlessness. If the patient becomes short of breath during activity, record this fact. Indicate how much activity he can tolerate before becoming short of breath and how long it takes for him to recover a normal breathing pattern after rest. If he has difficulty lying flat, note this too.

Finally, check for peripheral edema. Document its location, note any pitting, and record the degree of the pitting.

Cardiovascular System. Because pulmonary edema stresses the heart, document signs and symptoms of cardiac compromise. Record auscultation of heart sounds, noting decreased or abnormal sounds, such as S_3. Then document the quality of the pulse, which may be bounding in pulmonary edema. Be sure to document that you assessed for jugular vein distention too.

Document What You Do

To prevent your patient's condition from worsening, act quickly. Record your interventions as soon as possible after you implement them.

Airway, Breathing, and Circulation. Document that you assessed and ensured an adequate airway, breathing, and circulation

(ABCs). Make sure your documentation reflects that maintaining ABCs was your priority and preceded other interventions. Also document each time you assess the patient's vital signs, your notification of the physician about abnormal findings, his orders, and your actions. (See *Documenting your communications*.)

Record the time the patient was placed on a cardiac monitor and your explanation to him of the reason for the monitor.

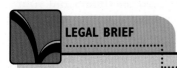

LEGAL BRIEF

DOCUMENTING YOUR COMMUNICATIONS

If your patient has pulmonary edema or another condition that requires quick assessment and intervention, you may have trouble finding the time to document every conversation you have with other health care team members. Recording such communications offers important legal protection if the patient or his family later files a lawsuit alleging malpractice.

Record What You Say, Not Just What You Do

Document not only what you do for your patient but also what you say pertaining to his care. Always document that you reported pertinent patient information to the physician and other health care team members, along with the time of notification and the person's name and response.

For example, suppose your patient's urine output has measured 20 ml for 2 consecutive hours and you've auscultated crackles in both lung bases with deep inspiration. Besides documenting these findings, note that you communicated them to the physician. Then record the interventions the physician orders, such as furosemide, 20 mg IV. Otherwise, the medical record would suggest only that you followed the physician's orders—not that you notified him of a significant change in your patient's condition.

Documenting notification time establishes the interval between your assessment of a significant finding and your report of that finding to the physician. This can prove crucial in a lawsuit involving suspected neglect, helping to show that you notified the physician promptly.

Record All Pertinent Communications

The physician isn't the only health care provider you work with. Record your communications with other health care team members too. For example, when a physical therapist works with your patient for the first time, document that you reported relevant information to the therapist, such as the patient's frequent episodes of vertigo.

As often as your facility requires, place a rhythm strip in his medical record. Be sure to label the strip with his name, the time and date, and the lead displayed. Also post a rhythm strip in the record any time his condition changes or an arrhythmia appears on the monitor. On each strip, mark the heart rate and rhythm, PR-interval and QRS-complex duration, and, if present, ST-segment elevation or depression. Document a significant change from one rhythm strip to the next. Then notify the physician, document your notification, and record his orders and your actions.

Also record the time chest x-rays were obtained to evaluate the patient's condition as well as interventions taken based on x-ray results.

Oxygenation. Document all actions you take to maintain adequate oxygenation—a primary outcome for a patient with pulmonary edema. Record your patient's baseline pulse oximetry reading, noting whether he was breathing room air or receiving supplemental oxygen at the time. Then document subsequent oximetry readings, including those taken after an increase in the oxygen flow rate, a change in the patient's condition, or initiation of a new intervention. Document other measures you take to improve oxygenation, such as placing the patient in high Fowler's position.

If the physician orders high-flow oxygen delivered by face mask—a typical intervention in pulmonary edema—document that you explained the reason for such oxygen administration and offered reassurance. (Wearing a face mask may heighten the patient's anxiety.)

Monitor and document vital sign measurements and pulse oximetry readings every hour, as appropriate, until values fall within normal limits. Then document these values as often as ordered or whenever the patient's condition changes. Also record arterial blood gas (ABG) levels from samples drawn after the patient was placed on oxygen, noting the oxygen flow rate.

Anxiety may amplify your patient's distress, so record all measures you take to decrease his anxiety, such as explaining procedures and speaking in a calm, reassuring tone. Note his response, along with signs and symptoms of decreasing or increasing anxiety.

Also document the emotional support you provide to the patient's family.

Drug and IV Therapy. A patient with pulmonary edema usually needs IV access for drug administration. Document the location of the IV site, date and time the IV line was inserted, name of the person who inserted it, catheter size, type and condition of dressing, and assessment of the site. Also note IV line patency and blood return.

Before administering a vasoactive drug, record the patient's vital sign measurements. After he receives the drug, document his response, especially noting his breathing pattern, urine output, and vital sign measurements.

If the physician prescribes morphine to relieve respiratory distress associated with pulmonary edema, be sure to document this. Then record the patient's response to morphine. Document other assessment findings that reflect the patient's comfort, such as a respiratory rate change, reports of increased comfort, and lack of facial grimacing.

Fluid Balance. Expect to administer diuretics to a patient with pulmonary edema. Record the name, dosage, and administration time and route of each diuretic you give. Monitor and document the patient's electrolyte levels during diuretic therapy. Record the time you notified the physician of abnormal values, the physician's response, and your actions.

Record fluid intake and output every hour during an acute episode of pulmonary edema and every 4 to 8 hours thereafter, as indicated. If a fluid imbalance occurs, if urine output falls below 30 ml/hour, or if output doesn't reflect a therapeutic response to the diuretic, document these findings, the time you notified the physician, orders given, and your actions.

Hemodynamic Monitoring. If your patient has a pulmonary artery catheter in place, document pulmonary artery pressure readings as often as ordered. Also record the date and time of catheter insertion, name of the physician who inserted it, how the patient tolerated the procedure, and ongoing observation of the site. If you detect a significant change in pulmonary artery readings or the patient's condition, document that you notified the physician, the time of notification, and your interventions.

Document What You Teach

Expect to tailor your teaching to the cause of pulmonary edema, such as heart failure. During an acute episode of pulmonary edema, provide teaching as you perform interventions. Document everything you teach. To refine your teaching plan, assess and record the patient's and family members' readiness to learn and their previous knowledge. Include the following topics in your teaching and documentation:

- heart and respiratory system anatomy and physiology
- disease process
- oxygen administration
- prescribed drugs, including their names, dosages, administration times and routes, adverse effects, and storage
- dietary and fluid restrictions
- treatment procedures
- diagnostic tests
- measures to reduce anxiety, such as drug administration and relaxation techniques
- oxygen conservation techniques, such as taking frequent rests
- signs and symptoms to report, such as increasing edema in the legs
- ways to prevent recurrences, including sodium and fluid restrictions and leg elevation when sitting

WHEN YOUR PATIENT HAS PULMONARY TUBERCULOSIS

Documenting your care for a patient with pulmonary tuberculosis (TB) can have far-reaching effects. Besides helping to ensure that your patient receives proper care, it can prevent the disease from being transmitted to others. By assessing and recording your patient's history, lifestyle, past treatments, and knowledge of TB and its transmission, you can evaluate her risk for developing active disease and infecting others. Your interventions and teaching can then address these risks.

Document What the Patient Tells You

When obtaining your patient's medical history, be sure to elicit and record information about past pulmonary or infectious diseases and other respiratory conditions. If she has undergone a tuberculin skin test (intradermal injection of purified protein derivative [PPD]), record the test date and result. If she had a positive PPD reaction, document other tests she has undergone, such as chest x-rays and sputum tests, and their results. Find out whether she has been treated for TB before. If she has, record the dates and duration of treatment, names of all prescribed drugs, and her compliance with treatment.

Then record current or recent symptoms your patient reports, including chronic cough, fever, chills, night sweats, bloody or purulent sputum, chest pain, weight loss, malaise, and anorexia.

Risk Factors. Elicit and document your patient's risk factors for TB, such as a family history of the disease. Describe her living arrangements, especially if she lives in an institution, community residence, nursing home, or shelter. Note whether she has spent time in prison, in a shelter, in the military, or as a homeless person. Record other risk factors, such as a history of alcoholism, IV drug use, and positive human immunodeficiency virus status.

Document other risk factors you uncover, such as advanced age, a job in health care or day care, recent travel outside the country, and a condition that increases the risk for TB (such as malnutrition, chemotherapy, steroid or immunosuppressive therapy, chronic renal failure, other chronic disease, and recent loss of more than 10% of body weight).

Document What You Assess

A patient who tests positive on a TB skin test doesn't necessarily have active TB. Your assessment can help determine her diagnosis and guide interventions.

When performing and documenting a complete nursing assessment, focus on the following expected abnormal findings:

- cough
- fever
- hemoptysis or purulent sputum
- adventitious breath sounds

- dyspnea
- hoarseness
- tachycardia
- poor nutritional status

Document What You Do

As soon as pulmonary TB is suspected—even before tests confirm the diagnosis—document that you have placed your patient in a double-door isolation room with negative-pressure ventilation. Record that you explained to her the reason for isolation and other interventions to prevent the transmission of TB.

Active TB cases must be reported to the local health authority. When the patient's diagnosis has been confirmed by diagnostic tests, document that her case has been reported and the name of the person or agency it was reported to. (See *Which diseases must be reported?*)

DID YOU KNOW?

WHICH DISEASES MUST BE REPORTED?
All states require health care workers to report tuberculosis cases. Most local or state health departments also require reporting of a wide range of other infectious diseases. In 2005, the National Notifiable Diseases Surveillance System (operated by the Centers for Disease Control and Prevention and the Council of State and Territorial Epidemiologists) issued the following list of reportable infectious diseases and conditions. This list may differ somewhat from your state's list. For a copy of state reporting requirements, contact your state department of health.

Acquired immunodeficiency
  syndrome
Anthrax
Arboviral neuroinvasive and
  non-neuroinvasive diseases
Botulism
Brucellosis
Chancroid
Chlamydia trachomatis, genital
  infections

Cholera
Coccidioidomycosis (regional)
Cryptosporidiosis
Cyclosporiasis
Diphtheria
Ehrlichiosis
Enterohemorrhagic
  Escherichia coli
Giardiasis
Gonorrhea

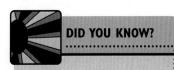

WHICH DISEASES MUST BE REPORTED?—cont'd

Haemophilus influenzae, invasive disease
Hansen disease (leprosy)
Hantavirus pulmonary syndrome
Hemolytic uremic syndrome, postdiarrheal
Hepatitis A
Hepatitis B
Hepatitis C
Human immunodeficiency virus (HIV) infection, adult
HIV infection, pediatric
Legionellosis
Listeriosis
Lyme disease
Malaria
Measles
Meningococcal disease
Mumps
Pertussis
Plague
Poliomyelitis, paralytic
Prevalence of tobacco use
Psittacosis
Rabies, animal
Rabies, human

Rocky Mountain spotted fever
Rubella
Rubella, congenital syndrome
Salmonellosis
Shigellosis
Smallpox
Streptococcal disease, invasive, group A
Streptococcal toxic shock syndrome
Streptococcus pneumoniae, drug-resistant invasive disease
Syphilis
Tetanus
Toxic shock syndrome
Trichinosis
Tuberculosis
Tularemia
Typhoid fever
Vancomycin-intermediate *Staphylococcus aureus* (VISA)
Vancomycin-resistant *S. aureus* (VRSA)
Varicella morbidity, deaths only
Yellow fever

Also record other measures you take to prevent disease transmission. Document that you taught family members and other visitors to wear an approved mask, keep the door closed, wash hands thoroughly, and limit contact with the patient.

If the patient must leave her isolation room for tests, document that she was wearing an approved mask when she left the room and that the personnel who administered the test were notified of her isolation status.

Drug and IV Therapy. Document the time prescribed anti-tubercular and antimycobacterial drugs were initiated, including drug names, dosages, and administration time and routes. Document the teaching you provide about drugs, including adverse effects and, if the patient is receiving rifampin, a possible change in urine color. Then observe for and record adverse reactions that occur.

If the physician orders IV fluids, document the time and date of IV line insertion, name of the person who inserted it, cannula size, infusion rate, infusion delivery device used, assessment of the IV site, and line patency. Also record each time you hang a new IV bag and perform tubing and dressing changes.

Oxygenation. Document your patient's baseline vital sign measurements, respiratory assessment findings, pulse oximetry readings, and arterial blood gas (ABG) levels. If the physician orders oxygen, document the time you initiated oxygen therapy, the flow rate, and the delivery device (such as a nasal cannula or face mask). If your patient has a history of chronic obstructive pulmonary disease, remember that this contraindicates the use of higher amounts of oxygen.

During oxygen therapy, monitor and document the patient's vital sign measurements and pulse oximetry readings every 1 to 2 hours, as appropriate, until these values fall within normal limits. Then note these values every 4 hours. Record ABG levels from samples drawn after oxygen therapy began, noting the flow rate the patient was receiving at the time.

If your patient has dyspnea or difficulty clearing secretions, document your actions to promote oxygenation and help her maintain a patent airway. Record your instructions on breathing techniques and your assistance in helping the patient turn, cough, and deep-breathe. Note that the head of her bed was elevated to promote easier breathing.

If the patient requires suctioning, document each suctioning session, your instructions about the procedure, the patient's tolerance, and proper care and disposal of suction equipment. Also record that you taught the patient about proper disposal of tissues she uses for secretions.

Notify the physician of significant findings or changes in the patient's status, along with the notification time, the physician's orders, and your interventions.

Diagnostic Tests. Log the names and results of all diagnostic tests the patient undergoes, such as sputum collection, PPD testing and anergy panel, and chest x-rays. Besides recording the date and time of the PPD test and anergy panel, document the test site location and the time when test results should be read.

When recording results of a TB skin test, describe the site in detail, expressing the induration in millimeters. (See *Using a ballpoint pen to measure PPD induration*.) Depending on your patient's risk factors for TB, you may need to notify the physician of significant induration. Document the time and details of notification and orders given, actions taken, or changes made in the treatment plan as a result.

Screening of Close Contacts. Before seeking treatment, your patient may have exposed family members, friends, and others to TB. Document that you helped her identify and contact anyone she may have exposed. After you report TB to your state agency, state officials will contact exposed individuals about getting tested for TB.

TIPS & ADVICE

USING A BALLPOINT PEN TO MEASURE PPD INDURATION

What's the best way to measure induration from a tuberculin skin test with purified protein derivative (PPD)? Researchers prefer the ballpoint pen method over palpation alone. To use this method, place the tip of a ballpoint pen 1 to 2 centimeters from the area of induration. Then gently roll the pen across the skin toward the center of the induration, making a small ink trail. When you meet resistance, lift the pen off the skin. Then repeat the procedure at another point on the opposite side of the induration. Measure the distance between the two end points, preferably using calipers; record the measurement in your patient's chart.

Document What You Teach

Documenting your teaching and the patient's understanding is crucial in preventing pulmonary TB transmission. Make sure that your teaching and documentation include the following topics:

- prescribed drugs, including their names, dosages, administration times and routes, adverse effects, and storage

- importance of complying with treatment for its duration
- nutrition
- hygiene and infection prevention, including handwashing
- proper disposal of sputum and tissues
- follow-up testing
- signs and symptoms to report
- testing of family members and close contacts.

WHEN YOUR PATIENT HAS SEVERE PAIN

For a patient in severe pain, developing the plan of care hinges on careful assessment, appropriate interventions, and thorough evaluation of the patient's response. (See *JCAHO standards for pain management*.) Documentation plays an important role in tailoring the plan to your patient's needs. It also communicates vital information to other health care team members so they can devise an effective pain-management plan.

Document What the Patient Tells You

Obtain and record a thorough health history from the patient. Include all possible sources of pain, such as chronic diseases, illnesses, and surgeries. Record his description of the circumstances when the pain first arose. Then elicit details about the pain, including its:
- onset
- location and radiation
- duration
- nature (such as sharp, dull, or stabbing)
- severity rated on a 0-to-10 scale, with 0 indicating no pain and 10 indicating the worst pain imaginable
- exacerbating factors
- relieving factors

Ask the patient whether the pain prevents him from performing certain motions or activities, interferes with activities of daily living, or decreases his quality of life. Also record what he tells you about his usual activity level, sleep pattern, and appetite.

Next, document your patient's use of analgesics, including over-the-counter preparations. Quoting the patient directly, record his perception of whether these drugs are effective or cause adverse effects. (See *How the courts view pain management*, pages 104-105.)

Then ask the patient to describe his use of alcohol and street drugs. Also find out whether he uses nonprescription drugs or other substances to control his pain. Finally, ask him about allergies to drugs and other substances. Document all responses carefully.

Document What You Assess

Record your findings from a thorough assessment. To avoid exacerbating the pain, be gentle when palpating, percussing, or auscultating the painful area.

First, document how well the patient can move the painful area, noting whether movement increases the pain. Describe weaknesses or functional limitations caused by the pain, and record diaphoresis or cool, clammy skin. Also record the patient's verbal response to pain, such as crying or shouting, and his nonverbal signs of pain, such as facial grimacing or guarding the painful area.

Next, measure and document the patient's vital signs. With severe pain, expect tachycardia, tachypnea, and hypertension. Assess whether the pain has distorted the patient's time perception. For instance, if he states, "My family left an hour ago," and you saw them leave 15 minutes earlier, document this alteration in time perception. Also record what you observe about his appetite. Finally, assess the patient's level of consciousness, keeping in mind that analgesics can produce sedation.

CASE LAW CLOSEUP

HOW THE COURTS VIEW PAIN MANAGEMENT
Pain management is increasingly becoming a legal battleground. For insight into the topic, review the following account of litigation in a North Carolina court.

Understanding the Case
Faison (administrix for the Estate of Henry James) *v. Hillhaven Corp. et al.*[1] questioned the management of pain control for Henry James, age 75. The case was filed after the patient's death and ultimately settled out of court, but the case remains relevant.

Mr. James had stage III adenocarcinoma of the prostate with metastasis to the lumbar sacral spine and left femur. In the hospital, he received radiation therapy. His level of pain was evaluated by the hospice unit staff, and he was given Roxanol (a liquid form of morphine sulfate), 150 mg every 3 to 4 hours as a scheduled drug. A nursing summary written on the day of discharge included a detailed schedule for his analgesic drug, and nurse's notes indicated that Mr. James's "pain was under control with Roxanol."

Ignoring Physician's Orders. After discharge, Mr. James was cared for briefly at home and then admitted to the Hillhaven Nursing Home with his usual orders for pain management. Family members had routinely given him Roxanol at home and later testified that they thought he was receiving it in the nursing home.

When Mr. James was admitted to the nursing home, the admitting physician noted that he had a poor prognosis and the short-term goal was to relieve pain. He ordered Roxanol, 150 mg every 3 to 4 hours around the clock; Tylenol, 3.25 mg, two tablets every 4 hours prn for pain and fever; and Darvocet-N, 100 mg every 4 hours prn for pain. After assessing Mr. James, the admitting nurse recorded that he was addicted to morphine and she intended to reduce his analgesic drug dosage and substitute a mild tranquilizer. Without consulting the admitting physician or family, she decided to wean the patient from Roxanol.

Investigating the Nursing Home. The North Carolina Department of Human Resources (DHR), investigating reports of possible deviations from required standards, interviewed Mr. James and reviewed his chart in April 1987. It determined that from February 2 to his discharge on February 24, 1987, he received analgesia intermittently, sometimes receiving three Roxanol doses over a 24-hour period and sometimes receiving none. DHR found that he received analgesic drugs a total of 60 times in those 23 days. It also found that these drugs, in the patient's words, "did no good." Concluding that the care rendered to Mr. James endangered his health, safety, and welfare, DHR fined the nursing home.

[1]Angarola, R: *Inappropriate Pain Management Results in High Injury Award (Letter),* J Pain Symptom Management 6(7):407, 1991.

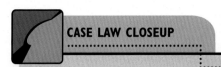

HOW THE COURTS VIEW PAIN MANAGEMENT—cont'd

The nursing director admitted that Roxanol was withheld from Mr. James. However, she testified that he requested analgesic drugs when he seemed to be having little or no pain. She said, "I did not want the patient to hurt, but I have seen patients much sicker, in more pain, and on less drug. The staff and I did not think he needed that much morphine."

The nursing home was cited for its lack of pain assessment. The only documentation was an occasional note describing the pain as "generalized" or "severe." Drug effectiveness was recorded as "good," "better," or "fair" in nurse's notes.

Issuing a Standard. In its final report, the North Carolina DHR set forth the following standard and accepted practice in the treatment of intractable pain:

- Assess the patient's pain and believe his assessment. Pain is subjective.
- Give pain drugs in doses high enough and frequent enough to control the pain.
- Treat the pain before it returns. This involves maintaining a constant blood level of the analgesic and giving the drug around the clock rather than prn.

How the Court Ruled

In a final order allowing a confidential settlement, the court noted that the plaintiff didn't allege that the defendants' conduct caused Mr. James's death, but that their conduct caused him increased pain and suffering. The court also noted that the defendants denied negligence or wrongdoing with respect to Mr. James's nursing care.

The Lesson Learned

Faison v. Hillhaven Corp. underscores the need for health care providers to evaluate pain control from the patient's perspective. Each patient's circumstances must guide the pain-control regimen. What might seem like an unusually high narcotic dose or frequent dosing schedule to the nurse might represent an effective pain-management regimen for that patient. Furthermore, all health care professionals must work together with the patient to provide effective pain relief. No nurse should decide on her own to ignore or change a physician's orders. If you disagree with an order, you must question the physician who gave it.

Federal Regulations and JCAHO Standards. Federal regulations now stipulate that nursing home patients have the right to an individualized plan of treatment, including pain control. Patients in other health care facilities have the same right under Joint Commission on Accreditation of Healthcare Organizations standards.

Document What You Do

To evaluate the effectiveness of interventions, assess and record the patient's pain characteristics before and after each intervention.

Drug Therapy. If the physician prescribes an analgesic, document that you have developed a drug administration schedule with the patient to help prevent his pain from becoming unbearable. For analgesics prescribed to combat breakthrough pain and for routine pain control, record the dosages and administration times and routes. Then, at a specified interval after administering an analgesic dose, assess and document the patient's pain, including his subjective rating of its severity on a 0-to-10 scale. If he tells you that his analgesic administration schedule is not effective, document your notification of this to the physician and record the orders you receive.

If the patient will use patient-controlled analgesia (PCA), document the programmed amount of the trial bolus dose and the time interval between boluses. Once the correct dose has been determined, record the programmed settings. Obtain and record your assessment findings every 2 hours for the first 8 hours after the patient starts using PCA. Document, too, that you provided instructions in using PCA and encouraged the patient to practice coughing and deep breathing to prevent respiratory complications. (See *Documenting the use of patient-controlled analgesia.*)

Also record adverse reactions to the drug, and describe the patient's alertness level after he receives each dose. Record, too, the safety measures you take to prevent injury, such as raising the side rails—especially if the patient is receiving narcotics.

Comfort Measures. Help the patient identify pain-relief strategies that have proved effective, and describe them in your documentation. Record the details of your discussions with him about the value of these practices to his overall health and long-term pain-management program. Document, too, assistance you give him to identify new strategies to decrease his pain. Record your observations and suggestions, as well as his response and willingness to try new therapies. As appropriate, add beneficial strategies to the plan of care.

If you provide instruction in guided imagery as part of pain management, document your teaching of this technique and the assistance you provide. Record his demonstrated understanding of your teaching and his reported comfort level after using guided imagery. Also describe distraction measures you provide, such as television or visitors, and record the patient's pain and comfort level during and after these measures.

Document that you have assisted the patient with relaxation techniques, such as music or meditation, to help manage his pain. Note whether he can demonstrate the techniques you've taught, and describe how these techniques affect his pain and comfort level.

Record factors that seem to make the pain worse. Note that you have shared your observations with the patient and helped him identify other factors to avoid, if appropriate. Describe in the record which position your patient finds most comfortable, and document each time you help him change position.

If the patient is receiving an analgesic drug, document that you encouraged him to accept the drug before the pain became unbearable. If indicated, also document your encouragement of patient activity and suggestions for getting adequate rest. Document your patient's activity tolerance as well.

External Pain-Relief Measures. Document external measures used to relieve pain, such as massage, transcutaneous electrical nerve stimulation, heat

CHARTING CHECKLIST

DOCUMENTING THE USE OF PATIENT-CONTROLLED ANALGESIA

If your patient is receiving patient-controlled analgesia, you're still responsible for documenting drug administration. Follow your facility's policy on proper documentation in this situation. Generally, record the following information in your notes at least every 4 hours:

- ❑ name and concentration of the prescribed drug
- ❑ exact dosage the patient is receiving (basal or continuous rate)
- ❑ dosage the patient receives when he self-administers a bolus
- ❑ minimum interval between self-administered boluses
- ❑ number of attempts the patient made to self-administer a bolus
- ❑ number of boluses the patient actually received
- ❑ cumulative dose delivered over the past 4 hours
- ❑ patient's subjective rating of pain severity on a 0-to-10 scale
- ❑ patient's respiratory rate and level of consciousness.

or cold application, and acupuncture. Document the patient's response to each measure, including his subjective pain rating before and after these measures.

Record the patient's activity tolerance after each nursing intervention for pain, such as positioning for comfort, reducing external stressors, encouraging verbalization of discomfort, and administering an analgesic. Also document the patient's rating of his pain before and after your interventions.

Emotional Support. Document the emotional support you provide to the patient and family. Include observations and discussions with them about effective coping mechanisms. Also describe the measures you take to decrease stressful stimuli, such as limiting visitors.

Document What You Teach

By thoroughly documenting your teaching plan, you can help your patient maintain effective pain control after discharge. Include the following topics in your teaching and documentation:

- prescribed drugs, including their names, dosages, administration times and routes, adverse effects, and storage
- use of drugs for breakthrough pain, as indicated
- use of PCA, if prescribed
- effective pain-control strategies, such as positioning, distraction, relaxation, guided imagery, and external measures
- signs and symptoms to report
- activity and rest guidelines
- factors that exacerbate pain
- healthy coping mechanisms
- realistic outcome criteria
- ways to promote proper sleep patterns
- avoidance of alcohol and substance abuse
- stress management
- importance of keeping in contact with the physician and complying with treatment
- resources for further information and support

WHEN YOUR PATIENT IS CONFUSED

When documenting care for a confused patient, you must show that you assessed for physiologic causes of her confusion, evaluated her behavior carefully, and checked for exacerbating factors. You also must indicate that you took measures to help orient her and ensure her safety.

Document What the Patient Tells You

If your confused patient isn't a reliable information source, try to obtain data about her health history and current condition from family members, friends, and medical records. Check all three sources closely for clues to the cause of her confusion. Note information about chronic illnesses, hospitalizations, and surgeries, as well as a history of neurologic problems, cerebrovascular accident, or transient ischemic attacks.

To discover whether an adverse drug effect, drug interaction, or inappropriate dosage is causing the patient's confusion, record the names of all drugs she uses, along with their dosages and administration times and routes.

Next, determine and record the patient's alcohol consumption pattern. Document information about her living situation, including the names of people who normally are with her during the day and at night and the names of social contacts and sources of support.

To help evaluate the patient's sleep pattern, find out whether she's exposed to natural light during the day. Such exposure aids time orientation and affects circadian rhythms. Disruption of circadian rhythms may reduce sleep, possibly causing confusion. Document how much sleep the patient usually gets, and describe her use of sedatives or other measures to promote sleep.

Also ask about sensory deficits, such as decreased visual acuity, hearing, and sensation. Describe corrective devices the patient uses, such as eyeglasses or a hearing aid, and record her perception of the effectiveness of these devices.

Document What You Assess

Because confusion can take many behavioral forms and stem from various physical causes, you'll need to perform and document a complete patient assessment. Include the following information.

Onset and Symptoms. If you notice that your patient becomes confused at certain times of day, document the behaviors, symptoms, and activities that occur at these times. Note whether the confusion has a gradual or sudden onset, and record the names, dosages, and administration times of drugs she received that day.

Determine whether the patient experiences weakness when confused. Assess for and document bilaterally equal hand grips and arm and leg strength. Note difficulty with coordinating fine and gross movements, and document speech abnormalities, such as garbled speech, word searching, aphasia, and difficulty articulating words. Also describe whether your patient is alert or lethargic. If she falls asleep frequently, record how long she can stay awake at one time and how easily you can arouse her from sleep.

Cognitive Functions. Record your assessment of the patient's orientation to time, place, situation, and person. Using direct quotes, document her answers to questions you ask when evaluating her reality orientation. When recording her ability to understand what others say, use measurable behaviors. Don't simply rely on her statement that she understands. For instance, document whether she can repeat instructions, follow commands appropriately, and demonstrate procedures taught to her.

Also record your assessment of her short-term, midrange, and long-term memory. Start by asking her to repeat several words you tell her, then ask what she did yesterday, and finally, question her about events that occurred many years ago.

Next, note whether the patient can focus on one activity for an extended period. In her own words, record inappropriate statements she makes; include a description of the circumstances. To make sure you didn't misinterpret her, ask her to explain her statement, and record her explanation.

If your patient exhibits abnormal behaviors or makes statements that suggest she's hallucinating, describe the specific behaviors and record her statements in her exact words. Document her emotional status too, noting anxiety, irritability, or depression. If her behavior suggests she may harm herself or others, document this behavior and the measures you take to ensure safety, such as providing one-to-one supervision.

Sensory Deficits. Document visual, hearing, or other sensory deficits you detect. Record exactly what the patient says and what you observe. For instance, you may write, "Patient states her hearing is adequate when wearing a hearing aid. She did not respond to her name when it was spoken in a normal volume from 2 feet away while she was wearing her hearing aid."

Document What You Do

Document interventions you take to keep your patient safe, decrease her confusion, and address its cause. Thorough documentation helps you detect factors that worsen or ease her confusion. If your patient is so confused that you question whether she's capable of consenting to treatment, notify the physician. (See *Is your patient competent,* page 112.)

Depending on the cause of the patient's confusion, you may need to document the interventions described below.

Frequent Observation and Orientation. Document your frequent observation of the patient to show that you assessed for changes in her condition and behavior. If she becomes disoriented, record the actions you take to orient her to reality, such as discussing current events, providing a clock and calendar, and calling her by name.

Document that you've promoted social contact to ease confusion that stems from isolation or loneliness. Also document that you encouraged family members and friends to visit. Try to arrange for continuity of nursing care so that she becomes familiar with the nursing staff, and document that you did so.

Safety Measures. Document the measures you use to safeguard the patient, such as keeping the side rails up, providing adequate nutrition, and assisting with elimination. If she becomes agitated or irritable, record your use of an appropriate technique to reduce her anxiety, such as distraction or simple redirection.

To document the frequency of checks you perform, you may want to use a flow sheet. Every 15 minutes, you or another

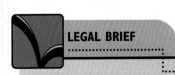

LEGAL BRIEF

IS YOUR PATIENT COMPETENT?

Legally, every adult is considered competent unless a judge finds otherwise in a formal hearing. A confused patient may be legally competent but unable to consent to treatment or otherwise participate in her treatment plan. If she can't understand the nature of her treatment, she's considered *clinically* incompetent or incapacitated.

Determining Clinical Competency and Capacity

In most facilities, the attending physician decides whether a patient is clinically incompetent or incapacitated. Nursing documentation of the patient's physical and psychosocial responses to therapy may play a major role in the physician's decision. Keep in mind that a patient may alternate between periods of clinical competency and periods of incompetence or incapacity. To determine clinical competency or capacity, the physician typically evaluates whether the patient can:

- make definitive decisions
- understand the information she's given
- engage in rational decision making and appreciate the possible outcomes of each option
- make a reasonable decision about her treatment

Murky Legal Waters

If the patient falls short in any area above, the physician usually tries to obtain consent from the next of kin or the patient's appointed health care decision maker. If the patient is legally competent, obtaining the consent of a surrogate may lead to a legal action for battery, based on unauthorized touching of the patient.

To clarify the issue, lawmakers are addressing the family's surrogate decision-making power. Typically, they favor granting such power if the family acts in good faith. Therefore, obtaining a surrogate's consent generally is considered safer than relying solely on the consent of a clinically incompetent patient.

Documenting Care

If you care for a clinically incompetent or incapacitated patient, obtain the names of all family members and identify the next of kin, family-appointed spokesperson, or surrogate decision maker to contact about treatment decisions. Also document conversations you have with these people. Record their names and telephone numbers in the medical record and your nursing documentation.

designated staff member should check the patient and fill out and initial the flow sheet.

If the patient recently consumed alcohol or used another psychoactive substance, document this information, along with your assessment for withdrawal symptoms, such as tremors, hypertension, tachycardia, and hallucinations. Also document interventions you perform to manage withdrawal symptoms.

Management of Stimulation. Document that you have provided or reduced environmental stimuli, as appropriate, to meet your patient's needs. For instance, if overstimulation exacerbates her confusion, document the measures you took to reduce it, such as turning off the television and avoiding loud talking. If some stimulation is beneficial to her mental status, document that you encouraged her to watch television or play a game. Record your patient's responses to the measures you provide. Also document that you've kept all instructions simple and direct.

Sensory and Communication Needs. If your patient has uncorrected sensory deficits, document that you provided assistance to correct them, such as helping her obtain eyeglasses or a hearing aid, if needed. If the patient resists efforts to correct sensory deficits, document that you provided additional measures to promote communication and understanding, such as a picture communication board, large-print reading materials, or a special telephone for the hearing-impaired. Record the effect of these measures on her confusion.

Drug Therapy. Document all drugs you administer and the patient's response. Note the dosages and administration times and routes. If you're giving a drug that could alter mental status, assess and document mental status findings before and after the patient receives the drug. If adverse reactions occur, describe them in the record, notify the physician, and document your notification.

Laboratory Test Results. Document electrolyte imbalances, abnormal arterial blood gas levels, nontherapeutic blood drug levels, and other laboratory data that could have a bearing on the patient's condition. Note that you reported the results to the physician, and describe orders he gives and interventions you take.

Document What You Teach

Teaching a confused patient and her family helps ensure safe, appropriate care while she's hospitalized and after discharge. When documenting the teaching plan you develop with them, take into account conditions in the home that could increase the patient's confusion. Also record the patient's and family members' readiness to learn.

When documenting your teaching, describe the teaching method used and the patient's and family members' responses to and understanding of your teaching. Include the following topics in your teaching and documentation:

- safety measures
- prescribed drugs, including their names, dosages, administration times and routes, adverse effects, and storage
- potential hazards of taking nonprescription or herbal preparations without consulting the physician
- importance of avoiding potential substances of abuse, such as alcohol
- signs and symptoms to report
- ways to monitor the patient's condition
- follow-up tests to check blood drug levels, if indicated
- nutrition
- importance of daily social contact and routine social activities
- appropriate stimuli, such as a newspaper, radio, clock, calendar, and television
- avoidance of drastic changes, such as rearrangement of furniture
- keeping the home clean and clutter-free
- effective ways to manage agitation and irritability
- resources for further information and support

WHEN YOUR PATIENT HAS A SEIZURE

Typically, a seizure is self-limited and poses no immediate threat to the patient's life. However, during a seizure, a patient may fall or aspirate gastric contents into the lungs. Also, status epilepticus (a series of uninterrupted seizures) may cause permanent brain damage or even death unless halted promptly by diazepam, phenobarbital, or another anticonvulsant drug. Your assessment and in-depth documentation of the patient's status and the actions you take to keep him safe can prove important to his diagnosis and treatment. For instance, your detailed record of his condition before, during, and after the seizure can help determine the seizure type and, possibly, its cause.

Document What the Patient Tells You

Ask your patient whether he's experienced a seizure before, and determine whether he's had other neurologic problems. Document his responses. Then record a history of diseases and conditions that increase the risk of seizures, such as hypoglycemia, head trauma, and alcohol or drug use.

If the patient has a history of seizures, document the date of the initial diagnosis and the current treatment plan, including prescribed drugs. Record the names, dosages, and administration frequency of anticonvulsants he's taking, along with the time of his last dose. If he reports a history of alcohol or drug use, document the substance, the time of his last use, and the amount he took.

Next, explore factors associated with previous seizures, such as lack of sleep and emotional distress. Document them in the patient's medical record. Then document nonspecific symptoms he reports just before the seizure, such as headache, mood changes, lethargy, and muscle spasms or jerking. Be sure to note the symptom's timing relative to the seizure. If the patient says he usually has an aura before a seizure, document his description of the aura in his exact words. For instance, he may describe a pungent smell, an unusual taste, nausea, indigestion, a rising or sinking feeling in his stomach, or a visual disturbance such as seeing flashing lights.

Document What You Assess

Besides offering valuable clues to the seizure type and its cause, accurate documentation of your patient's condition and behavior just before, during, and after the seizure provides baseline information that can help the health care team detect changes in his status. If you didn't witness the seizure, try to obtain information from someone who did.

Begin your documentation by describing events that preceded the seizure, such as an aura, outcry, or other behavior. Also record the following information:

- time the seizure began
- time it ended
- length of clonic and tonic phases, if present
- level of consciousness before, during, and after the seizure
- neurologic status
- pupil responses and arm and leg strength after the seizure
- specific body parts affected by the seizure
- vital signs during the seizure (if they can be assessed without harming the patient)
- vital signs after the seizure
- respiratory status, noting cyanosis and other signs of inadequate oxygenation
- urinary or bowel incontinence

The patient may receive care before the seizure ends, such as drugs to halt the seizure and position changes to prevent injury. Record these interventions. Also document the name, dosage, and administration time and route of the anticonvulsant given, and note its effectiveness in resolving the seizure.

Assessment After the Seizure. After the seizure ends, examine the patient for injuries sustained during the seizure, and assess his overall condition. Document your findings thoroughly. Depending on the seizure type and severity, he may display various behaviors immediately after the seizure. Besides documenting his level of consciousness, check for and record other signs and symptoms that occur. Expected findings after a seizure include:

- confusion
- emotional lability
- lethargy
- fatigue
- increased sensitivity to bright lights and noise
- amnesia related to the seizure

Continue to observe and document the patient's condition until he returns to his baseline status.

Document What You Do

To promote continuity of care throughout your patient's stay, record the interventions you take to maintain his safety before, during, and after the seizure.

Before the Seizure. If your patient has a history of seizures, arrange for him to have a room near the nurses' station for close observation. If his room assignment changes for this reason, record the move and the reason.

Then document that you've taken seizure precautions to prevent injury if a seizure occurs, such as:
- keeping the bed in a low position
- raising and padding the side rails
- placing the call button within easy reach
- keeping an emergency airway, supplemental oxygen, and suction equipment in the patient's room
- keeping resuscitation equipment and an emergency drug tray nearby

Document, too, that you instructed the patient to report an aura immediately.

During the Seizure. Record every action you take to safeguard the patient during the seizure. Generalized tonic-clonic seizures may warrant first aid for bruises, abrasions, and mouth or tooth injury. Other types of seizures (petit mal and focal seizures, for instance) may require minimal interventions. As appropriate, be sure to document these additional interventions:
- turning the patient to one side to maintain an open airway and prevent aspiration
- removing potentially dangerous objects from the area
- calling for assistance and requesting that the physician be notified
- staying at the patient's side until the seizure ends

Keep in mind that restraining a patient physically during a seizure is contraindicated because it may promote injury.

Notify the physician immediately to ensure timely and appropriate medical treatment. Document the information you communicate to the physician, along with the time of notification, orders he gives, your actions, and the patient's response to interventions. Report his response to the physician, and document that you did so.

If the physician prescribes an anticonvulsant or other drug, document each drug given, along with its dosage and administration time and route. If you administer a drug that can affect blood pressure, such as diazepam or phenobarbital, record the patient's blood pressure before and after he receives the drug.

When administering phenytoin, which can form a precipitate if it comes in contact with dextrose, document that you gave it through an IV line with normal saline solution and infused it at a rate slower than 50 mg/minute. Administering phenytoin at a faster rate can lead to life-threatening effects, such as cardiac arrest.

If the patient's seizure resulted from hypoglycemia, document that you gave dextrose 50% IV, as ordered. If your patient has a history of alcohol use or is experiencing alcohol withdrawal, document thiamine administration, if prescribed. Closely observe and record the patient's response to each drug you give.

After the Seizure.   After the seizure (in the postictal period), monitor the patient closely. Record his vital signs, level of consciousness, and neurologic status every 15 minutes. As needed, reorient and reassure him, and document these interventions. (See *How often should you reassess your patient?*)

Document What You Teach

When documenting your teaching, indicate your instructions to the patient and his family about preventing and managing seizures and dealing with the precipitating condition. Make sure your teaching and documentation include the following topics:

- myths and misconceptions about seizures
- prescribed drugs, including their names, dosages, administration times and routes, adverse effects, and storage
- importance of taking drugs exactly as prescribed
- need for regular monitoring of the anticonvulsant blood level
- need for regular dental care to treat trauma to the teeth, gums, and mouth
- importance of informing health care personnel, family members, and coworkers if an aura occurs and of immediately seeking safety

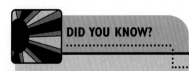

DID YOU KNOW?

HOW OFTEN SHOULD YOU REASSESS YOUR PATIENT?
The Joint Commission on Accreditation of Healthcare Organizations (JCAHO) has developed the following recommendations for patient reassessment. Keep in mind that these recommendations represent the *minimum* requirements. However, your patient may need more frequent reassessment.

Patient	When to Reassess
Same-day surgery patient	On return from postanesthesia unit and immediately before discharge
Stable patient in medical-surgical unit	Every 24 hours
Patient with decreasing neurologic status	Every 15 minutes
Patient in labor	Every 15 minutes
Patient with active GI bleeding	Continuously, on a one-to-one basis
Suicidal patient	Continuously, on a one-to-one basis
Patient in rehabilitation	Every 1 to 2 weeks
Long-term care patient	Monthly

- measures to help prevent seizures, such as getting adequate sleep, reducing stress, avoiding triggers (including video games, flashing lights, loud noises, and hyperventilation), avoiding alcohol and recreational drugs, consuming adequate fluids (especially when exercising), eating regular meals, and consulting the physician before dieting
- how to obtain medical alert identification
- resources for further information and support

Finally, document that you taught the patient about the status of his driver's license. When a patient has a seizure, the physician must inform the state motor vehicle department, which revokes the patient's license until the physician determines that the patient is seizure-free. Also document that the patient signed a statement verifying that he has been informed that he's not permitted to drive.

WHEN YOUR PATIENT HAS A CEREBROVASCULAR ACCIDENT

A patient who suffers a cerebrovascular accident (CVA, commonly called a stroke) may be in immediate danger of airway obstruction and further brain damage. To help ensure prompt treatment and develop an effective nursing plan of care, you must document her condition thoroughly and record her responses to rapid interventions. Your documentation provides a crucial record of events throughout the course of the patient's illness.

Not all patients who have had a CVA require similar care. The history and assessment findings you'll document and the interventions you'll perform depend on the brain area affected and the cause of the CVA. The most common causes include thrombosis, embolus, and intracerebral hemorrhage. Although diagnostic tests help identify the precipitating condition, timely and effective management hinges on precise nursing observation and documentation.

Document What the Patient Tells You

During the health history interview, obtain information about the patient's medical history and symptoms just before and during the CVA. If your patient can't communicate, interview family members and check medical records for relevant information.

Medical History. Document a history of hypertension, cerebral aneurysm, or a bleeding disorder because these conditions can cause intracerebral hemorrhage. Also record a history of rheumatic heart disease, endocarditis, posttraumatic valvular disease, open-heart surgery, atrial fibrillation, and other arrhythmias. These conditions suggest cerebral embolism as the cause of CVA. Then ask whether the patient has a history of peripheral vascular disease, hyperlipidemia, heart disease, diabetes mellitus, transient ischemic attacks, and trauma. Record the information you obtain.

Next, document the names and dosages of prescription and over-the-counter drugs the patient has been taking. If she's taking an antihypertensive or anticoagulant drug, find out when she last took it and in what dosage; record the answer.

Your patient's lifestyle may provide clues to the cause of her CVA. Documenting this information also promotes more effective rehabilitation planning. Gather as much data as possible about the patient's smoking history; dietary sodium, fat, and alcohol intake; daily activity level; and drug history.

Symptoms. Record information about the patient's condition during the days and hours that led up to the CVA. Ask family members whether the patient can't tell you herself. For example, document reports of headache, weakness, dizziness, confusion, memory disturbances, mood swings, tingling, numbness, poor muscle coordination, visual impairment (such as double vision), facial drooping, difficulty swallowing or talking, stiff neck, seizures, bowel or bladder incontinence, and bounding pulse.

Document What You Assess

Besides aiding diagnosis and treatment, the data you collect and document during your physical assessment help ensure continuity of care by providing a baseline for later comparison. When documenting your assessment, focus especially on the patient's respiratory, neurologic, and cardiovascular systems.

Respiratory System. Quickly check your patient for a patent airway and then take steps to maintain it. Measure her respiratory rate, pattern, and effort; evaluate her skin color; and review her pulse oximetry or arterial blood gas (ABG) analysis results. Immediately notify the physician of abnormalities or changes in the patient's status. Then document your findings and your notification of the physician, including the time of notification.

Neurologic System. Accurate documentation of your patient's neurologic status can help caregivers track her progress or deterioration. Record your frequent assessments of her level of consciousness. Remember, though, to document only specific and objective data, not interpretations of your findings. (See *Recording the level of consciousness: Objectivity counts,* page 122.)

Because hemiplegia is a common sign of CVA, assess for and document weakness, numbness, and tingling in the arms or legs. Report these problems to the physician promptly. Also check for

TIPS & ADVICE

RECORDING THE LEVEL OF CONSCIOUSNESS: OBJECTIVITY COUNTS

When documenting your patient's level of consciousness, include only specific, objective observations—not vague terms that one reader may interpret differently than another. For instance, if the patient is sitting up in bed talking with visitors, record this fact in detail. Don't state merely that she is "alert." If she is unresponsive with no reflexes, describe her that way rather than simply writing "comatose." For more hints, review the documentation dos and don'ts below.

Do Write	Don't Write
Awake and aware of environment. Interacting with visitors.	Alert.
Oriented to her name, place, and today's date, including year.	Appears to know where she is.
Sleeps when not stimulated. Easily aroused with verbal stimulation, and then is oriented to her name, place, and today's date.	Lethargic.
Aroused with difficulty. Requires physical versus verbal stimulation. Nonsensical verbal responses.	Obtunded.
Aroused only with painful stimuli. No verbal response.	Stuporous.
Reflex activity only with painful stimulation. Cannot be aroused.	Semicomatose.
No response or reflex reactions.	Comatose.

and record facial drooping, loss of voluntary movement, changes in reflexes, and speech difficulties. When documenting these findings, describe the specific areas of the body affected and the severity of the abnormality.

Next, evaluate for aphasia (defective language function). Remember that aphasia may be receptive, expressive, or mixed. To detect receptive aphasia (inability to understand language), assess the patient's ability to follow simple commands. To detect expressive aphasia (inability to express or form words), ask her to identify an object or a person. Document your findings, which may suggest that she has a specific type of aphasia or mixed aphasia (both types).

Cardiovascular System and Other Findings. Evaluate and document your patient's cardiovascular system. Measure and record her blood pressure; typically, a CVA increases blood pressure, requiring frequent monitoring and an antihypertensive drug. If you administer an antihypertensive, document its effectiveness. Be sure to notify the physician if you detect a drop in blood pressure, which may promote brain tissue ischemia or death or indicate continued life-threatening bleeding. Document your notification, including its time, the physician's orders, and your actions.

Then assess for a positive Homans' sign. This sign indicates deep vein thrombosis, a possible cause of the patient's CVA. Record your findings. Also monitor and document the patient's blood glucose level, which may increase as a result of steroid therapy to reduce cerebral edema caused by the CVA.

Document What You Do

Document all actions you take to maintain the patient's respiratory status and vital signs, prevent injury, prevent or manage CVA complications, and help her communicate her needs.

Respiratory Care. Monitor pulse oximetry readings and ABG levels, as ordered. Be sure to record all interventions you take to promote adequate oxygenation, such as:
- using an artificial airway, if needed
- positioning the patient to maintain a patent airway
- administering supplemental oxygen, if prescribed
- suctioning as needed, with hyperventilation of 100% oxygen before and after

If your patient's respiratory status declines, notify the physician at once. Then document the time of notification, time of the physician's response, and his orders.

If the patient requires endotracheal intubation and mechanical ventilation, document that you prepared her for this procedure. Once mechanical ventilation begins, record the ventilator settings, the patient's response to ventilation, and your frequent checks of ventilator function. Also record interventions you take to prevent pneumonia and counteract the effects of inactivity on the lungs, such as turning, frequent repositioning, and performing chest physiotherapy.

Vital Sign Checks. Measure and record the patient's vital signs every 2 to 4 hours, depending on the physician's orders, your facility's policy, and the patient's stability. Report abnormal vital sign measurements, including hypertension, hypotension, tachycardia, bradycardia, irregular heart rate, and a fever, to the physician. Document the time of notification and orders you receive.

Safety and Supportive and Restorative Care. A patient with a CVA requires comprehensive safety and supportive and restorative care—all of which you must document accurately. Document the safety measures you take and the supportive care measures you provide to maintain adequate activity, nutrition, hydration, hygiene, and elimination. They include:
- fluid intake and output measurements
- level of assistance provided for personal hygiene
- skin protection measures
- administration of gastric feedings, if ordered
- raising of the side rails and nearby placement of the call button
- use of a toileting schedule and other interventions to promote bowel function and avoid straining at stool

A CVA may leave your patient with paralysis and muscle weakness. Your interventions to address her impairments can help optimize her physical condition and rehabilitation. Document your efforts to preserve her muscle, skin, and tissue integrity, such as:
- repositioning her at least every 2 hours
- preventing pressure ulcers by turning the patient frequently and using pressure-relief devices, such as a special mattress and heel protectors
- performing passive range-of-motion exercises at least twice per shift to prevent muscle wasting and contractures
- applying antiembolism stockings, if ordered, to prevent complications related to prolonged bed rest
- using footboards, slings, splints, and braces as recommended by the physical or occupational therapist to prevent complications of prolonged immobility, such as footdrop, and to maintain correct body alignment

Communication. If your patient has aphasia, promote and document the methods you've provided to allow her to communicate her needs. Make sure your documentation reflects that you helped her select and use an appropriate method. Also document referrals to a speech, occupational, or physical therapist.

Document What You Teach

Teaching is a crucial aspect of care and rehabilitation for a patient who has had a CVA. To promote a positive attitude toward recovery, rehabilitation should start as early as possible. Direct your instructions to the family as well as the patient. Be sure to document that you covered the following topics:

- disease process
- ways to reduce risk factors for CVA recurrence
- signs and symptoms to report
- safety measures and devices to use at home, such as a shower chair
- adaptive measures to use when performing activities of daily living
- use of ambulatory aids, if needed
- home exercise program
- telephone numbers for home health agencies
- resources for further information and support

If a physical therapist or social worker presented some of this information, document that you reviewed and reinforced it with the patient and family.

WHEN YOUR PATIENT IS UNRESPONSIVE

An unresponsive patient must rely on caregivers to meet every need. No matter what condition led to his decreased level of consciousness (LOC), you and your colleagues must maintain his body functions. You'll need to document changes in his vital signs, neurologic function, and respiratory status; fluid intake and output; frequent repositioning; steps taken to ensure skin integrity and hygiene; and methods used to promote family interaction. Your thorough documentation supplies baseline information that may help the health care team detect subtle clues that the patient is deteriorating or improving.

Document What Sources Tell You

Your unresponsive patient can't provide health history information; you'll need to obtain data from family members, friends, and medical records. Document whatever you learn about the patient's medical history, accident and injury history, drug use, nutritional habits, sleep patterns, bowel and bladder patterns (including the date of his last bowel movement), living arrangements, support people, and available caregivers. This information will assist caregivers in supporting the patient's needs more appropriately.

Document What You Assess

Objective assessment is critical when your patient is unresponsive because he can't provide subjective input. Getting a clear picture of his baseline status can help the health care team establish a prognosis and track changes in his condition.

Neurologic System. Document improvements you detect in the patient's LOC, such as increased reflex withdrawal or purposeful withdrawal from painful stimulation. Note which body areas are involved in reflex withdrawal and purposeful withdrawal from painful stimulation. Record changes in pupil size and reaction to light, which may signal a change in neurologic status. Also document your close monitoring of his vital signs and your prompt notification of the physician if you detect significant changes. If appropriate, you may want to document your patient's neurologic status by using the Glasgow Coma Scale. (See *Using the Glasgow Coma Scale.*)

Airway Patency. Keep in mind that your unresponsive patient can't control his secretions effectively and is at risk for airway obstruction. To help prevent or identify problems that may lead to inadequate tissue oxygenation, frequently assess and document his respiratory rate, depth, and quality. Be sure to establish and maintain a patent airway, and note any secretions. Document breath sounds before and after suctioning. Record the frequency

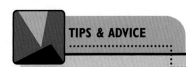

TIPS & ADVICE

USING THE GLASGOW COMA SCALE
To document your patient's level of consciousness (LOC), you may use the Glasgow Coma Scale (GCS), which assigns a numerical value to assessment findings. Originally used to evaluate patients' prognosis and recovery from head injuries, the GCS is now widely used to evaluate LOC. Test your patient's response to motor, verbal, and eye stimulation, using the scale shown below. Then total his score and document it, breaking the total into its components, such as M5, V3, E3 = GCS 11. Keep in mind that a patient who scores 15 points is fully awake, alert, and oriented; a patient who scores 3 points is deeply comatose. Because all health care team members will use the same scoring system, the patient's progress can be evaluated by comparing each new GCS score with the previous score.

Test	Score	Patient's Response
Motor Response	6	Follows commands
	5	Localizes pain on stimulus
	4	Withdraws from painful stimulus
	3	Shows abnormal flexion in response to pain
	2	Shows abnormal extension in response to pain
	1	No response
Verbal Response	5	Oriented
	4	Confused
	3	Inappropriate words
	2	Unintelligible sounds
	1	No response
Eye-Opening	4	Spontaneous
	3	Opens eyes on verbal command
	2	Opens eyes on painful stimulus
	1	No response

of suctioning, along with the results. Also monitor and record pulse oximetry readings and arterial blood gas analysis results, as ordered.

Skin and Tissue Integrity. Reduced blood flow, pressure on bony prominences during bed rest, inability to communicate discomfort, and dehydration can increase your unresponsive patient's risk for skin breakdown and its complications. Record your initial and ongoing assessment of the patient's skin and tissue integrity. In particular, note areas of redness, chafing, and other breakdown, especially in the most vulnerable areas, such as the sacrum, heels, toes, elbows, scapulae, and back of the head. Also assess the eyes and mouth for dryness and cracking caused by inadequate natural lubrication.

Fluid and Nutritional Status. Document the patient's fluid and nutritional intake to ensure that he receives sufficient fluids, calories, and protein. Assess and record his weight, skin turgor, and blood glucose level as well as the results of laboratory tests to monitor nutritional status.

Expect the physician to order gastric feedings or total parenteral nutrition. Document the feeding type, amount, and route; feeding times; and the patient's tolerance for the feedings. When administering parenteral nutrition, record your detailed assessment of the IV insertion site and the infusion rate.

Bowel and Bladder Function. Closely evaluate and document bladder and bowel function, which the unresponsive patient can't control. Accurately record his urine output and bowel movements. When documenting urine, include its amount, color, and any abnormalities, such as sediment and blood. When documenting bowel movements, include stool amount, color, consistency, and frequency. Also record abdominal assessment findings, such as active bowel sounds and abdominal distention or firmness.

Document What You Do

Primary nursing responsibilities for an unresponsive patient center on maintaining his respiratory status, skin integrity, nutritional status, bowel and bladder function, and safety. By documenting all actions you take, you help determine the need for changes in the nursing plan of care or the interdisciplinary treatment plan.

Respiratory Care. Record your measures to optimize gas exchange, including frequent patient repositioning to prevent aspiration. Also document the times when you give chest physiotherapy and the amount and characteristics of secretions you suction after each session. Document, too, that you raised the head of the bed slightly and hyperextended the patient's neck a bit to enhance gas exchange and keep abdominal organs from impinging on the diaphragm.

Skin Care. Maintaining an unresponsive patient's skin and tissue integrity is a challenging goal for the entire health care team. Frequent communication and collaboration among care-givers are crucial to managing problems that arise. Document the interventions you take to prevent breakdown over bony promi-nences, such as gently massaging high-risk areas. Record your use of pillows and blankets to maintain proper body alignment and prevent nerve and tissue damage. Also document that you performed passive range-of-motion (ROM) exercises to maintain muscle and joint integrity and increase blood flow. If a colleague helps you turn the patient or if you use a turning sheet or sliding board to avoid skin injury, document the protocol used.

Also record the hygiene measures you take to manage bowel or bladder incontinence, including use of barriers and emollients. Document that you performed oral care with soft brushes or swabs and applied lip balm to prevent cracking. If your patient lacks a blink reflex, obtain an order for eye ointments or drops to maintain eye moisture. Then document your actions.

Nutrition. Document your actions that ensure adequate nutrition. If you administer enteral feedings, record that you checked placement of the feeding tube before each feeding and elevated the patient's head and upper torso during and after the feeding. For intermittent feedings, measure and document the amount of residual feeding matter in the stomach before each feeding. For continuous feedings, record residual feeding matter every 4 to 6 hours. If the amount increases, document the inter-ventions you took.

If your patient is receiving parenteral nutrition, document that you assessed the IV line for patency and checked x-ray reports revealing line placement. Also document your care for the IV insertion site.

Bowel and Bladder Care. Document the interventions you take to promote bowel and bladder function. Include drugs you give to promote or slow peristalsis and enemas you administer, if prescribed. Record the results of these interventions. If the patient has an indwelling urinary catheter in place, document the catheter care you provide and the amount and appearance of the patient's urine.

Safety Measures. Document interventions you take to promote patient safety, including the use of side rails or soft restraints. If the patient is restless, record the measures you take to safeguard IV lines, feeding tubes, and other invasive devices.

Document What You Teach

Direct your teaching to the patient's family. Record your instructions about the purpose of all interventions and treatments. Also document that you encouraged family members to assist in caring for their loved one by teaching them to perform simple interventions. Record your instruction and their actions. If they will care for the patient after discharge, document that your teaching included the following topics:

- enteral feeding administration
- skin care
- frequent repositioning
- bowel and bladder care
- passive ROM exercises
- signs and symptoms to report
- names of home health agencies and local support groups

WHEN YOUR PATIENT ASPIRATES A TUBE FEEDING

Accidental aspiration of tube feeding matter into the lungs poses a serious risk. If it occurs, you must assess your patient's condition rapidly, take immediate corrective actions, and thoroughly document findings and interventions. Your documentation will stand as a record of the event and provide baseline information about the patient's condition and response to interventions.

Document What the Patient Tells You

Depending on your patient's condition, she may report symptoms that cause you to suspect aspiration. Document complaints of abdominal bloating or cramping, belching, regurgitation, and pain. These symptoms may indicate poor tolerance for the tube feeding and an increased risk for aspiration. Report these complaints to the physician, and document that you did so. Be sure to include the time of notification and the physician's response, and prepare to stop the tube feeding.

If your patient reports respiratory difficulty, such as shortness of breath and coughing, document that you stopped the tube feeding at once and notified the physician. These signs and symptoms indicate that aspiration has occurred or pneumonia is developing.

Document What You Assess

If you suspect or know that aspiration has occurred, document the patient's position in bed when you found her, along with the time you found her. (See *Block charting: A risky choice*, page 132.) Then rapidly but thoroughly assess her respiratory system, vital signs, and other factors.

Respiratory System and Oxygenation. Document the patient's respiratory rate and breath sounds. Note coughing, secretions, and use of accessory breathing muscles. If she coughs up secretions, document the color, amount, and odor. Obtain and record a pulse oximetry reading. Document the amount of supplemental oxygen, if any, the patient is receiving and the delivery device used, such as a face mask or cannula. To assess her oxygenation, evaluate and document the color of her skin, lips, and nail beds.

Vital Signs. Although impaired gas exchange is the most obvious consequence of tube feeding aspiration, your patient also may develop other complications, such as aspiration pneumonia and hypoxic bradycardia. To help detect these problems, measure and document her vital signs, including temperature, at least hourly for the first 4 hours after the incident and then every 3 to 4 hours. Report significant changes to the physician, and document your notification, time of notification, and the physician's orders.

....
LEGAL BRIEF

BLOCK CHARTING: A RISKY CHOICE

Have you ever been tempted to use block charting? Many nurses have. With this documentation style, you write a nurse's note for a broad range of time—say, 0900 to 1100—which lightens your charting burden somewhat.

The time that block charting saves may not be worth the legal problems that could arise if the patient's record becomes evidence in a lawsuit. Why? Block charting permits you to assign a wide range to the time when you assessed a particular change, implemented a certain intervention, or notified the physician of a patient problem. A patient's attorney could use your vague time frame to his advantage, scrutinizing each entry in the medical record for specific times. When he finds only a time range, he may contend that you failed to render timely care or that too much time elapsed between your detection of a problem and its correction.

How can you avoid this legal quagmire? Avoid block charting altogether. Instead, always record the date and time for each entry in your documentation and the date and exact times for specific assessment findings, interventions, and other actions.

Tube Placement. If you suspect that your patient has aspirated a tube feeding, check placement of the nasogastric (NG) tube. Record your findings and the method you used to check placement. If you discover that the NG tube is no longer in the stomach, record this and obtain an order from the physician to remove the tube. Then document the time the tube was removed.

If the feeding tube was inserted percutaneously into the stomach or jejunum, document its appearance at the insertion site and markings at the insertion point that indicate its position.

Residual Undigested Feedings. Check and document the color, amount, and consistency of undigested residual feeding matter in the patient's stomach. Compare your findings with those from previous checks.

Document What You Do

In your documentation, describe the prompt interventions you took to prevent serious consequences of tube feeding aspiration.

Immediate Actions. If you suspect that the patient has aspirated a tube feeding, immediately stop the feeding, keep the head of the bed elevated, and notify the physician. Document the time of the suspected aspiration, the actions you took, the patient's response, the name of the physician you notified, time of notification, and the physician's response.

Also record interventions you take to promote oxygenation, such as suctioning the airway.

Other Actions. If the physician orders discontinuation of the feeding tube, remove the tube. Then document this action and the patient's response. Obtain sputum specimens and record the source and the date and time you send them to the laboratory for culture and sensitivity testing.

The physician will prescribe antibiotics if he suspects pneumonia. When the results of the sputum culture and sensitivity tests are available, the physician will discontinue, maintain, or change antibiotic therapy, as indicated. Document the initiation of antibiotic therapy, if prescribed, and the patient's response. If a chest x-ray is taken, record the time and, when available, the results.

Document What You Teach

Your teaching and documentation for a patient who has aspirated a tube feeding should include the following topics:

- mechanism of tube feeding aspiration
- ways to prevent future aspiration
- possible complications, such as pneumonia
- prescribed drugs, including their names, dosages, administration times and routes, adverse effects, and storage
- purpose of ordered tests and treatments
- signs and symptoms to report

WHEN YOUR PATIENT HAS GI HEMORRHAGE

A patient may be admitted to your care with gastrointestinal (GI) hemorrhage from his home or may develop the problem while in your care. GI hemorrhage may be a complication of a disorder (such as a clotting problem) or a drug (such as an anticoagulant). Whatever the cause, your care begins with a rapid, careful assessment to determine the location and extent of bleeding and continues with life-saving interventions. At every step, be sure to document your findings and actions, as well as the patient's responses.

Document What the Patient Tells You

Review your patient's chart for a history of a disorder that increases the risk for hemorrhage from the upper or lower GI tract. If a careful history hasn't already been documented, record pertinent facts now. Specifically ask about a history of peptic ulcer disease, esophageal varices, diverticulitis, ulcerative colitis, and colon cancer. Record the patient's use of prescription and over-the-counter drugs, particularly noting such hemorrhage-inducing drugs as anticoagulants and nonsteroidal antiinflammatory drugs (NSAIDs).

Ask your patient whether he vomited blood (hematemesis), had rectal bleeding (hematochezia or melena), or both. Record the color of the blood, which may range from black and tarry to bright red and bloody in stool and may be bright red or the color and consistency of coffee grounds in vomitus. If rectal bleeding occurred, find out whether the blood was mixed with or followed the stool. Also have him estimate the amount of blood loss, such as a teaspoon or a cup. Document whether he noticed the blood in the toilet bowl or on toilet paper only.

Inquire about related symptoms, such as weakness, fatigue, nausea, vomiting, abdominal pain, and diarrhea. Ask whether the patient lost consciousness or felt faint. Record the onset and duration of each symptom, and the intensity, location, and quality of pain.

Find out whether the patient knows his blood type, but be sure to document the laboratory results of his blood typing. Ask whether he has ever had a transfusion, and document previous transfusion reactions

Document What You Assess

For a patient with GI hemorrhage, assess him quickly and stay alert for signs and symptoms of hypovolemia or hypovolemic shock. Even though this may be an emergency, remember to record the results of your rapid head-to-toe assessment.

Vital Signs. Immediately record the patient's vital signs, particularly noting fever, tachycardia, tachypnea, and hypotension. If possible, check the patient's blood pressure while he's supine, seated, and standing to check for orthostatic hypotension—an early warning sign of hypovolemia; record all measurements Also, calculate and document the pulse pressure. Compare it with previous calculations to detect narrowing.

Abdomen. Auscultate for bowel sounds and record their presence or absence and any hyperactivity. Observe for and document abdominal distention and pulsations. If the patient has localized abdominal pain, document its reported location in the appropriate quadrant. Record whether the pain is constant or intermittent and whether it's relieved by anything, such as the knee-chest position or antacid administration. Also document the type of pain, if possible. (See *Documenting types of abdominal pain*.)

TIPS & ADVICE

DOCUMENTING TYPES OF ABDOMINAL PAIN
When your patient reports abdominal pain, be sure to get a complete description of it. Then document and consider this data, which can help determine the type of pain and its probable cause, as shown below.

Description of Pain	Type of Pain	Probable Cause
Dull, diffuse, and intermittent; may eventually localize over the affected organ	Visceral	• Stretching or distention of the viscus of an abdominal organ • Damage to a hollow abdominal organ, such as the stomach
Intense, steady, and aching; usually localized	Somatic (or parietal)	• Damage or other stress in the abdominal wall, peritoneum, mesentery, or diaphragm
Sharp and well localized, but removed from its source	Referred	• Damage or other stress in the viscera, which travels along nerves to the skin

Fluid Balance. Assess for and document signs of hypovolemia. For example, record fluid intake and output hourly—or more frequently if needed. Also examine the patient's skin and nails. Check for pallor and coolness and delayed capillary refill in the nail beds, which can signal hypovolemia and anemia; document your findings.

Laboratory Test Results. Review and document the results of blood tests, such as a low hemoglobin level and hematocrit—possible signs of anemia from hemorrhage. Other noteworthy abnormal results may include a complete blood count that shows elevated reticulocyte levels, reduced platelet and red blood cell counts, and reduced red cell indices for normocytic, normochromic cells. If the serum iron level and total iron-binding capacity are decreased, record these findings and expect chronic bleeding. Make note of arterial blood gas analysis results that may indicate acidosis and hypoxemia, such as a low pH and oxygen saturation. For a patient with a nasogastric (NG) tube, check and record his serum electrolyte levels. Potassium is especially likely to be lost with GI hemorrhage.

If a stool specimen or any other sample was sent for analysis, record abnormal findings, such as blood in the stool.

Document What You Do

A patient with GI hemorrhage demands prompt attention, regardless of the severity of the hemorrhage. Your documentation of rapid interventions and their evaluation provides important details that can guide the patient's health care.

Frequent Monitoring. Document your patient's vital sign measurements every hour—or more often if he's unstable. Record changes in his temperature, heart and respiratory rates, and blood pressure. Plan to insert an indwelling urinary catheter. Then monitor and record fluid intake and output hourly to detect oliguria, which may indicate hypovolemia.

GI Care. As ordered, give the patient nothing by mouth (NPO). Following facility policy, flag his chart and other important documents to communicate his NPO status; also notify the dietary department. If the patient has upper GI bleeding, insert an NG tube. Note the size and type of the NG tube and record how it was secured. Then document your verification of correct tube placement according to facility policy (See *What's the best way to verify tube placement?*)

Record the amount of saline solution or other irrigant instilled through the NG tube, as well as the amount aspirated. Describe the aspirate's color and consistency, and note whether norepinephrine or another drug was instilled to constrict blood vessels and stop the bleeding.

If the physician suspects esophageal bleeding from a Mallory-Weiss tear (an esophageal injury caused by prolonged vomiting), assist with insertion of a chamber-balloon tube, such as a Sengstaken-Blakemore tube, to compress bleeding areas. Once the tube is in place, document your care for a patient with this type of tube, which should include the following:

- periodically deflating the balloon, as ordered, to prevent tissue necrosis
- suctioning the tube to avoid fluid accumulation
- keeping scissors at the bedside to cut and remove the tube if it deflates and migrates into the airway

DID YOU KNOW?

WHAT'S THE BEST WAY TO VERIFY TUBE PLACEMENT?

No doubt you understand the importance of verifying that a nasogastric (NG) tube is correctly positioned—in the stomach or duodenum—before you connect it to suction, infuse liquid nutrition, or inject saline. But did you know that verification by auscultating the epigastric area for the rush of injected air is *not* considered the best practice?

Recent studies show that abdominal x-rays and pH measurements of aspirated GI contents are superior ways to confirm tube placement. By documenting your use of at least one of these best practices, you help protect the patient from complications, such as pulmonary aspiration, and can protect yourself from legal problems.

Drug and IV Therapy. To maintain circulatory volume, administer IV fluids, such as lactated Ringer's or normal saline solution, through a large-bore catheter. If the patient has upper GI bleeding, the physician may order drugs, such as a histamine$_2$ (H$_2$) blocker, proton pump inhibitor, or antacid. If he has bleeding from a peptic ulcer caused by *Helicobacter pylori,* the physician may prescribe an antibiotic. Document your administration of these drugs and the patient's response to them.

If the patient needs blood transfusions, follow your facility's policies regarding what steps to take and how to document them. At a minimum, record the following actions:

- Before requesting blood from the blood bank, ensure that the patient has a keep-vein-open IV line, and record his baseline vital signs. If the patient has a history of febrile or allergic reactions to blood, premedicate him with acetaminophen, antihistamines, or both, as ordered.

- When requesting blood from the blood bank, provide the patient's name and medical identification number. This information becomes part of a permanent record in the blood bank.

- Ensure that a signed consent for transfusions is placed in the patient's medical record.

- To confirm compatibility, compare the ABO and Rh types listed on the bag label and blood bank forms to the types listed on the medical record. Note that this verification was done.

- Inspect the blood bag for leaks, and examine the blood for discoloration, excessive clots, and other abnormalities. Record the condition of the bag and its contents.

- At the bedside, enlist the help of another nurse to confirm the patient's identity (using his ID band) and to double-check the identifying information on the blood slip. Verify that the patient's name and medical record number match in both places, and sign or initial the slip to indicate that you did this.

- Stay with the patient for at least the first 15 minutes of the infusion to monitor for signs of a transfusion reaction. Record his vital signs during the first 15 minutes and then as often as required by facility policy until 1 hour after the transfusion is complete.

- Instruct the patient to report unexpected signs and symptoms, such as back pain or shortness of breath. If a transfusion reaction occurs, document your actions, such as stopping the transfusion.

Preparation for Invasive Tests and Treatments. Before your patient undergoes a procedure to diagnose or treat the source of bleeding, ensure that a signed consent form is placed in his medical record. Document that you removed dental bridges or dentures before the procedure. If you notice loose dentition, notify the physician and record it in the chart. Use a preoperative checklist to make sure you've taken all essential preoperative actions and to document them. If a colonoscopy is scheduled, record your administration of a bowel preparation, as prescribed. No matter what procedure is scheduled, document that you've confirmed the placement and patency of an IV line.

Nutrition. If your patient has chronic GI bleeding caused by a long-standing disorder, such as ulcerative colitis, expect him to be nutritionally depleted. If the physician orders bowel rest by keeping the patient NPO, work with the physician and dietitian to provide total parenteral nutrition (TPN). On a flow sheet, record the time you start the infusion and the rate and volume of the infusion. Document any adverse reactions, such as an allergic reaction to the TPN components. Chart the patient's blood glucose level every 6 hours or as ordered. Also document your use of aseptic technique to change catheter dressings and your close monitoring for signs of infection.

As the physician advances the patient's diet to clear liquids and then to solids, track how well your patient tolerates each dietary change. Plan to offer low-residue foods at first to prevent GI irritation.

Comfort Measures. A patient with GI hemorrhage is likely to have discomfort related to the disorder or its treatment. So be sure to provide and document all comfort measures. For example, if the patient has pain, nausea, or vomiting, administer prescribed analgesics and antiemetics and evaluate his response to them. If he has an NG tube, prepare his nostrils with a water-soluble lubricant and secure the tube so that it puts minimal pressure on the nostrils. Provide frequent mouth care by offering ice chips and lozenges, if permitted, and helping the patient brush his teeth. If he has frequent bloody stools, provide a bedside commode to help conserve energy and arrange for a private room, if possible.

Document What You Teach

Throughout the patient's hospitalization, document that you've informed him of his progress and care. Once your patient's condition is stable, prepare him for discharge by providing verbal and written instructions. In the chart, record that you covered the following areas in your teaching:

- disease process
- procedures and treatments
- activity limitations
- signs and symptoms to report
- prescribed drugs, including their names, dosages, administration times and routes, adverse effects, and storage
- IV therapy, including TPN, if prescribed
- dietary restrictions and supplementation
- follow-up appointments with the physician
- information on support groups for any chronic condition

WHEN YOUR PATIENT HAS HYPOGLYCEMIA

Defined as a low blood glucose level, hypoglycemia can lead to coma, irreversible brain damage, and death unless treated promptly and effectively. The condition occurs primarily in patients with insulin-dependent diabetes who don't eat enough food, who self-administer too much insulin, or who engage in unusual exertion. Other causes of hypoglycemia include cancer of the stomach, liver, or lung; adrenal gland hypofunction; malnutrition; liver dysfunction; alcoholism; and strenuous exercise.

To establish a foundation for the plan of care, focus your documentation on the patient's history of diabetes or other disorders, recent food and fluid intake, activity level, recent infections or emotional stress, and alcohol use. Be sure to document all physical assessment findings, laboratory test results, nursing interventions, and patient responses to interventions.

Document What the Patient Tells You

Most patients with diabetes experience warning symptoms of hypoglycemia. Ask your patient to describe how she has been feeling for the past few hours, and record her response in her

own words. If she noticed warning signs, try to determine—
and then document—exactly when they began and how they
progressed. Expect to document the following symptoms:
- nervousness or shakiness
- dizziness or feeling faint
- numbness or tingling in the hands and feet
- weakness
- diaphoresis
- hunger or nausea
- headache
- palpitations
- double vision

If the patient reports such symptoms, ask whether she has had
them before. If she has, find out whether she knows what caused
them. Record her responses in her exact words.

Document What You Assess

Although the patient's symptoms are important, you'll also need
to document objective signs of hypoglycemia. If you witnessed the
hypoglycemic episode, record your observation of:
- tremors
- personality changes, such as aggressiveness, stubbornness, nega-
  tivity, and depression
- decreased level of consciousness (LOC), such as confusion,
  difficulty speaking, delirium, seizures, and loss of consciousness
- poor coordination
- cold, clammy skin
- increased heart rate or a slow, bounding pulse
- increased respiratory rate

Document What You Do

Hypoglycemia can rapidly progress to neurologic compromise, so
you'll need to intervene immediately and notify the physician.
After verifying hypoglycemia, vary your interventions with the
patient's LOC.

Blood Glucose Level. If possible, immediately obtain a finger-
stick glucose level, using a portable blood glucose meter. Document
this action, the glucose reading, the name of the physician you

notified, and the time of notification. If the glucose meter displays a code for readings below a set glucose level (for instance, "LO" for a level below 40 mg/dl), document the displayed reading and its significance.

If you don't have immediate access to a glucose meter, document why you didn't perform this step, whom you notified of the patient's signs and symptoms, and your rationale for proceeding directly to treatment.

For the Conscious Patient. If you suspect or know that your patient is experiencing hypoglycemia, give her 15 g of a simple oral carbohydrate (such as juice, candy, dextrose, or honey) if she is conscious and can swallow. Document the type of carbohydrate you gave, the time you gave it, the amount the patient consumed, and her response. Record, too, that you stayed with her after this intervention. Be sure to report the patient's response to the physician, and document this action.

If you repeat testing of the patient's blood glucose level, document the time it was done, method used (finger-stick test or venipuncture sample), name of the physician you notified of the result, and time of notification.

For the Unresponsive Patient. If your patient is unresponsive and can't swallow, administer an IV carbohydrate (such as dextrose) or subcutaneous glucagon, as ordered, to raise her blood glucose level. If she already has IV access, document that you checked IV line patency.

If the patient has no existing IV access, obtain an order to start an IV line, and document the vein used, catheter size, and positive blood return. After administering the IV carbohydrate, document the amount you gave, the administration time, and the patient's response. Then recheck and document the patient's blood glucose level. Document the measurement method used and the name of the physician you notified.

If the physician prescribes repeat administration of the IV carbohydrate, again document the amount given, the administration time, and the patient's response. Repeat this cycle as ordered until the patient's blood glucose level stabilizes. Measure and record the patient's vital signs every 15 minutes until she regains consciousness.

Document What You Teach

Your patient may need comprehensive teaching to avoid future hypoglycemic episodes. If possible, instruct the patient and her family. Be sure to teach and document the following topics:

- cause of hypoglycemia
- importance of maintaining a normal blood glucose level
- signs and symptoms to recognize and actions to take
- safety measures
- importance of carrying an oral carbohydrate at all times
- sick day rules; ways to modify drug therapy when the patient can't eat
- importance of eating regular meals and snacks
- importance of wearing medical alert identification
- importance of having regular medical check-ups

WHEN YOUR PATIENT HAS HYPERGLYCEMIA

Defined as a high blood glucose level, hyperglycemia seldom poses an immediate threat until the glucose level exceeds 240 mg/dl. With extreme blood glucose level elevation, the patient's condition may rapidly progress to ketoacidosis, a potentially fatal metabolic disorder.

Although commonly caused by diabetes mellitus, hyperglycemia also may stem from Cushing's syndrome (pituitary dysfunction), physical stress (such as trauma, burns, and surgery), and certain drugs (including cortisone and thiazide diuretics). In a patient with diabetes, common causes of hyperglycemia include insufficient insulin dosage, dietary noncompliance, infection, and gastrointestinal (GI) illness.

To provide a basis for the nursing plan of care and the interdisciplinary treatment plan, first determine whether your patient has been diagnosed with diabetes. Then explore and document other aspects of his health history, including recent food intake,

CHARTING CHECKLIST

DOCUMENTING DIETARY ADHERENCE

Most patients with hyperglycemia follow a restricted diet to manage diabetes, but that doesn't mean your patient might not cheat occasionally. If you discover an "outlawed" snack at your patient's bedside, explain how the food will compromise his blood glucose regulation. Then offer him a snack that's on his diet plan.

Next, notify the physician of the incident and document:

❑ the food you found at the patient's bedside

❑ your teaching about dietary restrictions

❑ the patient's response to your teaching

❑ alternative snacks that you offered

❑ the name of the physician you notified

❑ the physician's response

infections, and physical injury. (See *Documenting dietary adherence*.)

Document What the Patient Tells You

Ask the patient how he has been feeling over the past few days, and record his response in his exact words. He may report these symptoms of hyperglycemia:
- weakness
- unusual thirst
- frequent urination
- anorexia
- vomiting
- drowsiness
- headache

Then find out whether he has had hyperglycemia before. If so, record the symptoms he experienced at that time.

Document What You Assess

Next, perform a physical examination. Expect to assess and document these signs and symptoms of hyperglycemia:
- flushed cheeks
- dry skin and mouth
- acetone (sweet) breath odor
- Kussmaul's breathing (fast, deep, labored respirations), especially if the blood glucose level exceeds 500 mg/dl
- weak, rapid pulse
- low blood pressure
- abdominal pain
- restlessness
- decreased level of consciousness (possibly unresponsiveness)
- electrolyte abnormalities, particularly potassium imbalance
- glucose and ketones in the urine
- signs of infection, such as a fever, increased pulse rate, and hot, dry skin that's flushed

Document What You Do

Besides documenting your rapid interventions, record the patient's responses to interventions to show that you took appropriate actions to reverse hyperglycemia.

Insulin Administration. The physician will probably prescribe insulin administration by continuous IV drip, insulin pump, or frequent subcutaneous injections of regular (short-acting) insulin. Record the delivery route used, the amount of insulin administered, and the patient's response.

Glucose Monitoring. As your patient responds to the insulin, check his blood glucose level frequently and document all readings. (See *Should a hospitalized patient check blood glucose levels with his home glucose meter?,* page 146.) Include in your notes the time the finger-stick test was done or the blood sample was drawn, name of the physician you notified, time of notification, and orders you received. For instance, the physician may prescribe additional insulin or may instruct you to adjust the rate of a continuous insulin infusion. Document that you implemented the physician's orders, and record your evaluation of the patient's response to the change in therapy.

Fluid and Electrolyte Balance. Document treatments the physician prescribes to correct dehydration and electrolyte imbalances, which typically are associated with hyperglycemia. Record IV fluid administration on the IV record or flow sheet, noting the solution type given and infusion rate. Remember to include IV fluid volume when documenting fluid intake and output.

Record the results of serum electrolyte tests, along with the name of the physician you reported them to, time of notification, and changes in treatment orders. If you administer electrolyte replacements, document the amount given, the delivery route, and the patient's response. Again, be sure to include this fluid volume in your patient's intake and output record.

Document What You Teach

Your patient and his family will require comprehensive teaching about hyperglycemia, especially its prevention and management. Be sure to teach about lifestyle modifications and management of

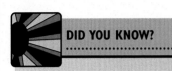

SHOULD A HOSPITALIZED PATIENT CHECK BLOOD GLUCOSE LEVELS WITH HIS HOME GLUCOSE METER?

Chances are that your patient with diabetes has years of experience at checking his blood glucose level with a home glucose meter. And he may strongly prefer using a particular model or brand. But should you allow him to continue checking his blood glucose level in the hospital, especially when clinical decisions may be based on the results? According to the Joint Commission on Accreditation of Healthcare Organizations, a patient can safely use his personal blood glucose meter in the hospital if:

- the practice is approved in writing by the hospital administration, prescribing physician, and laboratory director
- the patient's technique is deemed safe and accurate by a diabetes nurse educator
- the patient performs daily quality-control tests
- the meter's first reading is confirmed by a test result from the hospital laboratory
- any abnormal or unusual blood glucose level is confirmed by the hospital laboratory

To help ensure patient safety, all of the previous recommendations should be documented.

diabetic complications. In your notes, document that you covered the following topics:

- pathophysiology of the disorder
- mechanisms of hyperglycemia and ketoacidosis
- prescribed drugs, including their names, dosages, administration times and routes, adverse effects, and storage
- insulin administration, if indicated
- signs and symptoms of hypoglycemia and hyperglycemia, and actions to take if these conditions occur
- use of a home glucose monitor
- importance of regular glucose monitoring
- effect of diet, infection, stress, and exercise on the glucose level
- dietary restrictions
- foot care

- importance of seeing the physician regularly and having regular eye examinations
- resources for further information and support

WHEN YOUR PATIENT HAS ANAPHYLAXIS

An exaggerated and rapidly lethal allergic response, anaphylaxis requires quick assessment, emergency intervention, and accurate documentation of every aspect of your care. Once the acute crisis passes and the patient's condition stabilizes, the health care team must identify the substance that triggered the reaction. This will help prevent future episodes.

Document What the Patient Tells You

An anaphylactic reaction occurs when a person who was previously exposed to an allergen encounters it again. After anaphylaxis has been treated and your patient's condition stabilizes, try to pinpoint the cause of her reaction. For instance, ask her to list everything she has eaten or drunk in the past 24 hours; document this information. Find out whether she recently took prescription or over-the-counter drugs, and question her about recent contact with chemicals, plants, animals, or insects. Document her answers thoroughly.

Then find out whether the patient has known allergies or has had an unusual reaction in the past. If she reports that she's allergic to a particular substance, document her description of previous reactions. Also determine whether she has had a procedure that used contrast media. If she has, record this fact along with a description of any reaction she had. Document her answers in her own words, placing quotation marks around them.

Because subtle sensations may precede overt signs of anaphylaxis, document all symptoms the patient mentions—even vague ones. During an anaphylactic reaction, she may report:

- anxiety
- agitation

- flushing
- lightheadedness
- palpitations
- numbness and tingling of the hands, feet, or lips
- itchy palms and scalp
- air hunger or coughing
- chest tightness
- throat tightness or swelling
- throbbing in the ears
- abdominal cramping

Document What You Assess

After eliciting and recording the patient's symptoms, perform and document a physical examination. During an anaphylactic reaction, expect to find the following signs and symptoms:

- arrhythmias
- skin wheals, welts, or rashes
- shortness of breath
- wheezing or noisy breathing
- barking
- high-pitched cough
- sneezing
- decreased level of consciousness
- syncope, seizures, or unresponsiveness
- bowel or bladder incontinence
- angioedema (localized edema of the hands, feet, lips, eyelids, tongue, or genitalia)
- hypotension
- weak or rapid pulse
- pale skin
- diaphoresis

If you detect any of these abnormal findings, contact the physician immediately. Document the time of your notification and the physician's orders.

Document What You Do

A patient with anaphylaxis needs immediate treatment to avoid permanent tissue damage and death. Take steps to ensure an adequate airway and promote gas exchange. Then administer drugs, as prescribed. When time allows, document these actions and the patient's response.

Airway Maintenance and Gas Exchange. In anaphylaxis, respiratory distress (primarily caused by laryngeal edema) may be severe enough to warrant oropharyngeal intubation or tracheostomy. If your patient develops respiratory distress, prepare for intubation or emergency tracheostomy, and document these actions. If the physician prescribes supplemental oxygen, record the time oxygen therapy began, the flow rate, and the delivery device, such as a face mask or cannula.

Drug Therapy. Drug orders depend on the severity of the patient's condition. Expect to administer epinephrine and an antihistamine to reverse anaphylaxis; then document that you did so. If your patient is hypotensive, document that you gave a vasopressor and IV fluids, if prescribed, to replace lost plasma volume. If the physician prescribes a corticosteroid to reduce airway inflammation, record that you administered this drug. When documenting drug therapy, include each drug's name, dosage, administration time and route, and the patient's response.

Communication. In addition to documenting your communications with the physician, record that you reported your patient's anaphylactic reaction to appropriate departments in your facility. First, instruct the unit secretary to flag the patient's record and to note her allergy on the medication administration record and nursing plan of care. (See *Where should you document your patient's allergies?*) If the unit secretary

CHARTING CHECKLIST

WHERE SHOULD YOU DOCUMENT YOUR PATIENT'S ALLERGIES?

Duplicate documentation is often a necessary evil. But when it comes to recording a patient's allergies, most experts agree that duplication is a good thing. In fact, you probably can't document allergy information in too many places.

If your patient has a significant allergy history, verify that you've documented the pertinent information (including the patient's description of her allergic response) in all of these places:

❑ initial assessment form

❑ medication administration record

❑ nursing plan of care

❑ front of the patient's chart

❑ patient's identification bracelet

❑ physician admission orders

❑ pharmacy profile

❑ dietary profile

isn't immediately available, perform this extra documentation yourself rather than waiting for the secretary to return—and possibly risking a recurrence.

Also place an allergy identification bracelet on your patient's wrist, and report her anaphylactic reaction to the pharmacy, dietary department, blood bank, and respiratory services. Depending on your facility's policy, notify other departments as required.

Document What You Teach

You'll need to provide comprehensive teaching to help your patient avoid future anaphylactic reactions. Direct your teaching to the patient's family too, especially the members who are most likely to use an anaphylaxis kit. Include the following topics in your teaching, and document that you did so:
- name of the allergen, if known
- ways to avoid the allergen
- importance of telling family members, coworkers, and all health care providers about the patient's allergy history
- importance of obtaining medical alert identification
- use of an emergency anaphylaxis kit, especially if anaphylaxis resulted from an insect bite or sting

WHEN YOUR PATIENT HAS A TRANSFUSION REACTION

A patient who receives a blood transfusion is at risk for three types of transfusion reactions:
- *allergic*, stemming from a substance in donor blood to which the recipient is allergic
- *febrile*, a rare reaction caused by bacterial contamination
- *hemolytic*, resulting from administration of the wrong blood type

By recording your assessment findings, you can help identify the type of reaction, which in turn guides treatment for this serious condition. Accurate documentation also can prevent recurrence of a transfusion reaction.

Document What the Patient Tells You

Symptoms may be the earliest indicators of a transfusion reaction. Document that you instructed the patient to tell you immediately if he notices unusual sensations while receiving the transfusion. Then record statements he makes about how he feels during the transfusion. (See *Documenting transfusions: Covering all the bases,* page 152.)

A hemolytic reaction commonly causes signs and symptoms within 15 minutes after the transfusion begins. A febrile or allergic reaction may take longer to manifest. So be sure to record the time the transfusion started and the time the patient first reported symptoms.

During an *allergic* transfusion reaction, expect the patient to report:
- headache
- flushed feeling
- itching
- shortness of breath
- wheezing

For a *febrile* reaction, expect the patient to report:
- fever
- chills
- shaking

During a *hemolytic* reaction, expect the patient to report:
- chills
- shaking
- lower back pain
- shortness of breath
- chest pain
- flushed feeling
- nausea
- wheezing
- joint pain

Document What You Assess

Document all physical examination findings, and compare them with the baseline assessment you recorded before the transfusion began. During an *allergic* reaction, your physical examination may

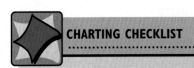

DOCUMENTING TRANSFUSIONS: COVERING ALL THE BASES

Whether your patient is receiving whole blood or a blood component, always document that proper identification (ID) procedures were used before the transfusion began. Then record all monitoring you performed during the procedure. Above all, follow your facility's protocol for specific instructions on documenting transfusions.

Before the Transfusion

Before you start the transfusion, document the following information:

- ❏ names of the two health care professionals who performed the pretransfusion ID check
- ❏ confirmation that the blood slips match the patient's name and medical record number on his ID band
- ❏ confirmation that the blood slips match the information on the blood bag describing the patient's and donor's blood groups, Rh factors, and blood bank identification number
- ❏ patient's vital signs

During the Transfusion

After you begin the transfusion, record the following data:

- ❏ time the transfusion began
- ❏ type and size of IV catheter used
- ❏ flow rate
- ❏ patient's vital signs at the start of transfusion and then as often as your facility requires
- ❏ use of a blood warming device
- ❏ abnormal symptoms the patient reports or abnormal signs you assess, along with the name of the physician you notified, time of notification, and his response

After the Transfusion

Once the transfusion ends, record the following information:

- ❏ time the transfusion was completed
- ❏ amount of blood or blood product transfused
- ❏ patient's vital signs

reveal dyspnea, increased respiratory rate, wheezing, flushed skin, and skin wheals. If your patient is having a *febrile* reaction, you detect fever. During a *hemolytic* reaction, your assessment may reveal:
- fever
- decreased urine output
- dyspnea
- increased respiratory rate
- jaundice or cyanosis
- low blood pressure
- increased pulse rate
- flushed skin
- vomiting
- diarrhea
- decreased level of consciousness
- wheezing

Document What You Do

If you suspect that your patient is experiencing a transfusion reaction, immediately discontinue the transfusion. Then notify the physician, documenting his name, time of notification, and his orders. Also record the time you stopped the transfusion and the amount of blood or blood product administered.

Next, follow the steps outlined in your facility's policy for a suspected transfusion reaction. Document the time you performed each step. Then implement the following interventions and document them thoroughly.

Close Monitoring. Measure and document the patient's vital signs frequently. Notify the physician of significant changes, and record the time of notification. Frequently assess the patient's respiratory function, recording your findings. Start monitoring fluid intake and output if you haven't done so already.

Drug and IV Therapy. Depending on your facility's policy, you may need to maintain the IV access used for the transfusion. If so, document that you did so. Then, if your patient has no other existing IV access, start a new IV line for drug or fluid administration. Document the time the new line was placed, its location, catheter size, and name of the person who placed it. Also document the drugs (such as epinephrine or diphenhydramine) and IV fluids the physician prescribes to treat the patient's symptoms. For IV fluids, document the solution type, dosage, and flow rate.

Laboratory Tests. According to your facility's policy, save all untransfused blood and the tubing used to administer it. Then send these supplies to the laboratory for testing. On the paperwork accompanying the blood container, complete the sections pertaining to a transfusion reaction. Place one copy in the medical record. Document your actions, recording the time you sent the blood and tubing to the laboratory.

Next, collect blood samples and urine specimens, as ordered, for testing to identify the cause of the transfusion reaction. Your facility's policy may require you to obtain several samples and specimens. Record the time each one was collected and sent to the laboratory. Document the patient's reaction on a blood transfusion reaction form and in your progress notes.

Document What You Teach

Document that you covered the following topics when teaching your patient who has had a transfusion reaction:
- what caused the reaction
- procedures he will undergo
- prescribed drugs, including their names, dosages, administration times and routes, adverse effects, and storage
- importance of reporting unusual signs and symptoms (which may indicate ineffective treatment of the reaction)
- reason for repetitive blood and urine testing
- importance of telling future health care providers about the reaction

WHEN YOUR PATIENT HAS HIV INFECTION

For a patient who tests positive for the human immunodeficiency virus (HIV), your documentation must include her risk factors for HIV infection, current signs and symptoms, treatments she's receiving, and her response to these treatments. This information helps the health care team determine whether her condition has progressed to acquired immunodeficiency syndrome (AIDS), which in turn guides medical management. (See *Drawing the line between HIV infection and AIDS*.)

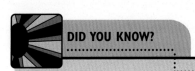

DID YOU KNOW?

DRAWING THE LINE BETWEEN HIV INFECTION AND AIDS

To determine whether human immunodeficiency virus (HIV) infection has progressed to acquired immunodeficiency syndrome (AIDS), the health care team checks for an *indicator condition*—an opportunistic infection, cancer, neurologic disorder, or other condition associated with AIDS.

The Centers for Disease Control and Prevention have identified at least 25 indicator conditions. An HIV-positive patient is officially diagnosed with AIDS if she develops one of these. Here's a list of some of the most common indicator conditions:

* severe immunosuppression with a CD4-T-cell count below 200 cells/μL
* HIV wasting syndrome, characterized by loss of at least 15% of normal body weight
* *Pneumocystis carinii* pneumonia, a serious lung infection that causes fever, fatigue, dry cough, shortness of breath, and weight loss
* esophageal candidiasis, a fungal infection that may lead to difficulty swallowing and subsequent malnutrition
* Kaposi's sarcoma, a neoplasm that causes bluish red skin nodules on the feet and legs that may spread to involve the entire body
* *Mycobacterium tuberculosis* infection, which may affect the lungs, brain, and spine and cause weakness, weight loss, fever, night sweats, cough, chest pain, and hemoptysis
* disseminated *Mycobacterium avium* complex, which may result in tuberculosis, fever, night sweats, weight loss, fatigue, stomach pain, and diarrhea
* toxoplasmosis of the brain (toxoplasmosis encephalitis), a serious infection that leads to headache, weakness, decreased cognition, fever, numbness, seizures, confusion, lethargy, and coma
* severe herpes simplex infection
* cytomegalovirus (CMV) retinitis with vision loss
* CMV disease affecting organs other than the liver, spleen, and lymph nodes

Document What the Patient Tells You

Document a thorough health history. Explore and record specific HIV risk factors that the patient identifies, such as:

- sexual contact with an infected person or with multiple partners of unknown infection status
- IV drug use
- past blood transfusions
- perinatal exposure to HIV

Assess the patient's knowledge of HIV infection and AIDS, and document this information. Record what she tells you about her drug regimen, and write down the names of every physician she sees. If she's receiving an antiviral or other drug, document the name and dosage of each drug. If she knows her latest CD4-T-cell count or viral load measurement, record these values along with the dates of the tests.

Then elicit information about the patient's symptoms. Typically, symptoms vary with the degree of HIV infection, antibody production, and CD4-T-cell destruction. Some HIV-positive patients don't show symptoms for up to 12 years. Others die within a few months of contracting the virus.

If your patient is in an early stage of HIV infection, expect to document the following symptoms:

- fever
- night sweats
- vague discomfort
- rashes
- joint pain

Keep in mind that these symptoms may develop before blood screening tests reveal HIV antibodies. Question the patient about the frequency of her symptoms and the approximate date of their onset; document her response.

As the number of viral particles in the blood increases, the patient may report such symptoms as:

- weight loss
- chills
- malaise
- fatigue

- chronic diarrhea
- headache or stiff neck

Record the approximate dates these symptoms began. Also note anything the patient says alleviates her symptoms.

Document What You Assess

Physical examination findings vary widely among patients with HIV infection. The findings you document will help the physician determine whether the patient's illness is in an early, intermediate, or advanced stage. Your physical examination may reveal:
- cachexia
- palpable lymph nodes
- rashes
- lesions
- pale mucous membranes
- white patches in the oral cavity (oral thrush)

In HIV-positive patients, abnormal laboratory test results typically include a decreased hemoglobin level and decreased platelet, white blood cell, and CD4-T-cell counts.

Document What You Do

Interventions for an HIV-positive patient focus on preventing opportunistic infections, managing symptoms, and monitoring laboratory test results. You'll also need to provide emotional support to the patient and family to help them cope with the physical and psychosocial implications of HIV infection.

Drug Therapy. If your patient is receiving antiviral, antibiotic, or other drugs, note each drug's name and dosage. Notify the physician of adverse effects, and document that you did so. As prescribed, administer drugs and other treatments to counteract adverse effects, and describe them in your documentation.

Your patient may receive an antiretroviral drug, such as zidovudine, didanosine, zalcitabine, lamivudine, or stavudine. These drugs slow disease progression. Document adverse effects, such as nausea, malaise, and fatigue, and your interventions to relieve them. Also record the use of protease inhibitors, such as saquinovir, ritonavir, or indinavir, which interfere with HIV replication.

Document adverse effects, such as nausea, diarrhea, and abdominal discomfort, and record your interventions to relieve them.

Also record that you administered drugs to combat opportunistic infections and HIV-associated cancers, if prescribed.

Other Measures. Document that you followed standard precautions while caring for your patient. Record her weight, caloric intake, and your interventions to promote optimal nutrition, such as offering a high-protein, high-calorie diet.

Record the measures you use to prevent skin breakdown, especially in the debilitated patient. If the patient develops neurologic deficits related to HIV infection, record the interventions you took to promote safety, such as keeping the side rails raised at all times.

Monitoring Laboratory Tests. Your patient's laboratory test results may indicate infection control or progression. Document the results of her current and previous CD4-T-cell counts. Keep in mind that a decreasing count signals worsening of the infection and, possibly, a heightened risk for certain opportunistic infections.

Also document the viral load measurement, which reflects the viral response to the drug regimen. A decreasing viral load indicates a successful regimen. An increasing viral load may indicate that the virus is becoming drug-resistant. Most likely, the physician will change the regimen.

Emotional Support. Document the concerns your patient and her family raise and their responses to other topics you discuss with them. Refer them to the social services department if they need additional counseling, and document your referral.

Document What You Teach

An HIV-positive patient needs comprehensive teaching to maintain optimal health, avoid opportunistic infections, remain emotionally stable, and prevent virus transmission to others. Document the teaching you provide on the following topics:

- pathophysiology of HIV infection
- opportunistic infections associated with HIV infection
- prevention of opportunistic infections
- prescribed drugs, including their names, dosages, administration times and routes, adverse effects, and storage

- signs and symptoms to report
- ways to prevent virus transmission, such as by practicing safer sex, avoiding needle sharing, and never donating blood
- importance of keeping regular medical appointments
- importance of having regular blood tests
- role of a balanced diet, adequate exercise, rest, and relaxation in optimizing health
- resources for further information and support

When teaching your patient about drug therapy, emphasize that she must take prescribed drugs exactly as scheduled. Tell her which drugs to take with foods and which to take on an empty stomach. Help her devise an administration schedule that won't dramatically alter her lifestyle. Be sure to document all discussions about drug therapy.

WHEN YOUR PATIENT HAS A PRESSURE ULCER

Also called a pressure sore, decubitus ulcer, or bed sore, a pressure ulcer is an ulceration of the skin and underlying tissue. It results from prolonged pressure, primarily on a bony prominence, and reflects ischemic tissue hypoxia. A pressure ulcer may take a long time to heal and demands meticulous care by all health care providers.

When documenting your nursing care, include the patient's risk factors for developing a pressure ulcer, your assessment findings and interventions, and the patient's response. This information helps the health care team evaluate the treatment regimen's effectiveness as healing progresses. (See *Documenting the plan of care,* pages 160-161.)

Document What the Patient Tells You

To determine when the pressure ulcer developed and to detect contributing health care problems, obtain and document a thorough history from your patient and family members. Ask them

DOCUMENTING THE PLAN OF CARE

The nursing plan of care is the road map you'll follow when providing and evaluating your care for a patient with a pressure ulcer or other health problem. The plan may involve nursing only, or it may encompass all health care team disciplines. The plan's components and format are described below.

Components

The plan of care must include at least the following:

- patient problems identified during the admission assessment and hospitalization
- expected outcomes, stated in measurable terms and specifying realistic target dates
- interventions to help the patient (and family, if appropriate) achieve the expected outcomes

You may also want to set aside an area on the patient's record where you document your periodic evaluations of his progress toward the outcomes and record the date his outcomes are met.

Traditional Plan of Care

Date	Problem	Expected Outcome	Interventions	Evaluation	Date Closed
1/14/06	Break in skin integrity - sacral wound	Wound size will decrease to 2 cm x 3 cm by 2/15/06. Wound will become more than 50% granulated by 2/15/06.	Wound care t.i.d. with half strength peroxide/ NSS. Pack with dry sterile gauze and cover with a dry sterile dressing.	1/21/06 -Wound 3 cm x 4 cm 30% granulated.	

Review dates	
Date	Signature
1/14/06	Betsy Small, RN
1/21/06	Patsy Clark, RN

Format

A nursing plan of care can take various forms. The two most common are the traditional and standardized plans.

The *traditional* plan of care usually has columns for each component, such as the date, patient problem, expected outcome, interventions, evaluation, and date closed. The nurse (or interdisciplinary team member) who completes the plan records each component in the appropriate column.

On a *standardized* plan, you list common problems along with expected outcomes and typical interventions. Blank spaces allow you to customize the plan. For instance, the target date for assessing more than 50% granulation tissue in a pressure ulcer is left blank so the expected date can be set according to the team's evaluation of the ulcer. In the intervention section, spaces are left blank so that the exact wound care regimen and frequency can be customized to the patient's needs.

Standardized Plan of Care	
Date *1/14/06*	Problem Break in skin integrity *sacral wound*
Target Date *2/15/06*	Expected outcomes Wound will decrease in size to *2 cm* by *3 cm* Wound will be more than *50%* granulated
1/14/06	Interventions Wound care *3* times a day using *half-strength peroxide/NSS. Pack with dry sterile gauze and cover with a dry sterile dressing.*

Review dates	
Date	Signature
1/14/06	*Betsy Small, RN*
1/21/06	*Patsy Clark, RN*

to describe any changes in the ulcer's size, appearance, drainage, and odor. Document their description accurately.

Then record your patient's complete medical history. Especially note risk factors for pressure ulcers, such as diabetes mellitus, peripheral vascular disease, immunosuppression, smoking, and delayed healing. Collect and document data about the patient's dietary habits to determine whether he's meeting his nutritional needs. Determine whether he has a history of incontinence, and document this information. Finally, ask about and record his usual daily routine, including his activity level. If he's bedridden, ask which positions he most often lies in.

Document What You Assess

When documenting your initial assessment, be as specific as you can, especially when describing the pressure ulcer's size, stage, appearance, drainage, and odor. Remember—your record provides a baseline for evaluating healing and gauging treatment effectiveness.

Wound Stage. In general, you should describe a pressure ulcer by its stage of tissue damage. However, you may not be able to stage it if thick, necrotic tissue obstructs your view of the underlying tissue. Whenever possible, assess the stage of the pressure ulcer according to this guide:

- *Stage I.* The ulcer affects the epidermal layer only. Intact skin displays redness that doesn't blanch and is unrelieved by removal of the pressure source. In dark-skinned patients, stage I produces discoloration, warmth, or induration.
- *Stage II.* The ulcer causes partial-thickness skin loss, affecting the epidermal layer and possibly the dermal layer. A superficial ulcer may appear as an abrasion, blister, or shallow crater. Minimal necrosis may be present.
- *Stage III.* The ulcer causes full-thickness skin loss. Damage or necrosis of subcutaneous tissue may reach (but not involve) the underlying fascia. Deep craters, undermining, and eschar may be present.
- *Stage IV.* A deep, craterlike ulcer produces destruction of the full thickness of the skin and deeper tissues. Muscle and bone may be exposed and damaged.

You may document wound appearance in a narrative format or by drawing a picture of the wound and labeling it appropriately.

When describing wound characteristics, include these features:
- precise location, using a landmark and direction when possible, such as "superior to the sacrum"
- diameter in millimeters or centimeters
- depth in millimeters or centimeters
- amount, color, and location of granulation tissue (moist, pink tissue that represents new growth)
- amount, color, and location of eschar (black or gray, scablike, crusty tissue covering the wound)
- amount, color, and location of necrotic tissue (dry, black tissue that represents tissue death)
- amount and description of drainage
- description of odor
- length and location of any undermining (cavity beneath the wound opening) or tunneling
- color and temperature of the surrounding skin
- pattern of any surrounding lesions, such as satellite or linear lesions

Describe the amounts of granulation tissue, eschar, and necrotic tissue in percentages of total wound tissue. For instance, if granulation tissue accounts for about half of the pressure sore, record this as "50% granulation."

Nutritional and Hydration Status. Adequate nutrition and fluid intake are crucial for pressure ulcer healing. To assess your patient's nutritional and hydration status, evaluate and document his skin's general appearance and turgor. Also record the results of serum albumin and total protein assays.

Document What You Do

Your interventions for a patient with a pressure ulcer focus on promoting healing and preventing further skin breakdown. Record each action you take and your patient's response. Also document interdisciplinary and collaborative consultations and interventions. (See *Pressure ulcers: When nursing documentation speaks, the courts listen,* pages 164-165.)

Wound Care. Detail the wound care regimen used, such as irrigation with normal saline solution and peroxide followed by wet-to-dry gauze dressings or use of an enzymatic debriding agent, absorptive gel, or other agent. To compare your findings

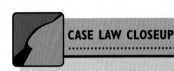

CASE LAW CLOSEUP

PRESSURE ULCERS: WHEN NURSING DOCUMENTATION SPEAKS, THE COURTS LISTEN

Whether your patient has a pressure ulcer or some other disorder, your documentation is just as important as the care it records. That's because it tells the court exactly what you have and haven't done for your patient. And as you'll see in this case, when documentation speaks, the courts listen.

Understanding the Case
NME Properties, Inc. v. Rudich[1] demonstrates the critical link between nursing care and its documentation for Mrs. Rudich, a nursing home patient with midstage Parkinson's disease. Because this patient had bowel and bladder incontinence, moderate to severe dementia, memory problems, and limited mobility, she depended totally on the nursing staff to meet her mobility, toileting, and bathing needs.

Two years after entering the nursing home, Mrs. Rudich was admitted to an acute care facility for colon cancer testing. After the tests results came back negative, she was readmitted to the nursing home. At that time, she had no pressure ulcers.

Two months later, nursing documentation showed a disturbing pattern of inattention to Mrs. Rudich's needs. She was not bathed daily; in fact, there was no documentation of her being bathed for 2 weeks. She required treatment for redness on her hip and buttocks. A few days later, a nurse noted that the patient had a stage II pressure ulcer on her coccyx. Then the ulcer continued to worsen, and Mrs. Rudich developed additional ulcers.

At that stage, the physician was notified of the patient's condition. After he diagnosed gangrenous stage IV ulcers in various locations, Mrs. Rudich was admitted to the acute care facility for treatment. Eventually, she was moved to the hospital's hospice unit, where she died of acute bronchopneumonia secondary to infected pressure ulcers.

Mrs. Rudich's family filed a lawsuit for negligent nursing care that resulted in the patient's untimely death.

How the Court Ruled
The court noted that it is the nurses' responsibility to complete pressure-ulcer reports; to document bathing, turning, dressing changes, and skin status changes; and to notify the physician of significant changes promptly. In Mrs. Rudich's case, the patient record held no documentation of competent nursing care despite clear evidence that her condition was deteriorating rapidly and significantly.

---

[1]*NME Properties, Inc. v. Rudich*, 2003 WL 289415 (Fla. App., February 12, 2003).

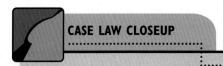

PRESSURE ULCERS: WHEN NURSING DOCUMENTATION SPEAKS, THE COURTS LISTEN—cont'd

Because the patient's care was so substandard, the court assessed punitive damages of $800,000 in addition to $150,000 as compensation for her conscious pain and suffering.

The Lesson Learned

Especially in cases of alleged substandard care, the court looks to the patient record for proof of nursing care. The fact that a 2-week period elapsed with no record of this patient's care infers that she received no care. The rapid development of stage II and IV ulcers supports this idea. Courts will continue to view a lack of documentation as evidence of a lack of nursing care, clearly reinforcing the old adage, "If it wasn't documented, it wasn't done."

more easily with those from earlier shifts, you may want to use a wound care flow sheet.

No matter which documentation form you use, be sure to describe the patient's response to each aspect of your care. Also document the name, dosage, and administration time and route of an analgesic, if prescribed.

If you notice significant changes in the pressure ulcer, notify the physician and document that you did so, along with the time of notification and his orders. Include in your documentation the actions you take as a result of new orders, such as changing the wound care regimen and sending specimens to the laboratory for culture and sensitivity testing.

Pressure Reduction. Depending on the pressure ulcer's stage and the patient's other risk factors for skin breakdown, expect to take steps to reduce pressure. For instance, you may need to provide an alternating-pressure mattress, apply heel and elbow protectors, and frequently reposition the patient. For a patient with several risk factors or a stage-IV pressure ulcer, you may need to use a specially designed mattress or bed system, such as an air-fluidized or low-air-loss bed. Document all interventions, noting the time they began and the patient's response.

Also maintain and document the basic pressure-reduction measures you use with all patients, such as frequent turning and repositioning, and good hygiene. If appropriate, obtain an overhead trapeze to assist in repositioning.

Interdisciplinary Collaboration. When developing a plan of care for a patient with a pressure ulcer, expect to consult the following health care team members:

- dietitian, for strategies on optimizing the patient's nutrition
- occupational therapist, for advice on frequent repositioning to maximize pressure relief
- enterostomal therapist, for evaluation of the wound care regimen's effectiveness
- medical social worker, for referrals and resource information to ensure continuity of care after discharge

Document your interactions with each person you consult, and record the collaborative strategies that arise from your discussions.

Document What You Teach

As you develop and document the teaching plan for your patient and his family, be sure to cover these essential topics:

- pathophysiology of pressure ulcers
- wound care regimen
- signs and symptoms to report
- importance of good hygiene and skin care
- nutrition and fluid requirements to promote healing
- use of pressure-reduction or pressure-relief devices
- importance of frequent repositioning

WHEN YOUR PATIENT HAS AN INFECTED WOUND

A wound infection—the most common type of wound complication—can become life-threatening without prompt, effective treatment. Documenting your wound assessment findings, skin care, and other interventions you implement establishes a baseline that the health care team can use to plan and evaluate patient care. (See *Decoding a case of ambiguous charting,* pages 167–168.)

Document What the Patient Tells You

Ask your patient when the wound first appeared and the circumstances surrounding it; record her response. Then find out about and document such details as the wound's cause, when the

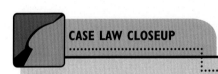

CASE LAW CLOSEUP

DECODING A CASE OF AMBIGUOUS CHARTING

Just as surgical preparation and wound care require meticulousness, so too does your charting of these actions. Documentation that's as precise and specific as possible reduces other health care professionals' guesswork when they need to know what has been done for your patient so far. And unambiguous documentation can be your best defense in a lawsuit.

Understanding the Case
Hutchins v. DCH Regional Medical Center[1] shows that potential risks associated with the ambiguous charting for Mr. Hutchins who was admitted for hemorrhoid surgery. Although the surgery was performed without incident, dermal tissue around the surgical site appeared infected a few days later. Mr. Hutchins subsequently developed respiratory problems related to infection with beta-hemolytic *Streptococcus.* He died of respiratory complications 34 days after the hemorrhoid surgery.

The patient's family sued the hospital for negligence that resulted in his untimely death. They claimed that the Mr. Hutchins' surgical preparation was substandard and directly led to the infection that he developed. The focus of their claim was this: the nurse who performed the surgical scrub documented that the surgical preparation took 8 minutes to do. A nursing expert for the family testified that, for this type of surgery, the standard of care required the nurse to scrub the anus, perineal area, buttocks, and back with povidone-iodine (Betadine) for 5 minutes and then paint the anus with povidone-iodine or a similar solution. The expert concluded that since the entire procedure was performed in 8 minutes, the full 5-minute scrub couldn't have been done.

[1]*Hutchins v. DCH Regional Medical Center, 770 So. 2d 49 (Alabama, 2000).*

Continued

CASE LAW CLOSEUP

DECODING A CASE OF AMBIGUOUS CHARTING—cont'd

How the Court Ruled

The nurse who performed the scrub testified in her own defense during the trial. She stated that charting an 8-minute scrub meant that she had spent 8 minutes on the Betadine scrub alone and that painting the surgical site with Betadine was *in addition to* the Betadine scrub. She further testified that it was her habit to chart the actual time of the scrub and not to document the time spent on other preparatory steps.

At the trial, the jury noted that the documentation was ambiguous, but held that the hospital wasn't liable because of the nurse's testimony. The Supreme Court of Alabama upheld the lower court's judgment. Although it noted that the nursing documentation was ambiguous on this critical point, it wouldn't alter the jury's decision.

The Lesson Learned

This case aptly illustrates the need for unambiguous charting. In fact, the nurse in this case could have avoided the lawsuit altogether if she'd been more precise in her documentation. However, she was fortunate because she was able to testify at the trial. In many cases, the nurse who charted the original entry is no longer available, and the only information the defense can present is the documentation in the patient's chart. If that had happened in this case, the patient's family probably would have been successful in their lawsuit.

wound occurred, and its early features. Encourage the patient to be specific when identifying the wound's size and appearance.

Document, too, medical treatment the patient has received for the wound, and note whether it was successful. If she's had more than one wound treatment regimen, determine what prompted the change. Then elicit and thoroughly document her current wound care regimen as well as the name of anyone who helps her with wound care.

Next, question the patient about her medical history. Be sure to record conditions that could impair healing, such as diabetes mellitus and immunosuppression. Also obtain information about drugs she's taking, including each one's name, dosage, and administration time and route. Flag any drug that could interfere with healing, such as a steroid or antirejection agent.

Because protein aids healing, question the patient about her usual diet, and document the foods she typically consumes. Also ask whether she has allergies, such as to foods or drugs. If so, note them in a prominent place in her record and anywhere else your facility requires.

In the patient's own words, record symptoms she reports that may indicate wound infection. Depending on whether the infection is localized or generalized, you may document the following symptoms:

- pain or tenderness at the wound site
- redness or swelling of the skin around the wound
- purulent (pus) or other drainage
- poor wound healing
- odor originating from the wound
- fever or chills
- weakness

Document What You Assess

Document all physical examination findings thoroughly, using a systematic approach. (See *Recording wound assessment findings*, page 170.) For consistency, encourage all health care team members to use the same format when documenting wound assessment findings.

Wound Appearance. Assess and document the size and stage of the wound. (See *When your patient has a pressure ulcer*, pages 159-166.) Then fully describe the wound edges, noting whether they adhere to the underlying tissue or have pockets or tunnels. Evaluate and record the wound color, and describe the color, amount, and odor of any drainage. Be sure to document whether the drainage descriptions are based on the wound or the dressing because some dressings, such as foams and hydrocolloids, can mask or change the odor of drainage. Also assess the type of tissue in the wound, documenting the percentage of granulation tissue, necrotic tissue, and eschar.

Next, evaluate and record the condition of the skin around the wound, noting whether it is red, warm, or swollen. Describe the presence and pattern of any lesions in the surrounding skin,

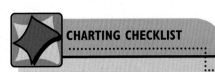

CHARTING CHECKLIST

RECORDING WOUND ASSESSMENT FINDINGS
When documenting a wound infection, be sure to cover the following information:

❑ *Wound stage.* Document the wound stage according to the level of tissue involved. In a stage I wound, the skin remains intact. In a stage II wound, you'll see open skin. A stage III wound involves the subcutaneous (fatty) layer. A stage IV wound extends to the muscle or bone.

❑ *Wound size.* Document wound size by describing the wound's length, width, and depth in millimeters or centimeters. If you don't have a ruler handy, compare the wound's size to that of a standard-size, common object, such as a coin.

❑ *Wound borders.* Evaluate and document the wound's borders, or edges, determining whether they are attached to the underlying skin or contain tunnels or pockets.

❑ *Wound color.* Document the wound's color. If it has several colors, describe the percentage of each color and note exactly where it is located within the wound.

❑ *Drainage.* Describe the color, amount, and odor of wound drainage.

❑ *Type of tissue.* Document the percentage of granulation and necrotic tissue and eschar

which can help identify a causative organism. For example, numerous satellite lesions around a larger central lesion are associated with a *Candida* infection. Also document tenderness the patient reports during palpation.

Then assess for and document other signs of infection, such as a fever and increased white blood cell or lymphocyte count. If the patient has undergone culture and sensitivity testing for wounds and blood, obtain and record the results.

Finally, document your observation of other conditions that could impair wound healing. For example, note whether the patient is obese or cachectic.

Document What You Do

Make sure your documentation for a patient with a wound infection reflects your frequent monitoring, meticulous wound care, and communication with the other health care team members. To provide a complete picture of the patient's treatment, document each drug you give and all specimens obtained for culture and sensitivity testing (along with their results).

Wound Care. Document wound cleaning or irrigation you perform, along with the name of the solution used, type of dressing applied, and the patient's tolerance of the procedure. If your facility's wound care protocol calls for wound packing, document the type and amount of packing used. When recording the amount, indicate the number of pieces of packing. For instance, write "two 7-inch pieces of gauze packing inserted." That way, subsequent caregivers will know how much packing to remove.

If you note a change in wound characteristics as you perform wound care, notify the physician and document the time of notification. Then, if the physician changes the patient's wound care regimen, record the details of these changes in your notes, along with the information that prompted the change.

Vital Signs and Cultures. Your patient's vital sign measurements and culture results reflect how well her body is fighting the infection. Record her heart rate and temperature every 2 to 4 hours. If a fever develops, administer acetaminophen or other antipyretic agent, as ordered. Document this action, along with the drug's name, dosage, and administration time. Then recheck and document the patient's temperature 2 hours later.

Record the date and time wound specimens were sent to the laboratory for culture and sensitivity testing, noting whether they were sent for aerobic or anaerobic cultures. When possible, send the specimens before antibiotic therapy begins, so that the drug won't alter test results. If the laboratory can provide a preliminary report after 24 hours, call for this report and document it in the patient's record. Then, when the final report is available, post it in the record and document that you notified the physician of the results.

Antibiotic Therapy. After the first culture specimens are sent to the laboratory, begin antibiotic therapy, as prescribed. Be sure to document the drug's name, dosage, and administration time and route. After giving the first dose, monitor the patient for adverse reactions. Document reactions that occur.

Keep in mind that many antibiotics require monitoring of the blood levels. If the physician orders such monitoring, record the time when blood samples were sent to the laboratory, noting whether they were sent for random or peak and trough antibiotic levels. Record the results when they become available, and document that you reported them to the physician. If he changes the regimen, record this change and the reason for it.

Promoting Healing. Along with the wound care regimen and antibiotic therapy, document the measures you took to promote healing. For instance, record the patient's dietary intake, specifying the type of food and amount of protein she consumes. Also document the percentage of meals she eats.

If you consult a dietitian, record this communication and resulting changes in the patient's diet or plan of care. If the physician prescribes nutritional supplements, document the time you gave them and how much of the supplements the patient consumed.

Unless contraindicated, encourage hydration. Document the provision of additional fluids and the patient's fluid intake.

Document What You Teach

In most cases, you'll instruct family members as well as the patient. Document that your teaching covered the following topics:
- physiology of wound healing
- signs and symptoms of healing
- signs and symptoms to report
- wound care regimen, including clean or aseptic technique
- prescribed drugs, including their names, dosages, administration times and routes, adverse effects, and storage
- which drugs to take with food
- nutrition and hydration measures
- infection-control measures to use at home
- telephone numbers of local home health agencies
- other resources for information and support

WHEN YOUR PATIENT HAS SEPSIS

When bacteria or other microorganisms enter the bloodstream, they may trigger a massive, systemic inflammatory response known as sepsis. If untreated, sepsis can progress to septic shock or death. Usually, sepsis develops as a complication of a disorder, such as pneumonia, or a procedure, such as indwelling catheter insertion. To spot the disorder early and monitor its progress or resolution, the health care team needs a detailed record of the initial signs of infection and all interventions, including patient teaching.

Document What the Patient Tells You

Ask about and record all signs of infection, which can vary with the source of the infection. For example, the patient may report localized signs and symptoms, including erythema, warmth, pain, and purulent drainage at the infection site, such as an IV insertion site. Or he may describe generalized signs and symptoms, such as weakness, malaise, flushing, fever, and rigors.

If your patient also has diabetes mellitus, he may tell you about increased blood glucose levels and insulin requirements. As the infection becomes systemic and progresses to sepsis, the patient or a family member may notice a decreased level of consciousness (LOC) or a behavior change, such as delirium. If so, record these changes in his status.

If known, document when the patient first noticed any signs or symptoms. Also note how they progressed or worsened. Record risk factors for sepsis, such as immunosuppressant therapy or chemotherapy. Document the patient's report of exposure to infection, and note any break in aseptic technique, such as improper wound care. Also, clearly document in the chart—and communicate to the health care team—any reported allergies, especially to antibiotics.

Document What You Assess

If you suspect sepsis, immediately record the patient's vital signs, staying especially alert for fever, tachycardia, tachypnea, and hypotension. Observe for obvious signs of infection, such as wound drainage, and record pertinent findings, such as drainage characteristics and the extent of erythema. Document any change in the patient's LOC or the presence of confusion. Perform a head-to-toe assessment and record your findings, particularly noting respiratory, cardiovascular, and other effects.

Respiratory System. Record the patient's respiratory rate and rhythm. Then auscultate his breath sounds and document abnormal sounds you hear, such as wheezes. If you detect areas of dullness on percussion, suspect consolidation and document your findings. If the patient has a cough, record whether it is dry or moist. For a productive cough, describe the amount of sputum produced and the sputum color, odor, and other characteristics. Observe for and record dyspnea as well as signs of hypoxemia, such as low oxygen saturation and cyanosis.

Cardiovascular System. Auscultate the patient's heart sounds, noting a murmur or other abnormal findings that may indicate vegetation on a valve. Also assess and record the amplitude of his peripheral pulses, which may be bounding. If he has continuous cardiac monitoring, note the presence of arrhythmias. If he's undergoing hemodynamic monitoring with a pulmonary artery or arterial catheter, record all measurements, including cardiac output and mean arterial pressure.

Laboratory Test Results. Record pertinent laboratory test data, such as an increased or decreased white blood cell count and bacteria in body fluids, such as the blood, wound drainage, urine, or sputum. Note an elevated blood glucose level, especially if a patient with diabetes mellitus. If sepsis progresses to septic shock, document indicators of organ damage, including elevated serum lactate, blood urea nitrogen, and creatinine levels and prolonged activated partial thromboplastin and prothrombin times. If the results of arterial blood gas analysis are available, record a low oxygen level or pH, which signal hypoxemia and metabolic acidosis, respectively.

Document What You Do

Record your interventions as you perform them to help show that you provided timely care—an important consideration in legal cases.

Frequent Monitoring. Record your patient's vital sign measurements every 4 hours or more frequently if he's unstable. Carefully document changes in temperature, heart or respiratory rate, and blood pressure. Write down hemodynamic measurements every hour or more often, as needed. Begin continuous pulse oximetry, and document the patient's oxygen saturation. After inserting an indwelling urinary catheter, monitor and record fluid intake and output every hour. Note oliguria, which may indicate renal insufficiency or failure.

Specimen Collection for Additional Tests. Before antibiotic therapy begins, obtain blood samples for culture and sensitivity testing. Record the number of samples and the times of collection and transmission to the laboratory. On the laboratory slip and the patient's chart, indicate the source of the samples, such as from a central venous catheter or a peripheral vein. Also document other specimens you collect for testing, which may include wound drainage, sputum, and urine. If you suspect an IV catheter may be the source of infection, remove the catheter and send its tip for analysis; document these actions.

Drug and IV Therapy. Immediately establish IV access with at least one large-bore IV catheter. Record the catheter size, location of the IV site, and any failed attempts at catheter placement in the vein. Document IV fluid administration, noting the type of solution (such as normal saline) and infusion rate. Also note whether the infusion flows by gravity alone or uses a pump.

If prescribed, give the patient acetaminophen or another antipyretic; document its administration as well as its effect on the patient's temperature.

Based on the results of culture and sensitivity testing, administer an IV antibiotic, antifungal, or antiviral, as prescribed. Because of the prevalence of antibiotic-resistant microorganisms, some antibiotics traditionally prescribed for specific bacteria may be ineffective. That's why documentation of the microorganism's antibiotic sensitivity is critical to effective treatment. Record the administration time of the first drug dose and any adverse reactions that may occur. If the patient has an adverse reaction, stop the drug and notify the physician and pharmacy; document these actions. Update all records to include the new allergy, and record your management of an anaphylactic reaction.

If the physician requires drug levels to be obtained, record the time when you send blood samples to the laboratory and clearly mark whether they are peak, trough, or random samples. Work with the physician to determine whether the patient is receiving the appropriate antimicrobial dosage; record any changes to the drug regimen. Remember: clear documentation of your interventions—and the patient's response to therapy—can help him receive the best treatment for his disorder.

If sepsis progresses to septic shock, the physician may prescribe a vasopressor, such as dopamine. Be sure to record the time this therapy begins, the dosage, and the administration site. Record the patient's vital signs every 15 minutes, as ordered, until he's stable. Then record his vital signs hourly or as directed by facility policy.

Oxygen Administration. If hypoxemia occurs, administer supplemental oxygen, as prescribed. Document the time you initiated oxygen therapy, the flow rate, and the delivery device (such as nasal cannula or face mask). Monitor and document pulse oximetry readings regularly.

If respiratory failure is imminent, prepare for endotracheal intubation and mechanical ventilation. Record who performed the intubation and when, the tube and cuff type and size, and the amount of air used to inflate the cuff. Document how far the tube was placed into the trachea, and mark the tube itself. Also note how you secured the tube in place. Record that tube placement was confirmed by chest x-ray and that you auscultated breath sounds equally and bilaterally. In addition, document the time mechanical ventilation began and the ventilator settings, such as the ventilation mode, fraction of inspired oxygen, and positive end expiratory pressure (PEEP). Your notation of these important facts can help confirm that you followed safe practice if complications arise.

Comfort Measures. To help reduce the patient's fever, use a hypothermia blanket or tepid baths, if indicated. Record the patient's response to your interventions. Also document the measures you take to reduce shivering and promote comfort, such as changing damp linens and clothes and adding or removing blankets to keep the patient's temperature between 97.7° and 100.4° F (36.5° and 38° C).

Document What You Teach

If the patient develops septic shock or is delirious, postpone most of your teaching until his condition stabilizes. Until then, regularly inform him and his family members of your actions and his progress. After the patient's condition has stabilized, prepare him for discharge and provide more extensive teaching. Document that you covered the following topics when teaching your patients who has had sepsis:

- disease process
- procedures and treatments
- activity limitations
- signs and symptoms to report
- drugs, including their names, dosages, administration times and routes, adverse effects, storage, and timing of dosages in relation to food
- home IV care, if prescribed
- temperature measurement and documentation
- infection-control measures

WHEN YOUR PATIENT HAS AN ADVERSE DRUG REACTION

A harmful, unintended reaction to a drug, an adverse drug reaction can vary from mild to severe. Some mild reactions are the expected adverse effects of a drug whose therapeutic benefit outweighs the slight discomfort it causes. However, a severe or acute adverse reaction can be deadly.

Whether your patient's adverse reaction is mild or life-threatening, your documentation plays an important role in the physician's appraisal of the situation and the drug manufacturer's evaluation of its product. Documenting your assessment findings and nursing interventions also provides a record of the care your patient received, which could become important if the adverse reaction leads to litigation.

Document What the Patient Tells You

Your patient may report a symptom that involves a single body system, such as a rash. Or she may report symptoms that involve multiple body systems, such as nausea, wheezing, and dizziness. Document her symptoms in her own words, placing quotation marks around them.

Central Nervous System. If the adverse reaction involves the central nervous system, your patient may report pain, hallucinations, vision disturbances, burning or tingling sensations, numbness, and weakness.

GI System. A patient with a GI adverse effect may report nausea, diarrhea, constipation, dry mouth, difficulty swallowing, metallic taste, abdominal pain or cramps, abdominal bloating, and heartburn.

Cardiovascular System. A patient experiencing a cardiovascular adverse reaction may report palpitations and chest pain.

Genitourinary System. A genitourinary adverse effect may cause painful or frequent urination, vaginal pain or itching and uterine cramps in a woman, and impotence in a man.

Integumentary System. A patient with an integumentary reaction may report rash, itching, burning, welts, and wheals.

Document What You Assess

Next, perform a physical examination, recording every finding in detail. Depending on the affected body system, expect to document these signs and symptoms of an adverse drug reaction:

- fever
- hypertension or hypotension
- heart rhythm disturbances, including premature ventricular contractions, widened QRS complexes, and ventricular fibrillation
- tachycardia or bradycardia
- adventitious breath sounds
- edema
- rash, hives, welts, wheals, flushed skin, or skin sloughing
- stomatitis, gingivitis, or oral lesions
- abdominal distention
- hyperactive or hypoactive bowel sounds
- decreased or absent urine output

Also document behavioral changes you observe, along with the time you first noticed them. For instance, record whether the patient seems restless, fatigued, hyperactive, irritable, overly talkative, or hostile. Document her level of consciousness too, especially noting confusion.

Document What You Do

If you suspect that your patient is experiencing a significant adverse drug reaction, you may need to stop the drug and evaluate her for emergent or urgent care needs. Consult the physician before discontinuing a drug.

Specific actions to take next depend on the seriousness of your assessment findings. If you must take emergency measures, such as cardiopulmonary resuscitation, document the time you called for emergency assistance and started your interventions.

If the situation is not an emergency, notify the physician. Document his name, time of notification, information you conveyed, and his response. Depending on the physician's orders, you may need to intervene by administering drugs and IV fluids and monitoring the patient closely. Document every action you take. (See *Reporting adverse reactions to the FDA,* page 180.)

Drug and IV Therapy. Document each drug the physician prescribes to treat the adverse reaction. Include the drug's name, dosage, and administration time and route as well as the patient's response. If you give supplemental oxygen, record the flow rate and delivery device used, such as a face mask or cannula, along with pulse oximetry readings.

If you administer prescribed IV fluids to treat an adverse reaction, such as hypotension, document the specific fluid given, its dosage, the infusion rate, and the delivery device.

Close Monitoring. Depending on the severity of the adverse reaction, measure the patient's vital signs every 15 minutes to 1 hour, or as ordered. Notify the physician of significant findings. Record the time of notification and his response. As ordered, send blood samples to the laboratory for immediate testing of drug levels if toxicity is suspected. Document this action and the time the samples were sent. Then record the results when they are available.

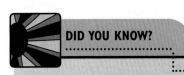

DID YOU KNOW?

REPORTING ADVERSE REACTIONS TO THE FDA

Through its MedWatch program, the Food and Drug Administration (FDA) collects data to evaluate potential problems with drugs, medical equipment, and special nutritional products. As a nurse, you can help identify potential concerns with the drugs you administer and the medical devices you use or monitor. To determine whether you should report your patient's adverse reaction to a drug or medical device to the FDA, ask yourself whether the drug or device may have caused:
- death, life-threatening illness, disability, or a congenital anomaly
- initial or prolonged hospitalization
- additional surgical or medical intervention to prevent a permanent injury

    Also ask yourself whether you believe that the drug or device:
- was defective or failed to function as intended
- had an inaccurate or unreadable label
- was involved in a packaging or product mix-up
- was contaminated or unstable
- contained particles (this applies to an injectable drug solution)

    If you can answer yes to any of these questions, report the reaction to the FDA. Remember—when you file a MedWatch form, you're *not* stating that the product definitely caused the problem. That's up to others to decide. The FDA will investigate the situation and report to you on any actions it takes. It will also protect your identity and the identities of your patient and employer.

How to File a Report

To file a MedWatch form, complete the sections that apply to your patient's situation. (Use a separate form for each patient.) You don't need to supply a lot of details. Just summarize the situation. You can submit your form to the FDA using the fax number or address printed on the form.

Reporting the Reaction. Once the patient's condition is stable, document that you notified the pharmacy of the patient's adverse reaction and updated the patient's medical record to reflect a new allergy or other adverse drug reaction. Depending on your facility's policy, you may also need to complete an incident report or a drug reaction report. Be aware that these forms are considered separate reports of the incident. In your documentation, don't mention that you submitted them.

Document What You Teach

After an adverse drug reaction, explain the reaction to the patient and the measures she and all of her health care providers must take to prevent a recurrence. Reassure her that other drugs should not cause the same reaction. Document that your teaching covered the following topics:
- pathophysiology of the adverse drug reaction
- name of the drug involved, including its generic name and all brand names
- importance of telling all health care providers, such as dentists, of the adverse reaction
- importance of wearing medical alert identification that specifies the drug involved.

WHEN YOUR PATIENT HAS IV INFILTRATION

Capable of causing permanent damage, IV infiltration occurs when an IV solution inadvertently enters the subcutaneous tissue. Depending on the IV agent involved, a patient may experience vesicant or nonvesicant infiltration. *Vesicant* infiltration destroys subcutaneous tissue and can lead to loss of an arm or leg. *Nonvesicant* infiltration may cause soft-tissue damage (such as phlebitis) as well as pain and infection. Documenting your assessment findings and rapid interventions shows that the situation was detected promptly and that the patient received appropriate treatment.

Document What the Patient Tells You

Symptoms of IV infiltration vary with the amount and type of IV fluid. To detect infiltration early, instruct your patient to report unusual feelings or sensations he experiences during an infusion. If infiltration occurs, expect to record the following symptoms:
- tight skin around the IV insertion site
- tenderness, pain, redness, swelling, or itching at the insertion site

- difficulty flexing or extending the affected arm or leg
- coolness of the affected arm or leg

Because vesicant solutions are highly irritating to the skin, your patient's report of pain may be the earliest sign of infiltration. Assess the site immediately and document the complaint. If you find no other signs of infiltration, yet the patient continues to report pain, record this fact in your notes. Then stop the infusion, notify the physician, and document both actions. If the patient continues to report pain after the vesicant infusion is halted, notify the physician. Record that you did so, along with the time of notification and the physician's orders.

Document What You Assess

Assess the IV site and surrounding tissues. Record all findings, including the dressing's condition and the skin's appearance and temperature. Also check for and document edema, noting the degree of any pitting. Next, measure the circumference of the affected arm or leg and compare it with the opposite arm or leg. Document the measurements.

If the IV solution has been infusing by gravity, assess the infusion rate and note whether the solution flows freely when the clamp is opened wide. Then apply pressure to the affected arm or leg above the IV insertion site and see whether the infusion stops flowing. Remove the IV bag from the pole and lower it below the level of the bed. Document whether you see blood return into the tubing, which suggests that infiltration hasn't occurred. Keep in mind that the absence of a blood return does not necessarily indicate an infiltration. (See *IV therapy: Recording the essentials*.)

If you've been administering the IV infusion by a pump or controller and the solution does not contain a drug, remove the tubing from the device and document the results of the test described above. With a drug such as potassium, temporarily disconnect and cap the tubing. Then check for a blood return, using a syringe and sterile normal saline solution. Document the outcome of your check.

Document What You Do

Preventing IV infiltration is the best intervention. Take appropriate preventive steps when beginning an infusion, and document

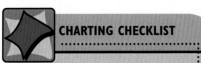

CHARTING CHECKLIST

IV THERAPY: RECORDING THE ESSENTIALS
When documenting your patient's IV therapy, you're not just creating a record of his care. You're also providing legal protection for you and your health care facility and supplying the information your employer needs for third-party reimbursement. Your documentation should address the following topics:
- ❏ type of IV solution administered
- ❏ number of venipuncture attempts made (if more than one) and assistance you obtained
- ❏ time the infusion began
- ❏ delivery device
- ❏ flow rate
- ❏ amount of solution infused
- ❏ appearance of the insertion site and dressing
- ❏ signs and symptoms of infiltration, including absence of blood return, sluggish infusion, and swelling, bruising, pain, redness, tightness, or coolness at or near the IV site
- ❏ signs and symptoms of infection, including fever, chills, pain, redness, and pus draining from the IV site
- ❏ your interventions to deal with the infiltration
- ❏ notification of the physician

You may document some of these items on an IV flow sheet. If you start a new IV line, change the tubing, or use a different IV site, record these actions on the IV flow sheet or in your documentation.

them in detail. If infiltration occurs, record all corrective interventions you perform.

Preventive Measures. Record all interventions to prevent the patient's IV cannula from slipping out of the vein. For instance, loosely secure his arm or leg on a board to prevent flexion if the IV insertion site is near a wrist or in a small vein that's sensitive to positioning. Securely tape a loop of the IV tubing next to the insertion site to serve as an anchor and help prevent catheter dislodgment. If your patient is restless or active, cover the site with stretch netting or a gauze wrap so that the tubing won't move at the insertion site.

Corrective Interventions. If infiltration occurs, immediately discontinue the infusion and notify the physician. Document the time of notification and the physician's instructions.

If the infiltrating substance isn't a vesicant, obtain an order to remove the catheter. For vesicant infiltration, leave the catheter in place so that an antidote can be infiltrated into the existing IV line. Document these actions, including their times and the patient's response.

If you removed the catheter, record this. Also document that you applied pressure to the insertion site, elevated the affected arm or leg, and applied ice to the insertion site, if indicated.

If appropriate, obtain an order to restart the IV infusion. Document the location of the new site, catheter size, name of the person who placed the new line, time of placement, and the patient's response.

Document What You Teach

Before administering an IV infusion, instruct the patient to report pain, swelling, leakage, and coolness at the IV site. Also document that your teaching included the following topics:

- signs and symptoms to report
- precautions to take to prevent accidental catheter dislodgment, such as avoiding bending the arm and making sudden arm movements
- intermittent heat application to the infiltration site to aid absorption of the infiltrated IV solution
- local wound care at the infiltration site

WHEN YOUR PATIENT HAS SURGERY

With more same-day surgeries being performed and shorter hospital stays for major surgery, you may find it a challenge to gather and document all the necessary patient information in the time allotted. Yet no matter how briefly you care for a patient, you must document *all* the care you provide. Besides serving as the basis for evaluating the plan of care, your documentation reflects the standard of care provided. This can prove important if the patient later sues you, other health care team members, or your health care facility. (See *Honestly avoiding fraudulent concealment,* pages 185–186.)

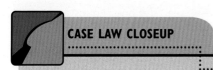

CASE LAW CLOSEUP

HONESTLY AVOIDING FRAUDULENT CONCEALMENT
Accidents can happen during surgery or even routine patient care. Yet your reaction to an accident and documentation of it can make the difference between maintaining your patient's trust and being sued for fraudulent concealment.

Understanding the Case
Kodadek v. Lieberman[1] shows exactly how forthright admission of a surgical accident involving a young boy undergoing a tonsillectomy avoided liability for fraudulent concealment. As the surgeon sutured a bleeding vessel, the needle tip broke off in the patient's tonsillar fossa. When the surgeon probed for the broken needle tip, the bleeding worsened. So he decided to leave the tip embedded in the tissue instead of retrieving it. An x-ray of the area was obtained, and the procedure was completed.

Afterward, the surgeon and the hospital's director of perioperative services (who was a nurse) met with the boy's parents. They explained that a small portion of the needle had broken off and was embedded in the child's tonsillar fossa, but assured the parents that this type of thing happened occasionally and would not be a problem for their son. The surgeon estimated that the broken needle tip was no more than 1/4-inch long. The parents indicated that they were satisfied with the surgical outcome and the explanation about the broken needle.

Then the hospital investigated the cause of the broken needle. The investigation revealed that the scrub technician had handed the surgeon a thinner needle than he had requested.

Later, the patient developed complications related to the needle fragment and required a second surgery to remove it. At that point, the parents brought a lawsuit for negligence.

---

[1] *Kodadek v. Lieberman, 545 S. E. 2d 25 (Ga. App., 2001).*

Continued

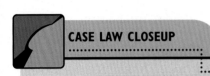

CASE LAW CLOSEUP

HONESTLY AVOIDING FRAUDULENT CONCEALMENT—cont'd

How the Court Ruled

Upon reviewing the patient record, the court noted that the operating room nurses didn't document that a needle had broken during the procedure, that an x-ray had been obtained, that the surgeon decided to leave the needle fragment in the tonsillar fossa, or that a needle other than the one requested had been handed to the surgeon to use. Although the parents were awarded $22,500 for negligence, they appealed the case, contending that the nurses had engaged in fraudulent concealment. Specifically, they cited the lack of nurse's notes regarding the entire incident and the follow-up care.

The court noted that a patient can sue a nurse or physician who fraudulently misinforms him or tries to conceal a mistake. Health care professionals have a duty not to deceive patients by covering up mistakes. Their relationship with patients is based on trust, which makes such conduct inappropriate.

Nevertheless, the court found no fraudulent concealment in this case. Although the parents were given information that later came to be partially untrue, they were told about the needle tip, which negated fraudulent concealment by the health care team. The court simply upheld the hospital's obligation to pay compensation for the nurse's negligence in selecting the wrong needle.

The Lesson Learned

This case underscores the importance of factually and accurately documenting events that occur, even if the facts place the nurse or physician in an unfavorable light. When charting, remember not to assign blame. Merely state what happened and tell how the patient was treated to ensure his safety. For example, record "The nurse handed the physician a size 3.0 silk on a cutting needle" instead of "The nurse gave the surgeon the wrong size needle."

Document What the Patient Tells You

Before surgery, document your patient's medical history. Ask her to describe previous health problems, treatments she received for them, and the effectiveness of those treatments. Then document the information she provides about previous surgeries and other medical procedures. Especially find out whether she has experienced an allergic reaction to a food, drug, anesthetic, contrast medium, or dye. If she has never been anesthetized, ask whether anyone in her family has experienced a reaction to an anesthetic.

Then determine whether she has had a problem with bleeding, such as easy bruising, blood in the urine or stool, and difficulty stopping a cut from bleeding. Also document the use of warfarin or nonsteroidal antiinflammatory drugs. These factors indicate that the patient may have bleeding problems during and after surgery.

Next, have the patient tell you what she knows about the scheduled procedure, and document her response. If she will go home shortly after surgery, record the type of transportation she will use and the name of the person who will accompany her. Also document whether someone will be at her home when she arrives or if she will be alone that night.

Next, ask the patient when she last ate or drank and what drugs (if any) she took that day. Record her reply in her own words. Then question her about any recent symptoms she has had, especially if they seem unrelated to the reason for her upcoming surgery. In particular, document shortness of breath, chest pain, nausea, anxiety, and urinary difficulties.

Record the date of the patient's last bowel movement, and indicate whether she moves her bowels regularly. Also document her usual activity level and daily routine, which may be disrupted during her recovery.

Ask the patient whether she has ever smoked. When documenting her answer, include the number of cigarettes per day she smokes or smoked. Also find out whether she regularly drinks alcohol or uses recreational drugs, and record her response. Document her use of assistive devices, such as a hearing aid, eyeglasses, and dentures. Finally, record the name of the patient's primary care physician.

During the Postoperative Period. After the patient returns from surgery, record reports of discomfort and other problems. Ask her to rate her pain's severity on a scale of 0 to 10, with 0 indicating no pain and 10 indicating the worst pain imaginable. Document her answer. Also record the following complaints:

- urinary urgency with inability to void
- shortness of breath

- chest pain
- nausea
- leg pain or cramping
- anxiety or fear

Document What You Assess

Perform a physical examination before and after surgery, and document your findings.

Preoperative Findings. Remember that your preoperative examination provides a baseline for later assessments. Notify the physician of abnormal findings, such as the following:

- hypertension or hypotension
- tachycardia or bradycardia
- fever
- abnormal breath sounds
- irregular heart rate
- abdominal firmness or distention
- cold or discolored arms or legs

Postoperative Findings. Document your postoperative physical examination findings, and then compare them with preoperative findings. Measure and record the patient's vital signs every 5 to 15 minutes for the first hour after surgery and then hourly. Auscultate her lungs, noting the rate, rhythm, and depth of respirations; document this data carefully. Then palpate her peripheral pulses, recording the strength of each pulse. Assess for and document pain on ankle dorsiflexion (Homans' sign).

Next, record the amount of urine in the drainage bag, if present. Use this measurement as a baseline when assessing urine output over the next several hours. Then auscultate and palpate the patient's abdomen, recording abdominal tone and the type of bowel sounds.

Document the appearance of the dressing and the area around the incision, including the amount and color of drainage or skin discoloration. Assess the insertion site for tubes, drains, and catheters, and record their appearance.

Review the patient's latest blood chemistry and hematology results. Notify the physician of abnormal values, and document that you did so.

Document What You Do

Document all interventions you perform before and after surgery. In your preoperative documentation, include the steps you took to prepare the patient for surgery. In your postoperative notes, record that you implemented all postoperative orders and helped the patient return to her baseline level of functioning.

Preoperative Interventions. Using the preoperative checklist, document that you made sure a consent form was signed. Record the patient's last set of vital sign measurements and then complete the checklist. Verify that the patient has the correct identification band and has removed all clothing, jewelry, and prosthetics, such as dentures and contact lenses. If she's allowed to keep her wedding ring on, place tape over it so that it won't become dislodged and possibly lost during surgery. Create an itemized list of other valuables and record the name of the person you gave them to. Take steps to ensure that the right patient is prepared for the right procedure on the right site. (See *Preventing wrong site, wrong procedure, and wrong person surgery,* page 190.)

Then administer the prescribed preoperative drugs, and document each drug's name, dosage, and administration time and route. After helping the patient transfer to a stretcher, review each item on the checklist. Then sign the checklist, write the time next to your signature, and place the checklist on the front of the medical record.

Postoperative Interventions. Measure and record your patient's vital signs as soon as she returns from the postanesthesia care unit (PACU). Compare the measurements you obtain with her preoperative, intraoperative, and PACU measurements. (Make sure that you've obtained a report from the PACU nurse.) Also document the patient's fluid intake, output, and loss.

Check the patient's dressings and drains with the PACU nurse, and document their appearance. Connect a suction device, if ordered, and document this action. Read and implement the physician's orders, recording each step you take. (See *Documenting perioperative care,* pages 191-192.)

Measure the patient's vital signs frequently, and notify the physician of significant changes. Document the name of the

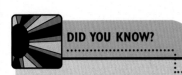

PREVENTING WRONG SITE, WRONG PROCEDURE, AND WRONG PERSON SURGERY

In 2004, the Joint Commission on Accreditation of Healthcare Organizations released guidelines for implementing the "Universal Protocol for Preventing Wrong Site, Wrong Procedure, and Wrong Person Surgery™" as part of its national safety goals. To help ensure that you're dealing with the correct site, procedure, and person in every surgery, follow theses guidelines:

• Preoperatively, verify the patient's identity as well as the correct surgical procedure and site for her. Involve the patient when she is awake, alert, and oriented. Also verify proper documentation of all items on the preoperative checklist.

• Whenever possible, have the surgeon make a mark with indelible ink near the operative site. (Keep in mind that this isn't possible for some procedures, such as dental surgery.) Make sure the mark clearly identifies the site.

• Call "time out" in the operating room before the procedure begins. Again verify the patient's identity and her surgical procedure and operative side and site. Also confirm proper positioning of the patient, availability of correct implants (if needed), presence of any special equipment, and adherence to any special requirements.

physician you notified, time of notification, information you conveyed, and orders he gave.

Continue to monitor and record fluid intake and output, and include relevant information from the PACU nurse on the flow sheet. When calculating fluid intake and output, make sure you account for all IV fluids and blood infused as well as drainage, emesis, and diarrhea.

Send blood samples to the laboratory for hematology and chemistry tests, as ordered. Document the time they were sent and, when available, the results. Compare the results with preoperative results, and notify the physician of significant changes.

Begin coughing and deep-breathing exercises, as ordered, using a pillow or folded blanket to splint the patient's incision during the exercises. Administer analgesics, if prescribed and needed.

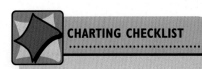

CHARTING CHECKLIST

DOCUMENTING PERIOPERATIVE CARE
Before your patient is transferred from the postanesthesia care unit to the surgery suite, review your documentation to make sure it addresses all important aspects of her medical and recent history, the surgery she has just undergone, her postanesthesia care, and her current condition.

Medical and Recent History
When documenting history information, be sure to include:
- ❏ the patient's medical and surgical history
- ❏ events leading to current surgery
- ❏ complications related to previous surgery or anesthesia (document this prominently at the front of the section)
- ❏ drug or food allergies
- ❏ current drugs and herbal supplements, such as ginkgo biloba
- ❏ tobacco use

Surgery
Surgery documentation should cover:
- ❏ type of procedure performed
- ❏ time the surgery began and ended
- ❏ type of anesthesia used
- ❏ duration of anesthesia
- ❏ range of the patient's vital signs during surgery
- ❏ name, dosage, and administration time and route of each drug administered
- ❏ fluid intake, output, and loss
- ❏ use of devices to stop blood flow to a particular area, such as a tourniquet
- ❏ type and location of drains, tubes, implants, and dressings left in place
- ❏ patient's tolerance of the procedure
- ❏ surgical complications

Continued

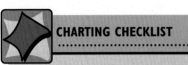

DOCUMENTING PERIOPERATIVE CARE—cont'd

Postanesthesia Period

During the postanesthesia period, you may document vital signs, assessment findings, and interventions on a postanesthesia flow sheet. No matter where you record the information, your documentation of the patient's postanesthesia course should include:

❑ vital signs

❑ level of consciousness

❑ skin color

❑ name, dosage, administration time and route of each analgesic or other drug given

❑ patient's respiratory status, including the time of endotracheal tube removal, use of supplemental oxygen, if ordered, and arterial blood gas levels or pulse oximetry readings

❑ unusual events or complications, such as vomiting, hypothermia, arrhythmias, swollen tongue, and postspinal headache

❑ interventions used to treat unusual events or complications above

Current Condition

At the end of your postanesthesia documentation, document the patient's current condition. Also include:

❑ vital signs

❑ level of consciousness

❑ interventions that will continue in the surgical unit

❑ If the patient is being discharged to home after same-day surgery, document additional pertinent findings, including:

❑ patient's ability to eat, walk, and urinate

❑ understanding of discharge instructions

Document each drug's name, dosage, and administration time and route as well as the patient's response. Also record that you applied antiembolism stockings, if ordered, and helped the patient perform leg and foot exercises. Finally, document that you provided emotional support to the patient and family.

Document What You Teach

Especially if your patient's stay will be abbreviated, you'll need to provide a great deal of teaching in a short time. Document that you instructed the patient and family on the following topics:
- coughing and deep-breathing exercises
- use of analgesics
- prescribed drugs, including their names, dosages, administration times and routes, adverse effects, and storage
- instructions for resuming previous drugs at home
- recommended activity level
- dietary recommendations or restrictions
- care of the incision and remaining drains
- use of antiembolism stockings, if ordered
- signs and symptoms to report
- dates and times of follow-up medical appointments

WHEN YOUR PATIENT HAS WOUND DEHISCENCE OR EVISCERATION

Wound dehiscence and evisceration are serious complications of wound healing. In dehiscence, the edges of a wound separate, exposing underlying tissue. Dehiscence may be partial, affecting only superficial tissue layers; or it may be complete, involving all tissue layers. Most commonly, dehiscence affects abdominal wounds from surgical incisions, when stress on the incision disrupts its integrity. This usually occurs 5 to 10 days after the wound is sutured. In evisceration, the intestines or other organs protrude through a gaping wound. If evisceration goes unrecognized or untreated, bowel strangulation and ischemia may occur.

For a patient with wound dehiscence or evisceration, careful documentation of your assessment findings interventions and his responses to treatment can help pave the way to a successful outcome. What's more, it can erase any doubt that he received prompt care for this complication.

Document What the Patient Tells You

Obtain a detailed preoperative health history to detect factors that can alert the health care team to potential postoperative complications. For example, review the history for preexisting conditions that increase the patient's risk for impaired wound healing, such as diabetes mellitus, asthma, emphysema, bronchitis, and anemia. Also record and review his drug history, particularly noting the use of corticosteroids or other immunosuppressants. These drugs can also delay or impair wound healing.

With the help of a registered dietitian, assess and document the patient's nutritional status. Also record if he's malnourished or above his ideal body weight. Either condition increases the risk for impaired wound healing.

When dehiscence or evisceration occurs, record what the patient tells you. Note reports of a sudden increase in pain or the sensation of the wound pulling, ripping, or giving way, especially after coughing or straining.

Document What You Assess

Carefully record your baseline assessment of the wound. For example, if you detect signs of infection, such as erythema, drainage, and warmth at the incision site, document these findings in your nurse's notes. Then discuss them with the physician and record your discussion. Because wound infection predisposes the patient to dehiscence and evisceration, take preventive measures, such as administering prescribed antibiotics. Be sure to document these measures and his response to them.

Wound. Whenever you suspect dehiscence or evisceration, document your assessment of the wound. Observe for separation of the wound edges, drainage (especially serous drainage), and protrusion of the viscera. Record pertinent findings.

Vital Signs and Pulse Oximetry. Record the patient's vital signs, particularly noting signs of shock related to tissue ischemia, infarction, or infection, such as decreased blood pressure and increased temperature and heart and respiratory rates. If you spot such signs, document them in your notes. Also assess the patient's oxygen saturation and document if it's less than 92%.

Tissue Perfusion. Document the quality of peripheral pulses, determining whether they're weak and thready or bounding. Record the color and temperature of the skin, especially if it's cool, clammy, and mottled. Note a decreased level of consciousness. Every hour, record the patient's fluid intake and output; document oliguria if it occurs.

Document What You Do

As soon as you recognize wound dehiscence or evisceration, document your immediate actions, such as assisting the patient to bed and reassuring him. Then record that you stayed with him and called for help as you intervened. Because the patient is likely to need surgery, also document all preoperative and postoperative interventions.

Immediate Interventions. Document that you helped the patient into a semi-Fowler's position with his knees slightly elevated to prevent further tissue tearing. If intestinal coils are protruding through the incision, make a note that you covered the wound with sterile, saline-moistened dressings. Then record that you started two large-bore IV catheters to administer the prescribed IV fluids and drugs. If the patient's oxygen saturation is low, document that you provided supplemental oxygen, as ordered.

Preoperative Interventions. If your patient is scheduled for surgery to repair wound dehiscence or evisceration, document that you gave him nothing by mouth. Also record your collection of preoperative blood samples, such as for blood typing and crossmatching, and submission of them to the laboratory. If ordered, obtain wound culture specimens and document that you sent them to the laboratory also. Before administering a preoperative sedative or analgesic, make sure that a consent form for surgery was signed and placed in the chart.

Postoperative Interventions. After surgery, record the patient's vital signs on the vital sign flow sheet every 4 hours or as ordered. Also document your administration of prescribed antibiotics, noting any adverse reactions. If blood or wound culture results reveal an infection with a specific organism, check its sensitivity to ensure that an effective antibiotic is prescribed. Regularly check the sutured wound for signs of infection, hematoma, or new signs of dehiscence or evisceration; note your findings.

If wound care is ordered, document the type of irrigant (if prescribed) and the dressings you use. Record your use of aseptic technique and the application of an abdominal binder, if needed.

Note that you taught the patient to splint his incision when coughing, deep breathing, and performing activities that require movement. Document that you helped the patient move and walk, unless contraindicated. Record any analgesia administered as well as the patient's response to it.

Record the presence or absence of bowel sounds, flatus, and bowel movements postoperatively. When advancing the patient's diet as ordered, document each change and how well he tolerates it.

Document What You Teach

As you prepare the patient for discharge, record your teaching, which should focus on promoting his recovery from surgery and preventing further complications. Document that you instructed your patient on the following topics:

- surgical procedures
- signs and symptoms to report
- prescribed drugs, including their names, dosages, administration times and routes, adverse effects, and storage
- wound care
- signs and symptoms to report, including signs of infection or impaired wound healing

- importance of adhering to the prescribed drug, activity, and diet regimen
- follow-up appointments with the physician, including one for suture removal, if needed
- follow-up diagnostic tests

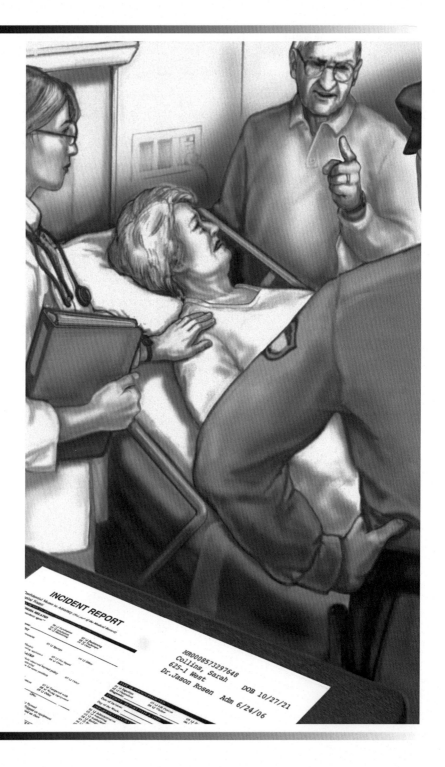

PART 2

Dealing with Challenging Patient Situations

T he patient's medical record serves two purposes. First, it identifies the patient and the primary reason for his admission. Second, it provides a dynamic history of the course of his treatment. The medical record has a third, equally important function: it provides a format for recording the care you provide in challenging situations, such as when a patient refuses treatment, threatens to harm someone, or brings contraband into his room.

Documenting such a situation is just as important as documenting a routine clinical situation. And because challenging situations can be complicated and fraught with legal peril, documenting them can be particularly difficult.

Challenging situations also tend to arise unexpectedly. Your documentation must show that you took steps to prevent the situation if possible. Being prepared can help reduce your legal exposure and safeguard your patient's health and rights.

How to Respond

Whether your patient refuses treatment, threatens to sue, or hides his prescribed drugs, your goals are to safeguard his well-being and protect his rights. These two basic goals may conflict in a challenging situation. For instance, if he threatens suicide, you may need to search his room for items he could use to harm himself. But while you conduct this search, you must uphold his right to privacy—and your documentation must show that you did so.

Your response in some situations also depends on state laws and your facility's policies and procedures, so be sure to review all the facts at your disposal. However, as you take pains to uphold regulations, don't lose sight of your special nursing role as empathetic caregiver. No matter how difficult your patient is or how complex the situation, always acknowledge his individual worth and offer skillful, compassionate care.

Communicate Therapeutically. To convey genuine concern and show that you understand your patient's feelings, communicate in a way that enhances a therapeutic relationship. For example, acknowledge him by name, restate what he has said to encourage him to elaborate or proceed, validate what he tells you, ask for clarification to prevent misunderstandings, and mirror his words. Avoid poor communication techniques: responding defensively, using clichés, belittling the patient, stereotyping, and offering inappropriate reassurance or advice.

What to Document

Remember the nursing adage: If it wasn't documented, it wasn't done. Clearly, documentation is the only proof of your actions. With the threat of malpractice lawsuits and many other legal, ethical, and fiscal issues facing health care providers, you can't afford to ignore this adage. Your documentation can save you—or sink you—if the care you provided is under scrutiny.

These days, in fact, you must think like a lawyer as well as a nurse. And you must document as if you expect lawyers, judges, and juries to read your words someday. In court, your best defense is comprehensive, accurate, and objective documentation. The evidence the medical record provides—or fails to provide—could determine your legal fate or your employer's.

Basic Facts to Document. In a challenging patient situation, many of the facts you'll document depend on the specifics involved. However, you must always document:

- pertinent patient statements, using direct quotes whenever possible rather than paraphrasing
- patient actions, recorded objectively
- names of people you notified about the situation, along with the times and results of notification (such as physician's instructions or advice from your facility's legal counsel)

- your actions in response to others' instructions
- patient assessment findings before, during, and after the incident
- names of others involved in the incident and their relationships to the patient

If required by your facility, also complete an incident report. Before submitting it, compare it closely with your nurse's notes and correct any discrepancies. Don't mention the incident report in the medical record.

Make sure you fill out other forms your facility requires, such as a special flow sheet. Also verify that the patient has signed any special forms required, such as a refusal-of-treatment form.

Special Concerns in Home Health Care

If you practice in the home health care setting, you may not have to deal with some of the challenging situations discussed in this part of the book. However, your patient may be more likely to refuse treatment, make a sexual advance, or threaten to harm himself than he would if he were in a facility.

At home, a patient is more comfortable and more in control— and may be more likely to behave inappropriately or irrationally. He may also be more concerned about protecting his rights.

What's more, you may not be able to ensure the patient's safety at home. This means that he's at higher risk for injury from falls, fire, medication errors, infection, and violence. To reduce these risks, you'll need to focus intensively on environmental and social factors during assessment, intervention, and documentation.

Going it Alone. Complete, accurate, and objective documentation plays a valuable role in home health nursing. You may be the only person with whom your patient has physical contact. You may find yourself alone with him at times, with no one to call for help or to witness the situation. If your patient sues you or your employer for improper care or violation of his rights, your documentation may be the only objective evidence that proves you acted in good faith and took the steps a reasonable, prudent nurse would.

Especially if you're the patient's sole caregiver, you can't afford to be haphazard when recording the care you provide. With no one to corroborate, clarify, or support your written statements about the patient's condition, treatment, and responses, your documentation must stand on its own.

WHEN YOUR PATIENT DOCUMENTS HER OWN CARE

Self-documentation can take many forms—from keeping a dietary log or describing warning signs of a headache to recording fingerstick blood glucose readings. A patient who documents self-care learns how to recognize patterns in her symptoms. This can help her adjust her treatment, if needed, after discharge. Self-documenting also may speed her recovery and expand her sense of empowerment, making her more likely to comply with therapy. (See *Self-documentation: Pros and cons.*)

The patient may use a narrative format or a preprinted form to record her information. Depending on state laws and facility policies, her documentation may or may not become a permanent part of her medical record.

How to Respond

Make sure you understand your role in self-documentation and the possible legal implications. Find out whether your facility requires the patient to sign a liability-release form. Then obtain a physician's order to include self-documentation in the plan of care. Having such an order on record may reduce your legal risk if the patient is injured or develops a complication as a result of self-documentation.

Next, develop a plan to teach the patient how to perform self-documentation. To determine what she should record, evaluate her treatment plan for areas that lend themselves to self-documentation, such as:

- level of pain
- blood glucose monitoring
- response to treatment
- ostomy care
- urine output
- dietary intake
- personal care activities, such as sitz baths, self-catheterization, and a self-administered bowel program

Make sure the physician's order spells out exactly what the patient should document. When teaching her, review the documentation forms she'll use. Provide oral and written instructions, and give her examples of the information she should record. As appropriate, include other professionals, such as a nutritionist or enterostomal therapist, in your teaching. Whenever possible, involve the patient's family too, so that they can lend support and encouragement. Tell the patient that self-documentation plays an important role in her treatment plan, and emphasize the importance of keeping accurate records.

Inform the rest of the health care team which areas the patient will document. This lets them know where to look for the information they need and gives them a chance to provide positive feedback to the patient.

Reviewing the Patient's Entries. After the patient completes her first entry, review it with her promptly. Praise her efforts, and make suggestions to improve her documentation, as needed. Review her next few entries too. Establish regular review times, and always provide as much feedback as possible. If her information leads to a change in her treatment plan, explain the connection so that she can see the value of her documentation.

....
DID YOU KNOW?

SELF-DOCUMENTATION: PROS AND CONS

Self-documentation can enhance your patient's treatment plan, but it has potential drawbacks too. Here are the facts you need to know about its advantages and disadvantages.

Advantages
Self-documentation can help:
- increase the patient's knowledge of her condition and its causes, symptoms, and treatment
- identify factors that trigger or exacerbate her condition
- yield more accurate symptom reporting because the patient records her symptoms in her own words
- improve compliance by involving the patient in her care

Disadvantages
Self-documentation may:
- demand extra time and commitment from you and the patient
- lead to incomplete, inaccurate, or misleading information if the patient doesn't fully grasp what or when to document or is too embarrassed to document the truth

What to Document

Record your involvement in the decision to have the patient use self-documentation and your discussion with the physician to obtain the self-documentation order. Include copies of release forms the patient has signed.

Also record your self-documentation teaching, detailing specific information you discussed. Place a copy of your written instructions in the medical record or describe them in your notes. Record, too, the patient's response to your teaching, your review sessions, and your suggestions to improve her documentation. Note that you informed other health care team members which information she'll document.

If the patient's documentation reveals an unusual, serious, or potentially serious finding, notify the physician. Then document your notification, including the physician's name and time of notification. Remember—failure to supervise and communicate could put you at risk legally.

If self-documentation will become part of the patient's permanent medical record, record information that contributed to a change in her treatment plan. For instance, if she documents her pain level and response to a prescribed drug, record her findings that led to a change in the drug selection or dosage or the administration schedule.

If her documentation won't become a permanent part of the medical record, transcribe the information she provides on a form that will go in her record. Note on this form that the information comes from the patient's records.

If your patient will continue documentation at home, note this in her discharge instructions. Give her the forms she needs, and document this action. Finally, tell her home care nurse which documentation system she will use so that the nurse can provide proper follow-up. Record that you gave the nurse this information.

WHEN YOUR PATIENT ASKS TO SEE HIS MEDICAL RECORD

Your patient may ask to see his medical record to find out more about his diagnosis, prognosis, and treatment options. Before you respond to his request, you need to understand state laws and your facility's policies. Most states allow patients to see their records but impose certain conditions to preserve confidentiality. A few states give patients direct access to their medical records without signed authorization.

Be aware that the patient's right to see his medical record doesn't extend to a family member or significant other unless that person has legal power of attorney. Also keep in mind that the record itself belongs to the health care professional or facility that generated it.

How to Respond

Usually, the patient must submit a written request to see his medical record and must specify which portions he wants to see. (See *Disclosing the record: When you don't need written authorization.*) If the patient is hospitalized when he makes the request, you're responsible for documenting the request and submitting it to the appropriate nurse administrator. If the patient has already been discharged, the medical records department is more likely to receive and process his request.

Before you release the record, confirm the patient's identity. Why? Occasionally, another person—an attorney, insurance

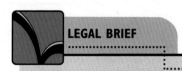

LEGAL BRIEF

DISCLOSING THE RECORD: WHEN YOU DON'T NEED WRITTEN AUTHORIZATION
You don't need written authorization to disclose the medical record if the patient, a family member, or his legal representative serves you or your facility with a subpoena, court order, or other legal document. Some states require advance notice for a disclosure request made by court order. If someone serves you with a legal document that requires disclosure of your patient's record, contact the appropriate nurse administrator or the facility's legal counsel or take other steps specified by facility policy to make sure no protective order has been issued. (A protective order might be issued if the requested part of the record was compiled for litigation, quality management, or peer review.)

Documenting the Disclosure
Document the nature of the legal order to disclose the record, your notification of the nurse administrator or legal counsel, instructions you received from that person, and actions you took in response.

company representative, or relative, for instance—may try to see a patient's medical record without his permission.

When releasing the record to the patient, take reasonable steps to keep it secure and to instruct the patient about its content. Keep in mind that, depending on your state's laws, the patient may be allowed to view only a portion of his record. If so, only give the patient the portion that's permissible to give, such as a laboratory test result. To maintain security, ask a nurse colleague or physician to attend as you supervise the patient's viewing of his record. If he views it in electronic form, make sure he doesn't see another patient's confidential records.

If you'll send a portion of the patient's record to him by facsimile (fax), keep the transmitted information confidential. Before faxing, find out whether your facility has specific policies about the use of fax machines to deliver medical records. Be sure to comply with these policies. To adhere to the Health Insurance Portability and Accountability Act, remove identifying information before faxing any medical records.

Explaining the Content. Depending on state laws, your patient may have the right to an explanation of the codes, symbols, and abbreviations in the medical record. Provide accurate explanations as needed.

Also, the patient may ask you to convert a document in his medical record to a form he can more easily read and understand. For example, he may request a typed version of a handwritten progress note or a film version of a computerized radiology image. State law governs which documents can be converted and under what circumstances and specifies how to document the request.

Handling Requests for Copies. In most states, your patient has the right to obtain paper copies of his medical record for his own use. Your facility may have the right to charge a reasonable fee for these copies before releasing them. To make sure legal and administrative protocols are followed, all requests for medical records must be processed through the medical records department (or responsible person).

Meeting Deadlines. If state law requires your facility to release the medical record within a certain number of days, inform the patient of any delay, the reason for the delay, and the date you expect his record to be available. Then document the reason for the delay, your explanation to the patient, and the date his medical record is expected to become available.

Denying Access. Your patient may be denied access to his record if disclosing it would harm him physically or emotionally or jeopardize another person's safety. For example, if he committed a violent crime, he might be denied access to his record if it contains the name of a witness whom he might try to harm.

If you suspect that disclosure could cause harm, discuss your concerns with the physician. Then document your discussion, the physician's response, your plan of action, and your implementation of the plan.

The health care provider may be able to deny access to a specific document in the record if:

- the document was created and used only for litigation, quality management, peer review, or research
- granting access would allow the patient to identify someone who provided confidential information
- access would violate a specific state law

If the patient is denied access to a portion of his record, his family or legal representative may be allowed to see that portion if the patient consents. Thoroughly document the reason for the denial, your explanation to the patient, and his response.

Responding to Requests for Correction. Your state's laws may require correction of the medical record if your patient thinks that it's inaccurate, confusing, or misleading. If he requests a correction, advise him to submit the request in writing. In most situations, the patient has the right to request an addendum to the record that corrects the information in it. Then make corrections according to your facility's policies and procedures.

What to Document

Document the following information if your patient or his authorized representative asks to see his medical record:

- method of request (oral or written); for an oral request, document that you instructed the patient to submit his request in writing
- type of information requested (such as admission records)

- name and address of the patient or other person to whom the information will be released, confirmation of this person's identity, and the patient's signed permission to disclose the record to this person
- portions of the record requested by the patient; if the record was photocopied, specify the number of pages given to the patient
- date the patient views or receives copies of the record
- names and credentials of people in attendance while the patient views the record, or name of the person making the record available if that's a different party
- requests your patient makes or questions he asks while viewing his record, and your responses
- your instruction to submit correction requests in writing, your receipt of a written request, and your response
- discussions about denying the patient's request for his medical record, reason for denial, names of people involved in the discussion, and plan of action formulated
- patient's physical and emotional status before, during, and after he sees his record

If the patient seems upset or angry while viewing his record, notify the physician. Document your notification, the plan of action formulated, and actions you took to implement the plan.

WHEN YOUR PATIENT'S MEDICAL RECORD ISN'T AVAILABLE

Whether your patient's medical record has accompanied her to a diagnostic procedure, is in use by a colleague, or is lost, you remain responsible for documenting the care you provide. Failure to document jeopardizes continuity of care, reimbursement, and your facility's accreditation. It also exposes you and your employer to legal risk if the patient sues over her health care.

An incomplete medical record implies improper nursing conduct or failure to provide care. A flow sheet with missing entries, a medical record without physician orders, and progress notes left blank for a given time range suggest that the patient received no care during the period in question—or that the record was tampered with.

How to Respond

If you know the medical record is with the patient in another part of the facility or in use by a colleague, wait until it returns to complete your documentation. But don't trust your memory. On a notepad, jot down the information you obtain each time you assess your patient, provide a treatment, administer a drug, or interact with the patient's physician or family members. Then, when the patient's record becomes available, document a complete note. A sample notepad entry might look like this:

2/18/06, 1400: A. Carson. c/o pain at IV site ® hand. No redness, swelling, or warmth. IV patent. Temp 98.6°F. Dressing dry and intact.

If the patient's record won't return until your shift ends or if you believe that it's lost or has been stolen, immediately notify the appropriate nurse administrator, risk manager, medical records department, and the patient's physician, or take other steps specified by your facility's procedure.

If you believe that the medical record is lost or has been stolen, create a new record. On the front, write "Substitute record." Document the current date and the time you created the substitute record and the reason for creating it. This will alert other staff members to the status of the original record and help explain time gaps. (See *Recollecting your documentation*, page 210.)

Try to recall whether the patient's original record contained signed consents, releases, "Do not resuscitate" orders, advance directives, or other special forms. If possible, obtain copies of these forms from the medical records department or the physician's office.

Then reconstruct the patient's record using these copies and copies of other original documents, such as medication sheets, physician's order sheets, and laboratory and radiology reports. Ask the physician's office for copies of the patient's history and physical findings and surgical consent forms.

LEGAL BRIEF

RECOLLECTING YOUR DOCUMENTATION

When making a substitute record, you may need to refer to a previous entry. Suppose, for example, you administered an analgesic drug and documented this intervention in the original record. Now you need to note the drug's effectiveness in the substitute record.

In this situation, create a temporary document. State that your previous notes are unavailable and that the information you're addressing is a "recollection of previous entries." This temporary document will explain discrepancies between the original record and your recollected notes if the original record turns up.

2/18/06, 1400: A. Carson. c/o pain at IV site ⓡ hand. No redness, swelling, or warmth. IV patent. Temp 98.6°F. Dressing dry and intact.

If you can't obtain copies, have the patient or her legal guardian sign new documents. On each new document, write "Substitute document, original unavailable." If you can't recall whether her record contained special documents, ask her, her family, or her physician.

Don't try to reconstruct your original nursing documentation. If the original record eventually turns up and shows discrepancies with your reconstructed notes, legal problems could ensue if the medical record ends up in court. If necessary, obtain another patient history to gather information about her allergies, past medical history, and other critical information.

Tell the patient that her medical record isn't available, but reassure her that you're taking steps to locate it.

What to Document

If the patient's record is temporarily unavailable in a known location, start a new page of nurse's notes or a new flow sheet. On this document, record the patient's name, identification number, admission date, physician, room number, and bed number. Then create an entry as you normally would. Record the date and time of the entry and each event you document, and number each page chronologically.

In your notes, state that your patient's record wasn't available and give the reason, if known. If your entry starts in the middle of a page—say, because of the particular documentation form your facility uses—draw an "X" through the blanks above your entry. Keep this temporary document in a safe place. Depending on your facility's protocols, you may need to start a temporary record or store your new notes in a designated location for loose documents.

When your patient's medical record becomes available, draw an "X" through blank areas, and file your temporary documentation sheets in sequence. Note the date and time the record returned to your unit. Then resume documenting in the usual way. Follow the same procedure for physician's order sheets, progress notes, medication administration records, flow sheets, and other forms with chronological entries.

If necessary, make a late entry. But don't ask other staff members to leave blank lines for your entry. And don't try to squeeze your entry between lines, at the end of a partially filled line, or in the margin. Instead, write the date and time of your late entry, label it "Late entry," and note the original date and time of the event you're documenting. State the reason for the late entry, such as "Record was unavailable," and note the date and time the record became unavailable. Record your late entry as soon as possible. Waiting too long could give a plaintiff's attorney reason to question your credibility.

Next, complete an incident report, describing the facts surrounding the missing record. Don't place this report in the patient's record or state in the record that you filed an incident report.

If you created a substitute record, document the names of the people you notified, the date and time of notification, and their response. Then document your actions related to the missing record.

Stolen Record. If you suspect that your patient's medical record has been stolen, document the names of the people you notified and their responses. Tell the patient that her record has been misplaced, and document her response. If an investigation proves her record was stolen, the facility's insurance carrier and legal counsel will determine whether and what the patient should be told about the theft.

Then complete an incident report, recording all relevant information. Next, describe the situation in writing on a separate sheet of paper. Name witnesses who can support your statements about theft of the record and your reconstruction of it. Include the names (if known) and physical descriptions of unauthorized individuals seen in the area around the time the record was last seen. Write the date and time on this document, and sign it. Make a copy for your records, and submit the original to the appropriate nurse administrator or the next person in the chain of command. Then take other steps specified by facility policy or procedure. Finally, contact your risk manager to ensure that the theft report was received.

WHEN YOUR PATIENT WITHHOLDS HIS MEDICAL HISTORY

Most patients willingly provide information about their health history because it makes them feel actively involved in their care. But occasionally, a patient refuses to cooperate. Perhaps he doesn't understand why you need the information or he's afraid it could reveal an interpersonal, psychological, or legal problem.

If you find yourself in this situation, resist the natural impulse to become annoyed and lose your objectivity. Keep in mind that the patient can't be forced to cooperate even if his refusal increases his risk for complications or injury. Every patient has the right to privacy and to withhold information he believes is personal and confidential. Besides, forcing the issue would destroy any hope of building a rapport. It could also get you in legal trouble.

How to Respond
During your first encounter with a patient, encourage cooperation by making a good impression. Your demeanor, word choice,

and tone of voice during the first few minutes set the stage for the rest of the interview and perhaps for all of your subsequent interactions with him. In fact, a patient's first contact with a nurse may influence his experiences with the entire health care team, for better or for worse. A bad experience may predispose him to filing a lawsuit if something goes wrong.

Begin the interview by explaining your role and the purpose of the interview. Tell the patient he doesn't have to answer questions that make him uncomfortable. This helps him believe that he's in control of the situation, which makes him more likely to cooperate.

If he cooperates initially but later refuses to provide specific information, respect his decision. Don't try to force him to answer by using threats, intimidation, or other fear tactics. Instead, ask yourself whether the information he's withholding could alter the plan of care or affect his well-being. If you believe that it wouldn't, move on to the next question. If you think that it would, try to find out why he has decided to withhold information. Perhaps he has misconstrued the question or doesn't understand why you need the information. As needed, provide clarification.

If your attempts to obtain information fail, consider asking a relative or friend of the patient to answer your questions. If this isn't feasible, move on to the next question and try to get the information from the physical examination, other health care professionals, or other documents.

If Your Patient Withholds All Information. What if your patient refuses to provide any history information? In a professional, caring manner, acknowledge his right not to divulge information. Then explain how his refusal may affect his well-being. Use easy-to-understand examples. For instance, tell him that the health care team must know if he's allergic to certain drugs so they can make sure he doesn't receive those drugs during his stay.

If your explanation fails to change his mind, end the interview and move on to the physical examination. Realize that his behavior probably isn't related to you personally. Chances are, he decided to withhold his medical history before he met you.

Then check with the appropriate nurse administrator. Depending on your facility's policy, the patient may be asked to sign a release-of-liability form.

If You Suspect Incompetency or a Serious Medical Condition. If you suspect that your patient isn't competent to make rational decisions or has a physical or mental problem that impairs his judgment or ability to communicate, contact the physician immediately. If the situation is an emergency and lack of history information could endanger the patient's life, try to obtain the crucial information you need from other sources.

If the patient's condition isn't life-threatening, provide appropriate care based on your initial and ongoing assessments. Assume that he has no unknown conditions, and treat him as you would any other patient. However, notify the physician as soon as possible. Also try to obtain the information you need from the patient's medical record.

What to Document

Your documentation must show that you tried to elicit information from your patient. Also document that you explained to him why the requested information was important, told him of his rights, and described the risks of withholding information. This indicates that you carried out your duties to inform and to keep your patient from harm while respecting his rights.

Document the patient's response and his understanding of your explanations. Also describe his physical and mental condition before and after the interview.

Record your objective assessment findings and the patient's statements, quoting him directly. Record your conversations with the appropriate nurse administrator, the physician, and the patient's family or legal guardian. Make clear exactly what you said to whom, when you said it, and that person's response. Also document your plan of care, nursing interventions, and resulting outcomes. (See *Planning care for an uncooperative patient.*) Make sure your documentation is consistent, complete, specific, and unbiased.

TIPS & ADVICE

PLANNING CARE FOR AN UNCOOPERATIVE PATIENT

If your patient withholds health history information, be sure to address this in your nursing plan of care. For instance, if appropriate, formulate the nursing diagnosis "High risk for injury related to unknown medical history" to alert your colleagues to the situation and to promote continuity of care.

Fill out an incident report and other documents your facility requires. Review the incident report closely to ensure that it mirrors the information in your nurse's notes. Don't refer to the incident report in the patient's record.

WHEN YOUR PATIENT REFUSES TREATMENT

A patient may refuse a specific procedure, such as a blood transfusion, or she may refuse all care. Except in unusual circumstances, you must honor a competent adult's refusal of treatment—even life-sustaining treatment. You also must honor a parent's or legal guardian's refusal of treatment for a minor, unless that treatment is lifesaving. However, if a parent or guardian chooses to withhold lifesaving treatment for a minor, your facility's legal counsel is likely to request a court order to provide that treatment. If your patient refuses treatment, review your facility's policies and procedures to determine under which circumstances her refusal may not be honored. (See *Must you always honor a treatment refusal?*, page 216.)

The right to refuse treatment is linked to the rights to informed consent and privacy and serves as the basis of advance directives and living wills. Although these rights may be at odds with your duty as a nurse to protect your patient from harm, you must respect your patient's wishes.

Types of Refusal. Treatment refusal can be express or implied. *Express* refusal, which can be verbal or written, is the patient's clear statement that she's unwilling to receive treatment. An express written refusal usually takes the form of an advance directive, living will, or release-from-liability form.

Implied refusal is conveyed by actions rather than words. For instance, suppose the physician orders blood tests, but when you ask the patient to keep her arm at her side so you can draw blood, she tightly flexes her arm at the elbow. Even though she

LEGAL BRIEF

MUST YOU ALWAYS HONOR A TREATMENT REFUSAL?
Depending on state laws and your facility's policies, a patient's right to refuse treatment may not be honored if:
- the treatment is for a communicable disease that threatens the life or health of others
- an innocent person may be harmed (for example, a fetus might die because the mother refuses a blood transfusion)
- the treatment would prevent the death of a patient who isn't terminally ill
- the refusal is from a minor (who isn't legally permitted to refuse treatment)
- the refusal violates your facility's ethical standards. For instance, you may not be required to administer foods or fluids forcibly if the patient refuses them and your facility opposes the refusal on ethical grounds. Your facility should request patient transfer to another facility that would honor her refusal.

   To determine whether your patient's situation falls into one of these categories, consult your facility's legal counsel.

hasn't refused the procedure verbally or in writing, her conduct indicates her implied refusal.

   Reasons for Refusal. A patient may refuse treatment because she lacks knowledge of her medical condition, misunderstands the treatment's benefits or risks, or believes that the treatment conflicts with her personal, cultural, or religious beliefs. Sometimes a patient's refusal stems from legal or clinical incompetency. If your patient is incompetent, a judge may have to decide whether she would have refused treatment were she competent.

How to Respond

Tell the patient you respect her right to refuse treatment. In a nonthreatening way, ask her why she's refusing it. If her answer reflects lack of understanding about her condition, treatment, or the consequences of refusal, provide teaching. However, don't use scare tactics to try to get her to change her mind.

If she continues to refuse treatment, notify her physician and the appropriate nurse administrator. Then follow your facility's protocol for dealing with treatment refusal. Unless the patient is violent or her treatment refusal could cause immediate harm to herself or others, don't try to restrain her. If you force treatment or use restraints, you may be charged with battery, false imprisonment, or violation of patient rights. Consult the physician about an appropriate plan of action. In the meantime, continue to provide the necessary care your patient allows.

Obtaining Informed Refusal. The physician will try to obtain the patient's informed refusal (release from liability). Similar to informed consent, informed refusal is a written statement acknowledging that the patient has received an explanation of the proposed treatment, reason for the treatment, and risks of not having the treatment.

Responsibility to obtain informed refusal rests with the physician. Be sure to document informed refusal in the medical record.

What to Document

Treatment refusal touches on emotional, legal, ethical, and clinical issues that demand careful documentation. If legal action is pursued, thorough documentation is your only proof that you did everything possible to keep your patient from harm while protecting her rights.

Suppose, for example, a pregnant patient is admitted with a dangerously high blood glucose level and a decreasing level of consciousness. Before losing consciousness, she refuses insulin. You administer the insulin anyway, believing that she and her fetus would die otherwise. In this case, you could be sued for not respecting the patient's right to refuse treatment.

When recording a patient's treatment refusal and your actions, include the following:

- date and time of her refusal
- specific treatment she refused
- names of people who witnessed or were involved in her decision and their relationships to the patient
- patient's physical and mental status at the time of refusal

- drugs or treatments she received in the 2 hours before refusal and her response
- presence and condition of medical equipment or devices being used by the patient
- statements you made to the patient and her response
- names of the physician, the appropriate nurse administrator, and other people you notified; times of notification; content of your discussions; and actions you took in response
- notation that the patient signed (or refused to sign) an informed refusal form
- existence of an advance directive or living will

Then complete an incident report that clearly details everything you stated in your notes. Before submitting the report, check it against your notes and correct any discrepancies. In the medical record, don't mention that you filed an incident report.

WHEN YOUR PATIENT IS NONCOMPLIANT

Noncompliance with the physician's orders or the nursing plan of care can frustrate the patient, his family, and everyone involved in his care. Noncompliance also poses a threat to his health if it allows his condition to worsen or increases his risk for complications.

Unless you deal with noncompliance properly, you may find yourself in legal jeopardy. The patient or his family could sue you and your employer on the grounds that he received inadequate teaching or monitoring or inappropriate treatment. The way you document the situation can prove crucial to your defense against these allegations.

How to Respond

If you suspect that your patient is noncompliant, review diagnostic test results and other evidence that supports your suspicion. During your discussion with the patient, remain nonjudgmental and avoid accusations. Simply state that you believe he hasn't been following the treatment plan. Then ask him directly whether this is correct. For instance, if he agreed to a 1,500-calorie American Diabetes Association diet but his blood glucose level measures 390 mg/dl several days later, ask him whether he has strayed from the diet.

Treat his response respectfully, keeping in mind that he has the right to refuse treatment. If he admits that he hasn't followed the treatment plan, find out why. If his answer reveals that the plan doesn't fit his lifestyle or habits, reevaluate the plan. Then, if necessary, try to adjust the plan to meet his needs.

For instance, suppose your patient admits that he hasn't complied with his self-medication program. You might say, "Thank you for telling me why you missed this morning's dose. I wasn't aware that you routinely sleep late. Let's work together with your physician to see whether we can change your dosage schedule." (See *Differentiating between compliance and adherence*, page 220.)

Be sure to reinforce the rationale behind the treatment plan. This helps the patient understand the importance of complying with it.

What to Document

Make sure your documentation includes the following:
- data used to evaluate the patient's adherence to the treatment plan, data sources, and the date you obtained the data
- content of your discussion with the patient
- patient's stated reason for noncompliance
- teaching you provided about the treatment plan, its importance, and possible consequences of noncompliance
- copies of written patient-education materials you provided
- patient's understanding of the teaching you provided
- objective and subjective findings from physical and mental status assessments
- treatment plan changes made to improve compliance
- your communication with other health care team members regarding the patient's compliance and treatment plan changes

If the patient's noncompliance leads to injury or increases his risk for injury, complete an incident report. Make sure the incident report agrees with your documentation in the patient's medical record. Don't mention in the record that you filed an incident report.

DIFFERENTIATING BETWEEN COMPLIANCE AND ADHERENCE
Compliance refers to acting in accordance with orders or giving in to others' demands. It implies obedience. *Adherence*, on the other hand, refers to continuing an agreed-upon treatment under limited supervision. It implies active participation and willing cooperation.

Do you want your patient simply to obey orders—or to actively participate in and willingly adhere to his plan of care? Asking a patient to give in to health care providers' demands may make him think that he has little control over his health or life. He may refuse to comply simply to regain some control.

Instead of forcing him to comply, promote his adherence to the treatment plan by including him when planning his care, encouraging him to participate in care decisions, and emphasizing his role in achieving a successful outcome. Then help him adhere to the treatment plan, even if that means adjusting it. After all, the best treatment plan is useless if your patient won't or can't follow it.

Documenting Your Partnership
In your documentation, indicate that you established a partnership with your patient to achieve compliance. Don't merely state that he is noncompliant. Instead, describe specific parts of the treatment plan he has or has not complied with. Use words such as "adhere to" and "follow" instead of "comply."

Finally, arrange for an appropriate health care professional to provide follow-up care to evaluate the patient's transition to the home, assess his compliance, and invite him to return to the health care facility for further education or treatment. Document this contact in the medical record. Also note referrals for home care, as appropriate.

WHEN YOUR PATIENT IS IN POLICE CUSTODY

When caring for a patient in police custody, you must take extra steps to protect her rights and the safety of everyone involved. Like any other patient, a patient in police custody has the right to health care—without discrimination based on her legal situation. She also has the rights to privacy, informed consent, refusal of treatment, and review of her medical record.

Once your patient's condition is stable in your facility, she will probably be transferred to a correctional setting. To promote continuity of care, you must accurately document her clinical condition and treatment. Your documentation must show that you took steps to safeguard her rights.

Because the state is responsible for ensuring the safety and well-being of a patient in custody, a police officer will supervise her 24 hours a day. Keep in mind that the officer is there to protect you and your colleagues as well as the patient. Don't let the officer's presence intimidate you.

How to Respond

Your interaction with the patient depends partly on why she's in your facility. Usually, a patient in custody receives health care outside a correctional facility for the following:

- laboratory tests, such as blood tests for drugs or alcohol and tests of other body fluids, hair, nails, or skin
- voluntary admission for medical or psychiatric care
- involuntary admission for psychiatric care (such as evaluation for legal reasons or to prevent her from harming herself or others)

For each type of visit, special considerations apply. Be sure to familiarize yourself with your facility's policies and procedures for caring for a patient in police custody.

Laboratory Tests. Usually, local law enforcement officials arrange in advance for laboratory tests for a patient in custody. If advance arrangements haven't been made, consult your facility's risk manager or legal counsel. Ask the police officer accompanying the patient to provide a written request for the tests, and obtain the patient's consent for them.

Then conduct a nursing triage assessment to determine whether the patient needs additional health care, and ask her directly whether she needs medical treatment. If you suspect that she needs emergency evaluation or treatment, inform the emergency department physician and obtain the patient's consent for treatment. If she refuses treatment, document her refusal. If she later needs treatment for an illness or if she dies of a condition that was present but not discovered during her visit, your facility could be at legal risk for failure to diagnose and treat.

Because the patient's samples and specimens are likely to become legal evidence, take precautions to ensure accurate collection and labeling. Attach a tracking slip to the sample or specimen container, and make sure everyone who handles it signs the slip. Never leave the container unattended. Such a break in the chain of evidence could give the patient's attorney cause to argue that it was tampered with. If necessary, deliver the container to the laboratory by hand. Make sure the receiving employee signs the tracking slip and knows that the container is legal evidence.

Voluntary Admission. If the patient was admitted to your facility voluntarily, expect the accompanying officer to question you about your interactions with her, the drugs she receives, and the procedures she undergoes. Answer such questions in a general way without divulging confidential information. For example, you can tell the officer that you're going to draw a blood sample, but don't say what the blood will be tested for.

Also review your state's laws regarding law enforcement officials' access to prisoners' medical records. These officials may need a court order to search or remove records from a patient's property. Or, in some states, they may be free to search through the medical record without a court order. Be aware, though, that an accompanying police officer seldom has the right to make decisions about the patient's care.

Keep in mind that no-publicity protocols may apply to a patient in custody. Check with the appropriate nurse administrator or risk manager before speaking with the media or other parties about your patient's presence in your facility or her status.

Involuntary Admission for Psychiatric Care. As determined by state law, your patient may be held for psychiatric care for a limited time without a court order. If the physician determines that she's mentally competent, she may refuse care. (See *When your patient refuses treatment,* pages 215-218.) Remember that a court order is required to hold a competent patient against her will, even if she's a prisoner. (See *Treating a patient in custody against her will,* page 223.)

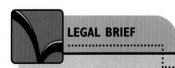

LEGAL BRIEF

TREATING A PATIENT IN CUSTODY AGAINST HER WILL
You may receive a court order to care for a patient in custody who has refused treatment. If so, make sure the order identifies your facility and the patient by name and specifies the procedure or treatment to be performed. Then ask your facility's legal counsel to review the order to determine whether it contains all necessary provisions and information.

If the Court Order Is Valid
If the legal counsel concludes that the court order is valid, tell the patient you understand she doesn't want the treatment but that the court order takes precedence over her wishes. Then document the following:
* name of the person who presented the court order
* name of the legal counsel who reviewed the order
* names of accompanying law enforcement personnel or attorneys
* interactions with the patient and your explanations of the court order and treatment
* patient's response to your explanations
* patient's response to the ordered treatment
    Place the original court order in the patient's medical record.

If the Court Order Is in Doubt
If the court order doesn't contain the required information, your legal counsel probably will advise you not to treat the patient. Document the counsel's advice—and follow it. Then record the:
* name of the person who presented the court order
* name of the legal counsel who reviewed and rejected the order
* names of accompanying law enforcement personnel or attorneys
    Place the original court order in the patient's medical record, and have the legal counsel document the reason for advising you not to honor it.

Patient Restrictions. A patient in police custody can't leave her room unless accompanied by a police officer. If she shares a room with another patient, the officer must stay in that room. Also, the patient is restricted when performing personal care and may be forbidden to have scissors, a razor, or other sharp items if she has a history of violent or suicidal behavior.

Give the patient as much privacy, autonomy, and participation in her care as the situation allows. Take steps to maintain her dignity. If she must wear handcuffs or other restraints when outside her room, try to conceal them.

Also take safety measures. Remove objects she could use to harm herself or others, such as sharps containers, unused needles, and IV supplies. Don't leave drugs in the room without a physician's order and permission from the supervising officer. Before admitting visitors, check with the supervising officer and review your facility's policy.

Patient Journals. A patient in custody may document her experience in the health care facility if state law allows. Her journal may address medical conditions, her response to treatment, and the names and addresses of health care providers with whom she interacts.

With the patient's permission, the health care team may use this journal to obtain valuable information about her medical history, such as allergies, previous diagnostic test results, and signs and symptoms. The journal may also reveal clues to her emotional status or her perception of health care providers. Be aware, too, that she may use the journal to support complaints of mistreatment.

What to Document

Document care for a patient in police custody as you would for any patient. Remember to record the police officer's presence and your interactions with the officer. Also describe unusual occurrences and your actions in response. Especially document circumstances that pose a potential threat to your patient, other patients, or staff members, such as the arrival of a visitor who becomes violent or forces himself into the patient's room. (Complete an incident report if this happens.)

If your patient keeps a journal during her stay, document this in your nurse's notes. If you use information from her journal to complete the nursing history and identify nursing care priorities, document the source of this information.

If you believe that the police officer or another person is trying to make decisions about your patient's medical care without legal authorization, notify the appropriate nurse administrator.

Then document this situation and your notification. Remember—
as the patient's advocate, you must protect her from physical and
emotional harm.

At discharge, thoroughly document the patient's condition
and instructions you gave about continuing her care in her next
setting. Such documentation can be crucial if she later asserts that
she was mistreated in your facility. Give a copy of your discharge
instructions to the patient and the accompanying officer. Record
that you did so, and write down the officer's name and badge
number.

WHEN YOUR PATIENT LEAVES AGAINST MEDICAL ADVICE

E very competent adult has the right to leave a health care facility against medical advice (AMA)—even in an emergency—
unless he poses a clear threat to himself or others. Usually, this
right also applies to a minor or a mentally impaired adult whose
parent or legal guardian wants to remove him from the facility,
unless abuse is suspected.

Typically, a patient leaves AMA because he doesn't understand his condition or treatment, has religious or cultural objec-
tions to medical care, or wants to exert control over his health
care. Less often, a patient leaves over a conflict with a nurse, some
other staff member, or another patient.

A patient who leaves AMA may be at increased risk for
complications and injuries. By taking the right actions and documenting them thoroughly, you can limit your legal exposure.

How to Respond

If your patient says that he intends to leave AMA, you must
protect his rights, make sure his decision is an informed one, and
prepare him for discharge to the extent possible. To strengthen his
sense of control and convey your respect, acknowledge his right
to leave.

Then, in a nonthreatening tone, ask why he wants to leave. Explore the situation using open-ended questions, giving him every chance to express his feelings. Teach the patient, as needed, to clarify his medical condition and ease fears about his treatment. Also explain the possible consequences of leaving AMA. Remind him that the treatment goals are his goals—not just those of the health care team.

Next, conduct a brief assessment if he allows this. Look for a possible medical cause for his behavior, such as poor oxygenation or a chemical imbalance. If he received drugs in the past 2 hours, realize that his behavior may reflect an adverse drug reaction. Also evaluate the patient's mental status to determine his orientation and emotional status. If you suspect that a chemical imbalance, an adverse drug reaction, or a mental or emotional disorder has caused incompetence, follow your facility's protocols and contact the appropriate nurse administrator immediately.

If you can't convince a competent patient to stay, follow your facility's AMA protocol. Alert the physician and the appropriate nurse administrator that the patient wants to leave. The physician is responsible for obtaining informed refusal of treatment. If he isn't available, follow the chain of command at your facility. If facility policy permits, contact the patient's relative or legal guardian to discuss his decision to leave AMA.

Don't try to restrain the patient chemically or mechanically, remove his clothing or other possessions, or take other steps that might violate his rights. If you detain a competent patient who poses no apparent threat of injury to himself or others, you may be charged with false imprisonment. (See *Understanding false imprisonment*.)

If the patient is connected to medical devices, remove those you can remove legally, such as a standard IV catheter. If he has a central line or other device that you can't remove, take all necessary steps to secure it. Then give him the medical supplies and equipment he needs for self-care, such as dressing materials or crutches, just as you would during a normal discharge.

If necessary, help the patient pack his belongings and put on his clothing. Teach him how to care for wounds or medical devices, provide verbal and written instructions for follow-up care, and have him sign a statement that he received and understands your instructions. Advise him to make an appointment to see his physician immediately after he leaves. Also arrange for an appropriate health care professional to contact him a few hours after he leaves to evaluate him and answer his questions.

Finally, tell the patient that he's welcome to return and that care is available if he needs it. Fully document the outcome of this contact to show you made every effort to ensure his health and safety.

What to Document

For a patient who leaves AMA, most facilities require completion of a specific form, such as a discharge AMA or refusal-of-treatment form. Obtaining the patient's signature (a physician responsibility) shows that the facility followed applicable standards of care and that the

DID YOU KNOW?

UNDERSTANDING FALSE IMPRISONMENT

By detaining a competent patient against his will, you run the risk of being sued or prosecuted for false imprisonment. The courts usually rule against health care facilities whose employees:
- use restraints without the consent of a competent patient
- threaten to hold a patient or his belongings because of unpaid bills
- refuse a patient's request to transfer to another facility
- lock away the patient's clothes, car keys, wallet, or other personal possessions
- house a competent patient in a locked wing

patient was fully aware of the implications of his decision. If your patient refuses to sign the form or leaves before one can be obtained, document this.

In your nurse's notes, detail the situation, including your actions and the outcome. Be sure to document:
- the patient's physical, emotional, and mental status at the time he decided to leave AMA
- his stated reason for leaving AMA
- names of the physician and facility administrator you notified, times of notification, content of your discussions with these individuals, their instructions, and your actions
- names of staff members or visitors who witnessed the patient's decision to leave AMA
- name of the staff member who informed the patient of the consequences of leaving and content of the discussion

- names of family members or friends who were notified of the patient's decision to leave AMA and time of notification
- discharge teaching, including instructions for follow-up care
- integrity and location of medical equipment or devices in place when the patient left
- medical supplies you gave the patient
- names of people who accompanied the patient when he left and instructions you gave

Also fill out an incident report, thoroughly describing the event from beginning to end. Make sure the information you write in the incident report mirrors your description in your nurse's notes. Don't mention the incident report in your notes.

Finally, review your nurse's notes, physician's orders, nursing flow sheets, medication administration records, and other documents to make sure they're accurate and comprehensive. Complete your documentation as soon as possible, while the event is fresh in your memory.

WHEN YOUR PATIENT THREATENS TO SUE

Any nurse who has direct patient contact may become the target of a patient's lawsuit. Because even a routine clinical situation can become an issue for litigation, some experts advise nurses to consider the possibility of a lawsuit during every patient interaction.

Your liability risk depends largely on the mistakes you make. A professional mistake can take the form of an error (an incorrect action) or an omission (failure to act when required). You're most likely to make a mistake when you're overworked or when you work back-to-back shifts.

Most patients who threaten to sue a health care provider perceive a potential or actual threat to their health, safety, or rights. However, not every patient sues when given the chance. Some patients are more likely to sue than others. (See *Spotting a lawsuit-prone patient.*) Besides becoming familiar with the profile of a lawsuit-prone patient, you need to learn how to respond to a patient's threat to sue—and how to document in a way that reduces your liability.

How to Respond

Take an actual or implied threat of a lawsuit seriously, and respond objectively and professionally. Don't try to determine whether the patient's threat is serious or whether she has a good case. For the moment, assume that she intends to sue and that her lawsuit could be legitimate.

All lawsuits start with filing a claim—a written or verbal complaint of perceived physical or emotional harm resulting

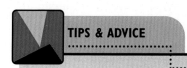

TIPS & ADVICE

SPOTTING A LAWSUIT-PRONE PATIENT
Some patients habitually express anger and dissatisfaction by threatening to sue. Typically, such patients are angry, dissatisfied, and resentful on admission. A few days into their stay, they may begin to think that they've lost control of their lives. This heightens their anger, dissatisfaction, and resentment and can turn a trivial event into an excuse for a lawsuit.

You may be able to identify a lawsuit-prone patient during your first encounter with her. Watch for—and document objectively—the following characteristic behaviors:
- She's uncooperative and makes countless excuses for her behavior. For example, she may refuse to provide health history information, angrily stating that she's already given it to several other people.
- She criticizes what you, your colleagues, and her physicians do and say.
- She uses criticism to try to turn you against a colleague.
- She makes hostile comments, such as, "If you stick me with that needle one more time, I'm going to hit you."
- She exhibits hostile or violent behavior, such as throwing objects.
- She depends on you and other nurses for virtually all her physical care, even though she's capable of performing it herself.
- She doesn't comply with treatment, yet blames caregivers for her medical condition.
- She takes offense at harmless comments.

from a health care provider's actions. If your patient files a claim, don't admit wrongdoing to her or to her relatives, friends, or attorneys. In fact, don't mention her claim or threat to sue when interacting with the patient. Any statement you make could become the basis for a lawsuit.

Instead, talk to your patient about her concerns, using therapeutic communication skills. Conduct a physical and emotional assessment, and if appropriate, provide teaching or other interventions necessary to address her concerns. Handling the situation this way shows her that you take her complaint seriously. It also gives her a sense of control over her situation and makes her think that she's more involved in her care.

Suppose, for example, you learn that your patient has threatened to sue because she thinks that she has received the wrong antihypertensive drug. You might say, "Mrs. Lewis, I understand your concern about your medication. Tell me what the capsule looked like and how it made you feel." Giving her this chance to express herself may help diffuse her anger.

After she responds, you might say, "Thank you for sharing this information with me. Your blood pressure reading hasn't changed. I'm confident that the pharmacy hasn't substituted a different brand of your medication, but I'll call the pharmacist just to be sure and I'll let you know what I find out."

If your patient's allegations involve you directly, consider having another nurse provide her care. If you must continue to care for her, don't try to make amends by giving her more attention. But don't try to avoid her either. Changing your level of care after she threatens to sue or files a claim could suggest that you're guilty of something.

Claim Investigation. As soon as you find out that your patient has filed a claim, notify the appropriate nurse administrator, the patient's physician, your facility's risk manager, and your personal malpractice insurer. Be ready for intensive questioning from each party as to what your patient said, your actions, and your objective and subjective assessment of the situation. If you believe that your mistake led to the patient's claim, admit this to the physician, the appropriate nurse administrator, your risk manager, and the insurance company—but not to your patient or her family, friends, or attorney. In fact, for you legal protection, avoid speaking about anything with the patient, her family, or her attorney.

However, don't be alarmed. You're not on trial. The insurance company will evaluate the seriousness of the patient's allegations and formulate the most appropriate plan of action.

Once the claim investigation is complete, you may hear nothing more about the incident. If the patient's claim is valid, your facility probably will try to negotiate a settlement to prevent the patient from filing a lawsuit. You probably won't be involved in settlement negotiations. If the patient doesn't settle or if your facility determines that her claim isn't valid, chances are nothing more will be done until she files a lawsuit.

Notifying Your Personal Insurance Carrier. If you carry individual nursing malpractice insurance, notify your insurance company as soon as you learn that you've been named in a suit. Depending on how your policy is written, failure to notify the insurance company of a lawsuit could reduce or nullify your coverage. Check your policy carefully because you may not need to report a threat of suit unless you're actually named.

What to Document

Your documentation provides valuable information for claim investigators and, if the case goes to trial, will serve as the core of your testimony. A patient may wait weeks, months, or even years to file a claim, so be sure to preserve all your original notes to help you recall the details of the incident. Also, if you keep a personal on-the-job journal to help defend yourself against lawsuits, make sure you understand the possible ramifications. (See *Personal journal: Help or hindrance in court?*, page 232.)

According to your facility's policy, document the following in your nurse's notes, progress notes, or other form:
- your patient's physical and mental status before, during, and after she threatened to sue or filed a claim
- your actions in response to your physical and mental assessment findings
- exact words (in quotes) used by the patient, her family members, or attorney during your discussions about overt or implied threats to sue or file a claim

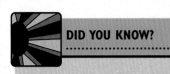

DID YOU KNOW?

PERSONAL JOURNAL: HELP OR HINDRANCE IN COURT?
Some nurses record workplace events in a personal journal in case they're sued. Lawyers disagree as to whether this practice is helpful or harmful. Some caution against it, warning that an opposing attorney could discredit the nurse if her private journal conflicts with the patient's medical record. Others believe that keeping a personal record of unusual events helps the nurse recall important details. If you decide to keep a journal, don't neglect your thorough, accurate documentation in the medical record. Remember that your documentation in the official record should stand on its own—and provide the full story.

If you choose to keep a personal journal, follow these guidelines:
- Keep it factual. Embellishing or lying will only lead to problems.
- Keep it objective. Documenting defamatory or nasty comments could embarrass you if your journal is subpoenaed by the court.
- Keep it safe. Store the journal in a secure place at home.
- Be truthful about its existence. If your attorney asks whether you keep personal notes, tell him you do. He'll review the journal to see whether it could cause you problems in court.

- statements that you and other participants made during these discussions
- names and relationships to the patient (if known) of people who witnessed or overheard your discussions about threats to sue or filing of a claim
- dates and times of specific events that the patient has threatened to sue over or has filed a claim about
- names of other staff members whom the patient said were involved in the incident
- names of people you notified of the patient's threat and time of notification
- patient actions that might have contributed to the incident, such as drugs brought from home, refusal to provide a thorough medical history, treatment refusal, and noncompliance
- presence of unauthorized items in the patient's room, such as a weapon, scalpel, syringes, or drugs

After you notify the appropriate people that the patient has threatened to sue or has filed a claim, don't document anything related to the claim investigation. For instance, don't mention interviews with insurance representatives, the facility's risk manager, or legal counsel unless instructed to do so. Check your facility's policy to find out whether you should file an incident report.

WHEN YOUR PATIENT MAKES A SEXUAL ADVANCE

The intimate nature of nursing practice makes you an easy target for a patient's unwanted sexual advance. Your inevitable physical contact with a patient may cause sexual arousal. Getting emotionally close to a patient, such as when you help him deal with emotional problems, also may contribute to sexual feelings.

An unwanted sexual advance (a type of sexual harassment that can take many form) violates the unspoken contract between nurse and patient. It also puts you in a precarious legal and ethical position. As a nurse, you must provide care without discrimination. Yet as an individual and a professional, you may be offended or feel threatened by your patient's advance. And as an employee, you have the right to work in a safe environment.

An unwanted sexual advance may have legal consequences unless handled properly. Depending on the situation, you could find yourself on either side of a lawsuit. If you refuse to care for the patient after his advance, he could file a claim against you or your employer for abandonment or for violating his rights or professional care standards. Or you could file a claim against him for sexual harassment, battery, or assault.

Defining the Problem. Legally, a sexual advance is unwanted physical, verbal, or other conduct that's sexually suggestive. A sexual advance may occur if your patient:
- deliberately touches you or exposes his genitals to you
- makes a sexually inappropriate gesture or comment or tells a sexual joke

- makes sexually suggestive comments about your appearance or behavior
- shows you a sexually explicit photograph or plays a sexually explicit audiotape or videotape in your presence
- makes an overt verbal or physical advance. For instance, he touches you and says, "Come to my room later tonight so we can be together."

Although you can't prevent every unwanted sexual advance, you can take steps to handle the situation properly if it occurs. For example, you may develop a basic plan for dealing with an unwanted sexual advance and practice your responses so that you can act automatically when the situation arises. You should also be prepared to document the situation to protect the interests of everyone involved.

How to Respond

Your best response to a patient's sexual advance is to stay calm and objective. If you lose your composure, you may react inappropriately, causing the situation to escalate.

If your patient makes a specific request with sexual overtones, simply say no. Then, in a professional, nonthreatening manner, explain that his behavior is inappropriate and that you won't tolerate it. Even if you find his behavior threatening or intimidating, don't tell him so. It could make him think that he has power over you.

Then report the incident to the appropriate nurse administrator and other staff members who care for the patient, including nurse colleagues, nursing assistants, mental health professionals, and the physician. Also notify your facility's risk manager.

Assess whether your safety may be at risk if you continue to care for the patient. If you believe that it would, contact the appropriate nurse administrator or ask another staff member to accompany you when you enter his room. Also review your facility's policy for refusing an assignment. Keep in mind that the patient could sue you for abandonment if you refuse to care for him— and you may lose in court if you have no objective evidence to support your refusal.

What to Document

When documenting a patient's sexual advance, be as accurate and clear as possible to protect yourself, your facility, and the patient. If your facility has policies and procedures for documenting sexually inappropriate behavior, follow those guidelines precisely.

In the nurse's notes, state exactly what the patient did or said that you considered inappropriate. Use direct quotes when recording patient statements that made you uncomfortable, and objectively describe offensive behavior. For example, if the patient stroked your hair, you might write, "While this nurse changed the dressing on the patient's right shoulder wound, patient reached up with his left hand and ran his fingers through this nurse's hair. After asking the patient to stop this activity, he repeated it three times. Patient was observed to be smiling and diaphoretic while engaged in this behavior."

Record, too, exactly what you said or did in response to the patient's advance, and describe how the patient reacted to your words or actions. Also document his physical and emotional status before, during, and after the incident. Note whether sexually related items (for instance, pornographic magazines or videotapes) were visible during the incident. If other people witnessed the sexual advance, record their names, credentials, and relationships to the patient, along with their statements about the incident. Also record the names of people you notified, instructions they gave, and your subsequent actions.

Describe the incident in the patient's nursing plan of care to alert other nurses to his behavior. Include interventions you used to prevent a recurrence, the patient's response to interventions, and your recommendations for actions to take if the situation recurs. Be sure to include the date and time in your entry and sign it.

If required by your facility, complete an incident report. Make sure the information in the report agrees with your nurse's notes.

As an optional, personal record, you may also write on a separate sheet all the facts of the incident as outlined in your nurse's notes. Include feelings you experienced as a result of the incident. Sign and date the note, and keep it in a safe place in case the incident leads to legal action.

WHEN YOUR PATIENT BECOMES HOSTILE

N o matter where you practice, you can occasionally be the target of a patient's temper tantrum or verbal abuse. If your specialty is psychiatric, emergency, or rehabilitation nursing or if you deal with workers' compensation or legal matters, you may encounter hostile patients often.

The line between hostile behavior and violence can be razor-thin. If not dealt with appropriately, hostility can rapidly escalate to violence and injury. When dealing with a hostile patient, virtually anything you say or do could provoke her into becoming violent.

When you care for a hostile patient, you have a duty to protect her from harm. But you also must protect yourself and others. Your response to a hostile patient and proper documentation of the situation can affect the well-being and legal status of all parties.

Types of Hostile Behavior. Hostile behavior can be verbal or physical. *Verbal* hostility includes shouting, name-calling, using profanities, and making condescending remarks. *Physical* hostility may include:
- breaking or throwing things
- taking personal property from other patients or staff members
- throwing, scattering, or spilling body fluids or excrement
- refusing treatment or diagnostic tests (See *When your patient refuses treatment,* pages 215-218.)

How to Respond

Using therapeutic communication, try to calm the patient. Keep in mind that what you say—and how you say it—can mean the difference between resolution and escalation of the situation. Remove potentially dangerous objects from the patient's reach. However, remember that you have no legal right to search her belongings without her consent. If you suspect that she has access to a dangerous object, tell the appropriate nurse administrator immediately and follow your facility's protocols.

Assessing the Situation. To gather information and develop an effective plan of action, conduct a physical and cognitive assessment to the extent the patient will allow. If you suspect that her hostile behavior could escalate rapidly to violence, ask a colleague to stay with you during the assessment.

Look for a physical explanation for her hostility, such as an injury, illness, or use of street drugs. Evaluate her psychosocial status to determine whether anxiety is at the root of her hostility. For instance, perhaps she is seriously ill and feels a lack of control over her body. Or maybe she has financial concerns or family problems.

After completing these assessments, survey the immediate surroundings for cleaning supplies, unauthorized substances, and other equipment or devices the patient might have tampered with, creating a safety hazard. As you conduct this inspection, refrain from making threats or accusations. Remember—your words and behavior must convey trust, caring, and respect.

Using Behavioral Interventions. Consider using behavioral modification strategies to calm the patient. Begin by acknowledging the situation. For instance, you might say, "Mrs. Benson, when you throw things, it makes me think you're trying to make me angry. I'd like to talk with you about what's happening between us." Then give her an opportunity to voice her feelings, but don't let her start screaming or otherwise lose control.

Set firm limits. Calmly and clearly tell the patient to stop the hostile behavior. If she ignores your request, summon help. Don't try to reason with her; this may worsen the situation. Instead, reinforce good behavior, providing positive feedback when she controls her hostility. Make sure your interventions don't constitute patient abuse or neglect or infringement of the patient's rights.

Notify your patient's family and legal representatives of the patient's hostile behavior. If family members are present, teach them how to use behavioral interventions to calm her when staff members aren't available.

Taking More Drastic Measures. If your patient's hostility escalates to violence, call for help immediately. If necessary, contact security personnel. Also notify the physician and the appropriate nurse supervisor. Don't leave the patient alone unless you believe that you're in imminent danger of harm.

Consider applying restraints only as a last resort. If you do restrain the patient, be sure to follow your facility's policies and procedures. (See *When your patient must be restrained,* pages 244-251.)

What to Document

Your documentation must show that you acted in good faith, took all possible measures to control the situation, maintained nursing standards, and respected your patient's rights. Document the patient's hostile speech or behavior in detail, quoting her directly when possible and describing her hostile behavior objectively. (See *Facts only, please.*) Also document findings from your physical, cognitive, psychosocial, and environmental assessments, and record the names and credentials of people who witnessed or were involved in the incident.

Document the plan you developed to deal with your patient's hostility, along with the rationale for the plan. Then describe how you implemented the plan and how your patient responded to interventions. If you applied restraints, make sure your documentation indicates that you complied with facility policies and procedures. If you removed the patient's personal belongings, explain your rationale for doing this and describe the location of these items.

Record the names of everyone you notified, times of notification, instructions you received, and actions you took in response. As appropriate, complete an incident report, making sure it agrees with your nurse's notes.

Then update the patient's nursing plan of care to inform your colleagues of the patient's hostile behavior. In the plan, describe successful interventions as well as those that failed to decrease her hostility. Also record orders you received from the physician to calm the patient. Flag your patient's medical record to alert personnel from other departments to the patient's special needs.

As a precaution, record the events on a separate piece of paper for your own reference. Keep this record in a safe place. You may need it later if legal action is brought. Finally, make sure everyone who comes in contact with the patient knows what to

TIPS & ADVICE

FACTS ONLY, PLEASE
Objectivity is a crucial documentation skill. Recording assumptions and other subjective information will do more harm than good in court. Document only what you can see, hear, feel, or smell. And always keep your language neutral.

Avoid Assumptions
Suppose you see a food tray and its contents on the floor when you enter your patient's room. Would you assume it got there because the patient threw it, even though you didn't see her throw it? If so, you're making an assumption. If you document this assumption and later testify about the incident in court, an attorney could discredit you by showing that your notes represented conjecture, not fact.

Instead of documenting your assumption about how the food tray ended up on the floor, describe only the location and condition of the tray, dishes, silverware, and food when you entered the room.

Eliminate Bias
Using words with negative connotations can spell trouble. Avoid terms that convey a negative attitude toward your patient, such as "complainer," "abusive," "obstinate," "drunk," "obnoxious," and "disagreeable." Using these terms gives the impression that you disliked the patient and thus provided substandard care. A patient who sees herself described this way in her medical record may sue for libel or defamation of character—especially if she's already unhappy with her care.

Rather than labeling your patient, describe only her behavior and record only her exact words, placing quotation marks around them.

do if she becomes hostile again. Document your communications and update your patient's nursing plan of care.

WHEN YOUR PATIENT THREATENS TO HARM SOMEONE

A patient's threat to harm someone could indicate that he's hostile or about to become violent. If your patient makes such a threat, you must take prompt action to stop him from carrying it out. Keep in mind that although your primary responsibility is to your patient, you must protect the welfare of other patients, staff members, and visitors.

A threat to cause harm can be blatant or subtle and can be delivered verbally or through gestures. For instance, a patient may threaten harm by showing a closed fist or by making punching or strangling motions with his hands.

Recognize that a threat is a precursor to violence. Remember, too, that verbal aggression and agitation may precede threats and violent behavior. Your patient may signal his intent to cause harm by demonstrating generalized anger or agitation. For example, he might channel his dissatisfaction with the care he's receiving by threatening to harm his wife, who initiated his involuntary commitment to the psychiatric unit. Even a simple statement that he dislikes another person could represent a conscious or subconscious threat to harm that person.

Agitation, characterized by excessive, repetitive, uncontrollable, nonproductive activity, may accompany or precede a threat. Physical signs of agitation are easy to spot and may include pacing, hand wringing, fidgeting, and attempting to remove or damage medical devices. Verbal signs of agitation may be less apparent. They include telling lies about someone and constantly repeating the same story, statement, or word.

You can't always predict whether your patient could become violent. Just as you use standard infection precautions with all patients, you must treat every patient as potentially violent. This will prepare you to act promptly and objectively if your patient threatens to harm someone. (See *Reporting a patient's threat: Breach of confidentiality?*)

How to Respond

After taking immediate steps to protect yourself and others, evaluate the patient's physical and psychosocial status. If you sense that he may harm you, ask another staff member to stand near you during the assessment. If the patient threatens you, you may want to request that a colleague care for him. (See *When your patient becomes hostile,* pages 236-239.)

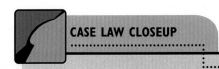

CASE LAW CLOSEUP

REPORTING A PATIENT'S THREAT: BREACH OF CONFIDENTIALITY?
Courts remain divided on whether health care providers must protect the confidentiality of threats against named individuals or reveal these threats to protect the intended victims. A Delaware case, described below, provides some guidance. Because laws vary, be sure to familiarize yourself with the laws in your state.

Understanding the Case
State v. Bright[1] concerns a veteran who was receiving outpatient therapy for chronic alcohol abuse. Over the previous 20 years, he had been diagnosed with bipolar disorder and was receiving therapy for that condition. His therapist knew he had killed his brother and been found not guilty by reason of insanity. The patient had repeatedly told the therapist that he intended to kill his ex-wife, who was in hiding in another state because of his harassment, intimidation, and threats.

During one therapy session, the patient told the therapist that he was leaving town that evening to find his ex-wife and kill her. The therapist called the local police and the police in the town where the ex-wife was thought to be living. The police apprehended the patient about 2 miles from the ex-wife's residence. They found duct tape and a newly purchased knife in his car. He was charged with making terrorist threats and attempted murder.

How the Court Ruled
At trial, the patient's attorney argued that his client's confidentiality was violated when the therapist called the local authorities and that the case should be dismissed for lack of evidence.

However, the court praised the therapist's actions and found that he hadn't violated the patient's confidentiality when he reported his threat to law enforcement officers. The court relied on the patient's previous actions, his state of mind at the time of his last therapy session, and his previous threats against his ex-wife as evidence that he was capable of enacting his threat. It also noted that he had repeatedly violated an injunction to stay away from her. The court found the patient guilty of attempted murder.

The Lesson Learned
This case encourages psychologists, psychiatrists, therapists, and other mental health workers to warn intended victims when a patient makes threats against them—especially when the patient has the ability to carry out his threats. The case also reminds nurses to take expressed threats seriously and ensure that appropriate health care providers are made aware of the threats.

[1] *State v. Bright,* 683 A. 2d 1055 (Del. Super. 1996).

During your assessment, check for a physical or psychosocial reason for the patient's behavior, such as dementia, brain injury, epilepsy, a developmental disability, schizophrenia, depression, a personality or anxiety disorder, or a substance abuse problem. Also assess for physical disorders that can cause a chemical imbalance that leads to confusion, agitation, and aggression.

After you complete the assessment, immediately discuss your findings with the physician and develop a plan of action. Consider using such interventions as:

- behavioral modification
- treatment of the underlying medical condition
- drug or dosage adjustment, if needed
- environmental controls, such as prohibiting visits by people the patient has threatened, reducing the noise level, and removing items he could use to cause physical harm

Protecting the Intended Victim. If a patient threatens to harm a specific person, instruct that person to leave the area at once. If the intended victim isn't in the facility, arrange a meeting with the appropriate nurse administrator, a mental health professional, your facility's risk manager, and the physician to discuss the best way to inform that person of the patient's threat.

Notifying Others. If you haven't already done so, report the situation to the appropriate nurse administrator, your facility's risk manager, the security department, and other health care team members. Tell them about interventions that have proved successful in dealing with the patient's behavior.

Upholding Patient Rights. Like all patients, your patient who makes threats has the right to privacy, confidentiality, and treatment refusal. Even if you dislike his behavior, you must convey caring, trust, and respect when interacting with him.

What to Document

Your documentation serves as the only objective evidence that you followed nursing standards and took steps to prevent harm to all involved. In your nurse's notes, describe the incident in detail. Record the patient's threat in his own words, along with statements made by people who heard his threat. Also detail the patient's threatening behavior. (See *Describing a threat.*)

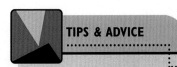

TIPS & ADVICE

DESCRIBING A THREAT

If your patient makes a threat, your documentation must show that you did everything possible to protect him, his intended victim, and other parties involved. Here's an example of a nurse's note detailing the behavior of a hostile patient and describing nursing interventions.

3/19/06 0830: Observed patient walking back and forth in his room. Patient's wife was present in the room, sitting in a chair near the door. Patient's activity was causing tension on the central line IV tubing. This nurse instructed the patient to return to bed to avoid dislodging his central line. Repeated instruction three times over 5 minutes. Patient continued the activity without verbalization. Patient did not make eye contact with this nurse. After the third instruction to sit down, patient's wife stated, "Jim, please sit down." At 0835, immediately after wife's request, patient walked to the nightstand to the right of his bed, reached into the drawer with his right hand, and retrieved a pocket knife. He then opened the knife to expose the blade, pointed the blade at his wife, and took two steps toward her. This nurse immediately instructed patient's wife to leave and instructed patient to put down the knife. At 0836, immediately after verbal instructions, this nurse called security. As his wife passed through the doorway, patient loudly told his wife, "I'm going to kill you." Patient was observed to be trembling and diaphoretic. Wife left the room. Patient continued pacing and repeating the threat. Nurse remained in the doorway and repeated instruction to sit down. Patient did not respond to instruction. Security guards arrived at 0837, restrained patient, and removed knife. Dr. Symington notified at 0840 and returned call at 0845. Dr. Symington prescribed lorazepam 1 mg to be given I.M., which was done at 0850. Wife was unable to be located via visual search of the unit and facility-wide page. Nursing supervisor notified of incident at 0850.   -Jane Williams, RN

Record the names of people you notified, times of notification, and actions you took.

Then document the incident in the patient's nursing plan of care. Include instructions from the physician, security personnel, and your facility's risk manager as well as your recommendations for specific interventions.

Complete an incident report, making sure the information you write reflects your nurse's notes exactly. Finally, make sure all staff members and other appropriate people are aware of the patient's threat and have been instructed how to deal with the situation.

WHEN YOUR PATIENT MUST BE RESTRAINED

M any patients are at high risk for injury because they're confused, hostile, or agitated. In some cases, the best— perhaps only—way to protect your patient or the health care team is to restrain her. Restraints also can be used to help manage unexpected dangerous behaviors, such as violence; to help provide care as part of an approved protocol, such as for a sedated patient who could injure herself by removing a tube; or to comply with standard practice.

Restraint refers not only to the use of physical restraining devices but also to chemical treatments and environmental interventions that restrict a patient's freedom of movement. Commonly, restraints are used when:
- the patient is at high risk for self-harm or is a threat to others
- alternative methods of protecting the patient or others have failed
- a written order is placed in the medical record. (See *Ordering restraints: How to comply with JCAHO regulations.*)

Physical restraints include straps, vests, mitts, seat belts, side rails, and special beds with high, padded walls. A cast, continuous passive motion machine, or medical device that controls or limits

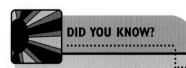

DID YOU KNOW?

ORDERING RESTRAINTS: HOW TO COMPLY WITH JCAHO REGULATIONS
Applying restraints to a patient can put you in legal jeopardy if the patient's chart doesn't have an order for them. To comply with the restraint regulations of the Joint Commission on Accreditation of Healthcare Organizations (JCAHO), follow these guidelines:

- Verify that the chart contains a written order for restraints from a licensed independent practitioner (LIP), such as a physician, nurse practitioner, or physician's assistant.
- If a change in the patient's condition, such as the sudden onset of delirium, constitutes the emergency, notify the LIP immediately. In an emergency related to an existing problem, such as dementia, notify the LIP within 12 hours of restraint application and obtain a verbal or written order for restraints.
- Make sure the LIP evaluates the patient and supplies a written order with 24 hours of initiating the use of restraints.
- Ensure that a new order is placed in the chart every 24 hours, if restraints remain necessary.
- If restraints are used to manage a behavioral health problem, obtain a new order every 4 hours if the patient is age 18 or older, every 2 hours if she's age 9 to 17, or every hour if she's under age 9.
  Never accept a prn order for restraints to be used as needed.

movement can be a physical restraint if the patient can't free herself from it. *Chemical* restraints include such drugs as diazepam, haloperidol, and lorazepam, which reduce the patient's level of consciousness or impair her motor function. *Environmental* restraints include:

- measures that prevent a patient from obtaining her clothing, car keys, or mobility device
- confinement in a locked room
- behavioral modification strategies that encourage or discourage a certain behavior—for instance, refusing to let the patient leave her room or the facility unless she controls her angry outbursts

Restraints can cause more problems than they prevent. Physical and chemical restraints can lead to falls, damage to skin and soft tissues, respiratory impairment, neurologic and orthopedic injury, and death. Environmental restraints can cause harm if the patient tries to overcome them. For example, a patient whose wheelchair is deliberately kept out of her room may fall when trying to walk unassisted. The use of any type of restraints can result in the loss of dignity, causing emotional harm. For these reasons, consider using restraints only as a last resort.

Legal Risks. Besides potentially harming the patient physically and emotionally, restraints can expose you and other caregivers to legal risk if used in a way that violates patient rights. Restraining a patient inappropriately also can lead to a charge of false imprisonment. (See *Understanding false imprisonment*, page 227.)

Failure to use restraints when indicated may violate standards of nursing practice. Besides understanding when to use restraints, you need to know how to document properly. Your documentation must accurately describe your patient's safety risk and show that you followed the correct procedure when using restraints.

How to Respond

When weighing the benefits and risks of using restraints, conduct a complete physical and cognitive assessment. Consider applying restraints only if the patient poses a threat to herself or others.

Next, assess the potential risk of applying restraints by evaluating the patient's skin, bone structure, and ability to summon help. For example, if your patient has skin tears and is receiving a corticosteroid, leather restraints could promote skin breakdown. If she has respiratory distress, a vest restraint could restrict her breathing.

If needed, consult another staff member for advice. For instance, a physical or occupational therapist may be able to suggest an alternative to restraining the patient, such as:
- placing her in a Craig bed or other special bed
- keeping the call button within easy reach and making sure she knows how to use it
- equipping the bed with an alarm that will sound if she tries to get out of bed unsupervised
- increasing the frequency of physical and cognitive assessments

If your evaluation indicates that restraint is the only feasible option, determine the most appropriate type of restraint to use. If the patient has soft, fragile skin, consider gauze restraints or hand mitts rather than leather or traditional wrist restraints, which could tear the skin. Snug leather restraints, on the other hand, may be the best choice if the patient is violent or keeps trying to remove her endotracheal tube.

Before applying the restraint, discuss its use with the patient and her family or legal guardian. Also consider your facility's policies and procedures. Be aware that except in an emergency, you must obtain a physician's order and informed consent to apply restraints. In most facilities, the physician's order must state the type of restraint to use, when to apply it, duration of use, and frequency of assessments during restraint. (See *How restraints hold up in court*, pages 247-248.)

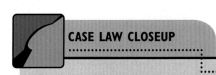

CASE LAW CLOSEUP

HOW RESTRAINTS HOLD UP IN COURT
Although often a last resort, sometimes using restraints is the appropriate action. In the case examined here, the court found that nursing documentation supported emergency use of restraints to protect an agitated patient and the people around him.

Understanding the Case
White v. State of Washington[1] concerns a nursing home resident who had grown increasingly agitated. He had a history of burning himself by putting lit cigarettes in his pants pocket and of trying to eat objects, such as plastic pudding containers. He also scratched himself repeatedly.

On the day in question, he was more agitated than usual and was quickly becoming a threat to himself and other residents. The nursing staff decided to place him in a Posey vest to "prevent self-harm," according to their notes. The vest was in use for a short time while the nursing staff contacted the medical director.

[1] *White v. State of Washington*, 929 P.2d 396 (Wash. 1996).

Continued

CASE LAW CLOSEUP

HOW RESTRAINTS HOLD UP IN COURT—cont'd
The medical director declined to order physical restraints on an ongoing basis. The patient received a drug as prescribed by the medical director, and the Posey vest was immediately removed. In his notes, the medical director stated that use of the Posey vest was an appropriate emergency measure, but that the patient's individualized plan would be reevaluated and other measures taken to prevent continued agitation. Use of the Posey vest caused no injury to the patient, and no one in the home was injured.

How the Court Ruled
In a suit brought by a former staff member over substandard care and patient abuse by the staff, the Supreme Court of Washington noted that the nurses' temporary use of a restraining device was promptly reviewed by the medical director. The court also noted that the nursing home had a sound policy of allowing nurses to use their professional judgment about applying physical restraints in an emergency to prevent patients from harming themselves.

The court commended the nurses for thoroughly documenting their use of restraints and their rationale and ruled that the temporary restraint they applied did not constitute patient abuse.

The Lesson Learned
The court based its conclusion on two critical points, both of which apply to nursing documentation in emergencies:
- The nurses' documentation showed that they carefully weighed the need for restraints and the patient's continuing agitation, which failed to subside with use of more conventional interventions. These observations, which the nurses recorded, led them to consider and apply the Posey vest.
- The nurses immediately notified the medical director of the situation, documented this fact, and removed the restraints when instructed.

If you must restrain a patient in an emergency, your documentation should reflect the same attention to details. Always record why such an intervention became necessary, the name of the physician you contacted, physician's orders you received, and your subsequent actions. Your documentation must show that your patient received competent care.

Assessing the Patient. If possible, place a restrained patient in a room easily seen from the nurses' station. Keep the door open so that you can see and hear her if she tries to remove the restraints or calls for help.

If your facility has no established protocol for the type and frequency of assessments during restraint, check the patient at least every 15 minutes. When using physical restraints, assess the patient's skin each time you check on her—especially those areas in direct contact with the restraints. Also evaluate her circulation, motion, and sensation.

Evaluate the patient's physical and cognitive status to determine whether the restraints are still necessary and to detect injuries resulting from their use. Because restraints limit mobility, make sure all the patient's needs are met and that she has an appropriate mechanism to summon help.

In the patient's room, place signs that provide specific instructions on the use of restraints, and notify other staff members of the conditions for their use. To ensure continuity of care, review your colleagues' documentation to determine whether they're using the restraints as ordered.

Closely review physical and cognitive assessment findings obtained by the nurse on the previous shift. Follow up on findings that suggest a possible complication from the use of the restraints. For instance, if the patient has leather wrist restraints, evaluate your colleagues' findings from circulation, motion, and sensation assessments to detect significant changes from baseline.

What to Document

In most facilities, the patient or legal guardian must sign a consent form before restraints can be applied. Obtaining informed consent reduces your legal exposure. (Be aware that consent can be revoked verbally or in writing at any time.) Document that you provided the patient and family with thorough information about the type of restraints to be used, their purpose, duration of use, and actions you'll take to help the patient stay as independent as possible during restraint.

Also document the use of restraints. Describe the type of restraint you recommended and your rationale. Note specific patient behaviors that support your rationale.

If you must apply restraints in an emergency, document your assessment of the situation, measures you took before restraints were applied, and your patient's response to those measures. Record the name of the physician who gave the verbal order for restraints and the names of witnesses (noting their relationships to the patient). Record the time and date of your contact with the physician, content of the discussion, instructions you received, and actions you took in response.

Document prerestraint physical and cognitive findings and your ongoing assessments, interventions, and recommendations during restraint. Be as specific as possible. For instance, instead of merely stating that you checked the patient's circulation, record actual findings, such as "warm skin and strong distal pulse." Also record the times you released or loosened the restraints to rotate them or allow the patient some supervised activity. If you gave the patient a special device to call for assistance or take care of personal needs, document this action. (See *Documenting assessment findings during restraint.*)

If your facility has a special flow sheet to use when documenting care for a restrained patient, be sure to record your specific findings in the blanks provided, in addition to using check marks. If the flow sheet doesn't have blanks, record your findings in the narrative portion of the nurse's notes, progress record, or other appropriate form.

In the nursing plan of care, record specific outcomes and interventions for the use of restraints. Include outcomes that must be achieved before restraints can be discontinued. If you suspect that a staff member may have failed to restrain the patient as ordered, discuss the situation with the appropriate nurse administrator and the physician. If required by your facility, complete an incident report stating that restraints weren't applied when indicated or ordered. Be objective. Report the facts only and don't blame a particular staff member. Don't mention violations of the standard of care in your patient's medical record because this could lead to legal problems if the allegations prove to be false.

CHARTING CHECKLIST

DOCUMENTING ASSESSMENT FINDINGS DURING RESTRAINT
If your patient must be restrained, assess her every hour and document the:
- ❏ type of restraint in use
- ❏ reason for the restraint
- ❏ education provided to the patient and her family about the need for restraints, the expected duration of their use, and the best way to summon help, if needed
- ❏ patient's position
- ❏ condition of the patient's skin, especially at pressure areas
- ❏ circulation to the arms and legs
- ❏ reapplication of restraints, if needed
- ❏ other safety precautions in use
- ❏ assistance to the bathroom or offers of this
- ❏ assistance to eat or drink or offers of this
- ❏ reevaluation of the continuing need for restraint
- ❏ observation that the restraints aren't restricting breathing

Recording Less Frequent Assessments
Every 1 to 2 hours, record that the restraints were released for 5 to 10 minutes to reduce pressure and promote circulation. Every 2 hours, note that range-of-motion exercises were performed. At least once per shift, record that you explained to the patient that restraints are for her safety. As appropriate, document that you tried or considered alternatives to restraints.

WHEN YOUR PATIENT IS ANXIOUS

Many people feel anxious or intimidated in a medical setting. So when your patient is hospitalized, he's likely to feel mild anxiety related to pain, embarrassment, loss of control, or complications of his disorder. However, high anxiety may interfere with his ability to provide critical information for the medical record or to understand your teaching about treatments or discharge.

That's why prompt recognition and management of anxiety is vital to effective care. It's also why careful documentation of your care and instructions plays such an important role in communicating effectively with an anxious patient and his caregivers.

How to Respond

When your patient is hospitalized, mild anxiety can be useful because it helps him focus on answering questions and following instructions and gives him the energy to carry on. If he's like most patients, your empathy and reassurance are enough to keep his mild anxiety from escalating and to promote cooperation. To convey empathy, tell the patient you understand his stress and will provide support for him. For instance, you may say, "I know this experience can seem overwhelming, but I'll be here to help you. Now take a deep breath and try to relax."

However, don't try to calm the patient with reassuring statements that may not be true, such as "Everything will be all right." False reassurances can jeopardize his trust in you and the other health care team members.

Managing a Patient with Moderate to Severe Anxiety. If your patient is moderately anxious, guide him through breathing or relaxation exercises, recording their use in your notes. When he's calmer, start the interview with an open-ended question to invite him to begin talking. Then proceed as appropriate.

If he's extremely anxious, ask the physician about the need for a psychiatric consultation and record his referral. The patient may need an antianxiety drug to reduce his anxiety before you can provide care. If so, give it as ordered and document its administration and effects.

Modifying Patient Care. When taking a health history, document the anxious patient's medical problems and drug use carefully. If possible, examine his medical record first and use the information to guide him through the health history when anxiety makes him forgetful. For example, if the record shows that he was taking aspirin daily, but he neglects to mention it because of high anxiety, prompt him with a statement such as, "I noticed that your record said you were taking one aspirin tablet a day. Is that still true?"

An anxious patient may worry that a physical examination or treatment will cause pain or embarrassment or reveal a serious illness. To help minimize his anxiety, be sure to maintain privacy. Close the door and draw the curtain. Don't allow others to enter the room without the patient's permission. However, if a family member or friend seems to calm the patient, try to allow this person to stay with him during your care. Make a note of anyone who remains with the patient during examinations and treatments.

Then when providing care, expose only the body area you need to examine and cover it promptly when you're finished. Before examining the patient or administering a treatment, prepare him by stating what you're going to do. Prior to auscultating his lungs, for example, you could say, "Now I'm going to place my stethoscope on your back and listen to your lungs. It might feel a little cold." That way, you'll avoid startling him and keep him involved in the examination.

When you must perform a painful treatment, don't gloss over its potential discomfort. Instead, let the patient know what to expect and how you'll help him cope. For example, say something like, "You may feel a ripping or pulling sensation when I remove the dressing. If it gets too painful, let me know and we can take a break. Or I can remove it quickly if you'd rather get it over with sooner." In your nurse's notes, document how well the patient tolerated the procedure and whether you were able to complete it without stopping. If the patient requested a break to help him cope, make a note of that too.

If you need extra time for a certain part of the examination, such as heart sound auscultation, tell the patient you're going to spend a few minutes listening to his heart. Otherwise, he may become anxious, fearing that the additional time spent listening to his heart means that something is wrong. After you finish listening, reassure him as appropriate with a statement such as, "Your heartbeat is regular and strong," but don't give false reassurance. If you discover an abnormality, control your facial expression and verbal response and calmly record your finding. Otherwise, the patient may become alarmed.

When teaching an anxious patient, provide written information whenever possible because high anxiety can prevent him from absorbing your instructions. Document your actions and the patient's response to them.

What to Document

When you are caring for an anxious patient, documenting the details of your care and patient teaching can make the difference between a smooth hospital stay and a rocky one caused by miscommunication. Be sure to record details in these areas:

- patient's anxiety level with objective findings, including pressured speech and subjective statements, such as "I'm so nervous"
- anxiety-reduction interventions, such as relaxation exercises, and his response to them
- information from the patient, such as his recall of drugs used at home, and the method you used to verify this information
- patient care modifications, including special measures to ensure privacy
- presence of family members or friends—and whether they're calming or anxiety-provoking for the patient
- all patient teaching, including the provision of written instructions

WHEN YOUR PATIENT THREATENS SUICIDE

You can expect to care for a suicidal patient at some time no matter where you work. If you fail to identify and document a patient's threat of suicide and she then harms herself, you could be sued for violating standards of nursing care.

Some patients have suicidal thoughts before they seek health care. Others become acutely depressed during their hospital stay. Any patient who is old enough to understand what suicide is and who has the physical and mental capacity to carry out a threat should be considered at risk. To limit your legal exposure, you need to know how to deal with a suicide threat and how to document the situation properly.

How to Respond

If your patient threatens suicide or you suspect that she's at high risk for suicide, perform a physical and psychosocial assessment. Watch for clues to suicidal ideation—thoughts of suicide without definite intent. (See *Suicidal intent: Gauging the seriousness*, page 256.)

During the assessment, try to establish a rapport. If your patient is comfortable with you, she may be more willing to express suicidal thoughts and feelings verbally rather than carry out her threat.

Keep in mind that some suicide threats are expressed nonverbally. Also be aware that a patient who's depressed, cognitively impaired, or receiving a drug such as meperidine or morphine may hide her suicidal thoughts and feelings.

If you notice scars (especially on the patient's wrists), ask what caused them. If her explanation is inconsistent with her health history, consider that the scars may have been caused by a previous suicide attempt.

Also check the patient's history for recent suicide attempts. Patients with a history of suicide attempts and hospitalizations for suicidal ideation or self-destructive behavior are at high risk. Others at high risk include:

- depressed patients
- postpartum women
- elderly patients
- patients recovering from anesthesia
- patients with a newly diagnosed debilitating or life-threatening disease
- patients who have experienced a major trauma
- those with psychiatric disorders, interpersonal problems, chronic illnesses, or a history of substance abuse
- patients with organic brain dysfunction, such as from head injury, epilepsy, dementia, or mental retardation
- those with renal failure or certain other hemodynamic imbalances

During the interview, note negative self-talk or verbalization of hopelessness or helplessness. Evaluate the patient's recent behavior for sudden changes in activity, giving away of personal possessions, refusal of non–life-sustaining treatment or tests, refusal of food and fluids, and tampering with medical devices. Be aware

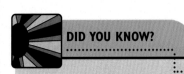

SUICIDAL INTENT: GAUGING THE SERIOUSNESS

If your patient expresses suicidal thoughts or if you suspect that she's suicidal, use these guidelines to evaluate the seriousness of her intent.

Suicidal Ideation

Suicidal ideation refers to direct or indirect thoughts of suicide or self-injury expressed verbally or through writing or art without definite intent or action.

Suicide Threat

More serious than suicidal ideation, a suicide threat is a direct verbal or written expression of intent to commit suicide without action. Typically, it's accompanied by angry outbursts, emotional lability, social withdrawal, attitude changes, or decreased work or school performance.

A person who makes a suicide threat may or may not verbalize a suicide plan. Sometimes the threat is expressed only through nonverbal behaviors, such as neglecting personal hygiene and withdrawing from social interactions.

Suicidal Gesture

More serious than a suicide threat, a suicidal gesture is a physical expression of intent used to attract attention but carried out in a way that causes no serious injury. For instance, the patient may take several over-the-counter sleeping pills, knowing that this will cause symptoms and attract attention but won't kill her.

Keep in mind that a suicidal gesture is designed to influence, control, or manipulate. It may be a precursor of a suicide attempt.

Suicide Attempt

A suicide attempt is a serious action by a person who intends to harm herself or end her life. Often, an attempt represents a final plea for help. The person may plan her attempt so as to cause a significant risk for injury or death. The final outcome depends on the method used and the time elapsed between the attempt and treatment. If your patient cuts her wrist, for example, her chance for survival depends on the wound's severity and the interval before her wound is treated.

that a quadriplegic who has a tracheostomy and can't speak may communicate suicidal feelings through facial gestures or crying. She may even try to hold her breath in an attempt to kill herself.

Because a suicide threat can be blatant or subtle, evaluate your patient's statements and behaviors for hidden meaning as well as overt intent. Realize, too, that a patient who has made a firm decision to commit suicide may not tell you for fear you'll try to stop her.

If appropriate, ask the patient directly whether she's thinking of killing herself. Don't worry that your question will give her the idea to commit suicide. On the contrary, it will allow her the chance to express her feelings, help you determine the extent of her depression, and show your concern for her welfare.

When Your Patient Makes a Direct Threat. If your patient makes an overt suicide threat, obtain the help of a mental health professional and contact the physician right away. But be discreet. If the patient suspects that you're calling for help, she may try to leave or make an immediate suicide attempt.

While waiting for assistance to arrive, keep the patient talking. Make her conscious of her identity by repeating her name, and try to help her identify the reason for her suicidal feelings. If she begins to calm down and seems capable of rational thought, offer constructive help with her problem. If your efforts fail to calm her or if she makes gestures that suggest an immediate suicide attempt, you may need to restrain her physically. Secure the environment by removing objects or drugs she could use to harm herself. Supervise her continuously until the immediate danger of suicide passes.

Inform the appropriate nurse administrator, other health care team members, and the facility's risk manager of the situation. With the physician, discuss plans for speaking with family members and friends. Realize that the patient's loved ones may feel guilt, shame, and self-blame for failing to recognize her dire emotional state.

What to Document

When documenting a patient's suicide threat, remember these goals:
* to inform other health care team members of the patient's threat so that they can take steps to protect her

- to limit your legal exposure and that of your colleagues and employer (See *Responding to a suicide threat: A court victory for nurses.*)

In your nurse's notes, describe the details of the patient's suicide threat. Quote the patient directly when appropriate, and cite gestures or behaviors that indicated or suggested her suicidal intent. Be sure to document your physical and psychosocial assessment findings.

Then record your interventions and the patient's response. Describe her immediate environment, your removal of items she could use to harm herself, and the current location of those items. If visitors were present during or just before her suicide threat, document what you know about their interaction with her. Include their names and relationships to her, if known. Also record the names and credentials of the physician and other people you notified, time of notification, instructions you received, and actions you took in response.

Next, update your patient's nursing plan of care to inform your colleagues of her suicide threat. Describe interventions that succeeded in calming her as well as those that had no effect or exacerbated her behavior. In the plan, record new orders from

CASE LAW CLOSEUP

RESPONDING TO A SUICIDE THREAT: A COURT VICTORY FOR NURSES

As the following case shows, careful documentation of your steps to protect a suicidal patient—and your rationales—may defeat a wrongful death action.

Understanding the Case

In *Sabol v. Richmond Heights General Hospital,*[1] a patient was admitted to the intensive care unit of an Ohio hospital after taking a deliberate drug overdose. Although a hospital psychologist strongly recommended that the patient immediately be transferred to a psychiatric facility, Richmond Heights General accepted his admission to stabilize his physical condition, on the condition that he be transferred to the psychiatric facility as soon as feasible. Lack of insurance coverage delayed the transfer.

---

[1] *Sabol v. Richmond Heights General Hospital,* 676 N.E.2d 958 (Ohio App. 1996).

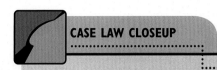

CASE LAW CLOSEUP

RESPONDING TO A SUICIDE THREAT: A COURT VICTORY FOR NURSES—cont'd
While in Richmond Heights General, the patient became increasingly paranoid and delusional, threatening suicide and promising, "I'll do it right this time." One nurse sat at his bedside trying to calm him. The nursing staff discussed restraining him in bed but decided against it, fearing it would make him even more paranoid and agitated. They documented their decision and its rationale.

The patient got out of bed, knocked down the nurse at his bedside, fought his way past two other nurses trying to stop him, and ran off the unit. He then kicked out a third-story window and jumped, fracturing his arm and sustaining other relatively minor injuries. The patient's family sued the nursing staff, hospital, and hospital board of directors, claiming that negligent nursing care had led to his injuries.

How the Court Ruled
The Appellate Court of Ohio ruled that the nurses hadn't been negligent in caring for this patient and weren't legally liable for his injuries. Their actions, the court found, "were fully consistent with basic professional standards of practice for medical-surgical nurses in an acute care hospital. They did not have, nor were they expected to have, specialized psychiatric training and would not be judged as if they did."[2]

The Lesson Learned
This case shows that a nurse who recognizes a patient's potential for suicide and acts appropriately given her expertise and setting has met applicable standards of care. Because the nurses thoroughly documented their actions and rationales, the court found that they understood the severity of the situation and tried to prevent further patient injury in an acceptable manner. This case shows that documenting the "why" of nursing actions is as important as documenting the "what."

---

[2]*Ibid.,* at 562.

the physician and recommendations or instructions from mental health professionals.

Finally, review your facility's policies and procedures on documenting suicidal behavior. Complete an incident report and other required documents. Make sure what you write on these forms agrees with your nurse's notes.

WHEN YOUR PATIENT ACCIDENTALLY INJURES HIMSELF

No matter how many precautions you take to prevent patient injuries, accidents do happen. Some patients who sustain injuries in health care facilities may try to find fault with the care they received, even though their own actions led to the accident. In fact, most legal claims against nurses result from personal injuries to patients. In hospitals, falls, scrapes, cuts, bruises, lacerations, and burns are the most common patient injuries.

When evaluating a personal injury claim, the court focuses on whether care providers took adequate preventive steps and treated the patient promptly and effectively after the injury. Therefore, risk assessment can help prevent injuries, but it's only part of the picture. You also must know how to intervene if an accident occurs and how to document the incident defensively. (See *After the accident: Taking effective notes*, pages 261-262.)

How to Respond

With all patients, assess for physical factors that increase the risk for injury, such as illnesses and injuries that reduce mobility. Keep in mind that elderly patients with reduced mobility are at especially high risk for injury, as are those with vision or hearing impairments, head injuries, orthopedic problems, epilepsy, and developmental disabilities. Also be aware that IV lines, catheters, and some other medical devices limit movement and that a restrained patient may incur an injury if he tries to overcome the restraint.

Next, check for psychological and cognitive risk factors, such as depression, suicidal ideation, impaired problem-solving skills, poor judgment, confusion, and effects of street, over-the-counter, or prescribed drugs.

Then assess for socioeconomic risk factors. For instance, if your patient is illiterate, he may accidentally take an overdose when self-administering a prescribed drug. If he can't afford footwear that provides adequate support and traction, he may easily slip on the floor.

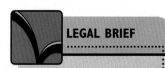

LEGAL BRIEF

AFTER THE ACCIDENT: TAKING EFFECTIVE NOTES

A patient who brings legal action over an accidental injury has the burden of proof. To prove you're responsible for his injury, he must show that he sustained an injury, that nursing standards of care weren't met, that you could have foreseen and prevented the injury, and that your actions or lack of actions caused the injury or resulted in complications from it.

Your documentation will tell the story. Be as accurate and explicit as possible in your notes and all reports you submit. To help protect yourself and your facility, document the items listed below, which are followed by examples.

Patient's condition before accident (include physical and psychological assessments)

1930: Mr. Wilson awake and watching TV. Ambulated back to bed with assistance of one person. Commented on sad story shown on news program. ® leg dressing dry and intact. Call button secured to bed. Side rails elevated, bed in low position.

Events preceding accident

1940: Heard loud thud from room 411. On entering room, found Mr. Wilson on floor next to bed.

Mechanism of injury, as witnessed by you or reported to you by patient or another witness

Patient stated, "I was trying to get to the bathroom and fell."

Patient's response to accident

Patient attempted to stand up as nurse entered room. Expressed anger at having fallen.

Contributing factors or other circumstances

Puddle of liquid noted on floor next to bed. Overturned water pitcher next to puddle.

Patient's condition after accident (include complete physical, psychological, and environmental assessment)

Patient suffered 2-cm superficial skin tear to ® forearm. Blood noted on ® front corner of nightstand. Patient complaining of burning sensation at injury site, denies any other pain. Speech is clear and coherent. No other skin breaks noted. Mr. Wilson can move without restriction or pain. ® leg dressing remains intact.

Continued

LEGAL BRIEF

AFTER THE ACCIDENT: TAKING EFFECTIVE NOTES—cont'd
Your actions in response to accident

> *With Mr. Wilson seated on floor, assessed for other injuries. Assisted patient back to bed. Cleaned ℞ forearm wound with soap and water, patted dry, applied transparent sterile dressing. Call button on bed near ℞ hand.*

Names and credentials of people who witnessed accident or were notified (as appropriate, include their relationship to patient)

> *No one in room with Mr. Wilson at time of fall. After stabilizing patient, notified Dr. Weston and Nancy Brown (nursing supervisor) of incident.*

Preventive measures implemented as result of accident

> *Instructed patient on importance of calling for assistance to ambulate to bathroom. Updated plan of care to reflect need for frequent patient checks to offer assistance to bathroom. Instituted fall prevention protocol.*

Finally, evaluate for religious or cultural customs that could result in injury. If your patient's religion involves incense burning, for example, he could be at risk for burns.

Environmental Assessment. Check for environmental conditions that could lead to an accident. Note whether equipment or furnishings in your patient's environment pose the risk for injury. Environmental hazards include a bedside wheelchair with brakes that aren't engaged or footrests that are extended. (The patient could suffer injury when trying to get into or out of the wheelchair.) A rolling bedside table can lead to injury if your patient uses it to stabilize himself when getting up.

Hot foods, cigarettes, eating utensils, nail trimmers, razors, curling irons, and scissors may injure a patient with reduced mobility. Your patient with a psychological or cognitive dysfunction may be injured if flowers, potted plants, glassware, or objects with sharp edges are left within reach.

Postaccident Interventions. You can't predict or prevent every accident, but your interventions after an accident can affect the ultimate outcome. If your patient injures himself, treat the injury as if it could be life-threatening, no matter how minor it seems. Begin by checking his airway, breathing, and circulation (ABCs). If necessary, start cardiopulmonary resuscitation and have someone call for help.

Once the patient's ABCs are stabilized, perform a rapid head-to-toe assessment, moving the patient only if necessary. Determine whether he's in pain. If he can't speak or comprehend what you're saying, look for nonverbal signs of pain. Then thoroughly assess for skin breaks and other objective signs of injury, such as bruising or deformity of a body part.

Find out whether the patient's cognitive status has changed since the previous assessment. Then evaluate the immediate environment for the possible cause of the injury. Make a mental note of the patient's position when you found him and the condition and location of devices in use at the time of the accident. Also note the placement of furniture and other large objects.

If the injury occurred in the patient's room, check the bed rails, bed height, and call button location. Inspect the condition of the floor, room lighting, and the status of safety devices in use. But don't disturb anything in the immediate accident area unless it interferes with your ability to provide immediate care. Otherwise, your notes may not match your colleagues' and nurse administrator's documentation, which could cause problems during a formal investigation.

Subsequent actions depend on the severity of the patient's injury. If you're sure it's safe to move him or if a physician gives permission, assist him to a chair or back to bed, as appropriate. Make sure he's comfortable and address his immediate needs and concerns. Place the call button within his reach, and tell him to use it if he experiences new symptoms or if a preexisting symptom worsens.

Notify the patient's physician, if you haven't already done so, along with the appropriate nurse administrator and your facility's risk manager. Then carry out their instructions.

Next, inform the patient's family or legal guardian of the accident and the actions you've taken. Limit your discussion to the facts. Don't speculate on the possible cause of the accident.

If you suspect that your actions or those of another staff member caused or contributed to the accident, don't admit this to anyone except the physician, appropriate nurse administrator, legal counsel, or risk manager.

For the next 48 hours, increase the frequency and intensity of your assessments to detect injury complications. Remember: an injury that seems minor at first may lead to extensive damage if complications occur. For example, a superficial scratch or paper cut on a finger can lead to a serious infection—and ultimately amputation—unless treated promptly.

To prevent recurrence of the accident, provide patient teaching as needed. Convey caring, trust, and respect when interacting with the patient. This may reduce the chance that he'll initiate a lawsuit.

What to Document

Document the following information after a patient injury:
- assessment findings before and after the accident
- events immediately preceding the accident
- mechanism of injury
- patient's response to the accident
- factors that contributed to the accident
- actions you took in response to the accident
- names and credentials of people who witnessed or were notified of the accident
- measures taken to prevent a recurrence
- measures you implemented to prevent the accident from recurring

For each of these items, provide complete details. Keep in mind that if the accident results in a lawsuit, the court will look for deviations from the standard of care before, during, and after the injury. (See *How documentation prevents liability in accidental injury cases,* pages 265-266.)

Also complete an incident report according to your facility's protocol, and submit it to the appropriate nurse administrator. If you performed special interventions to deal with your patient's injury or risk for injury, inform other staff members of them. Post signs at the bedside describing safety instructions to follow, such as keeping the bed in a low position.

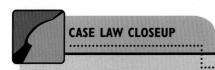

CASE LAW CLOSEUP

HOW DOCUMENTATION PREVENTS LIABILITY IN ACCIDENTAL INJURY CASES
When a patient accidentally injures herself, your care of her before, during, and after the incident can reduce your liability. So can your documentation of that care, as you'll see in the following case.

Understanding the Case
Curtis v. Columbia Doctors' Hospital of Opelousas[1] reveals the importance of documentation related to self-injury when a patient takes matters into her own hands instead of relying on her nurses. Ten days after total knee replacement surgery, Mrs. Curtis fell and reinjured her knee while in the rehabilitation unit of the hospital. She immediately received corrective surgery, but then developed an infection and other complications that required additional surgery and hospitalization. She sued the hospital and nursing staff for negligence, claiming that they failed to use her side rails and allowed her to roll out of bed and fall.

For 6 days before the patient's fall, nurse's notes indicated that she was fully aware of the need to call and wait for assistance when ambulating. The notes further documented that Mrs. Curtis understood the safety teaching that the nurses frequently reminded her of. This was evidence by the fact that she regularly used the call bell to summon assistance, received assistance when ambulating, and didn't try to get out of bed and use the bathroom by herself.

Written at 10:00 and 11:00 P.M., the last nurse's notes before Mrs. Curtis' fall showed arrows pointing up, indicating the side rail position. The nurse who came upon the patient documented that Mrs. Curtis was found on the floor near the bathroom door, about 6 or 7 feet from the bed.

How the Court Ruled
The court acknowledged that the nursing staff would have been guilty of negligence if they had kept the side rails down and let the patient roll out of bed and fall, but it ruled that those actions didn't happen in this case. The nurse's notes clearly demonstrated that the side rails were up and that Mrs. Curtis was closer to the bathroom than her bed. These facts allowed only one conclusion: The patient had attempted to get up and use the bathroom by herself.

The court further noted that nursing negligence does not exist when a patient has the capacity to know better, has been taught to know better, understands her limitations, knows that she must ask nurses for assistance, and knows that she will receive assistance if requested, but nevertheless tries to do something by herself that results in injury.

---

[1]*Curtis v. Columbia Doctors' Hospital of Opelousas, 2003 WL 22961359 (La. App., December 17, 2003)*

Continued

CASE LAW CLOSEUP

HOW DOCUMENTATION PREVENTS LIABILITY IN ACCIDENTAL INJURY CASES—cont'd
The lesson learned
This case illuminates the need for nurses to document various points. Based on the nurse's notes, the court recognized that the nurses regularly reinforced Mrs. Curtis' education about the need to ask and wait for assistance with ambulating. On these points, the notes validated her comprehension of their teaching: she regularly used the call bell and waited for assistance and did not attempt to use the bathroom by herself.

The documentation also showed that the side rails were up. Remember that the court doesn't care whether this type of information is recorded on a checklist or written longhand in nurse's notes. The mere fact that it was documented is the critical factor.

Finally, the nurse's notes recorded exactly where the patient was found after she fell. If Mrs. Curtis had rolled out of bed as she contended, she would have been close to the bed—not several feet away.

WHEN YOUR PATIENT IS CAUGHT SMOKING

Despite the health risks associated with smoking, some patients want to smoke in the health care facility. The uncertainty and unfamiliarity of hospitalization may intensify this urge. If your patient smokes, your duty to protect her rights may conflict with your duty to safeguard her well-being.

Most health care facilities prohibit smoking or restrict it to designated areas. Besides jeopardizing the patient's health, smoking puts other patients, facility employees, and visitors at risk from secondhand smoke. Smoking may also lead to an explosion if it occurs near high-concentration oxygen, such as that delivered by nasal cannula or mask. Or it may start a fire accidentally if the patient drops a cigarette or partially extinguishes one. Cigarette smoke can even trigger an asthma attack in a susceptible person nearby.

If a smoking-related accident occurs, a patient who smokes even though she knows it's prohibited may be held responsible for contributory negligence. (See *Understanding contributory and comparative negligence*, page 268.) If you permit a cognitively impaired patient to smoke, you and your facility could share the blame.

How to Respond

Discuss your facility's smoking policy with the patient on admission and reinforce it in writing. If your facility has smoking areas, review the smoking areas, restrictions, and guidelines with her. Ensure that these areas are clearly marked and that "No smoking" signs are posted on doors and above beds of patients who are receiving oxygen. Also make sure that the smoking guidelines are posted in a clearly visible location on the floor or unit.

Then assess your patient's cognitive and neurologic status to determine whether she can smoke unsupervised. Ask the physician to record the number of cigarettes permitted and the amount of supervision required.

If you find your patient smoking in a no-smoking area, calmly remind her of facility policy and guidelines. Explain that for everyone's safety, she may smoke only in designated areas. Provide a safe way to extinguish her cigarette, and offer to escort her to the smoking area. If she has difficulty walking, plan to have someone take her to a smoking area at prearranged times of day.

Also counsel her to stop smoking, and provide information on options and resources for smoking cessation. If she decides she can't stop at this time, be supportive. Otherwise, you may alienate her and discourage her from turning to you for support when she's ready to quit.

If Your Facility Prohibits Smoking. A patient may become upset and angry when she learns that cigarette smoking is not permitted anywhere in the facility. Especially if she's had serious health problems, she may see the no-smoking policy as one more aspect of her life that she can't control.

LEGAL BRIEF

UNDERSTANDING CONTRIBUTORY AND COMPARATIVE NEGLIGENCE
If your patient's actions lead to her injuries, she may not be able to win a lawsuit against the health care facility or its employees. For example, a patient who smokes in a health care facility although she knows it's not permitted may fail to recover damages if she sues over a resulting injury.

Contributory Negligence
In some jurisdictions, the patient can be held at least partly responsible for injuring herself under the doctrine of contributory negligence. A health care facility or provider may assert contributory negligence as a defense if the patient knowingly and willfully failed to follow the physician's orders, such as by getting out of bed without an attendant, lowering the side rails, or refusing prescribed drugs. When this defense is used, the court considers the circumstances and the patient's mental status.

Comparative Negligence
Because contributory negligence usually bars the patient from recovering damages, other jurisdictions use comparative negligence when the patient and defendant share negligence. After comparing the negligence of the plaintiff and defendant, the court awards damages to the plaintiff based on the relative degree of negligence it finds.

Explain the reasons behind the no-smoking policy, and explore the patient's options. If appropriate, escort her outside the building to smoke. Discuss the possibility of stopping smoking, and offer to talk to the physician about nicotine replacement therapy.

If Your Patient Has a Cognitive or Neurologic Impairment. Smoking poses added dangers for a patient with a cognitive or neurologic impairment. If you believe that your patient can't smoke safely unless supervised, discuss your concerns with the physician. If the physician agrees, talk to the patient and her family about your concerns and use their responses and ideas to develop a plan of action. For instance, consider making a contract with the patient to provide supervised smoking periods at designated times if she lets you keep her cigarettes.

What to Document

Record the instructions you gave the patient on admission about the facility's smoking policy. When obtaining the patient's health history, document her usual pattern of tobacco use and your discussion with her about stopping smoking.

If you find your patient smoking in a no-smoking area or anywhere in a no-smoking facility, record:

- when and where you found her smoking
- your notification of the physician
- your explanation of the facility's policy
- your instruction on the dangers of smoking and discussion of smoking-cessation options
- the patient's response to your teaching
- the plan of action you develop with her

In the nursing plan of care, include the contract you and the patient made so that other caregivers can use a consistent approach. If the patient agrees to consider quitting smoking, document your suggestions on quitting and your teaching about signs and symptoms of nicotine withdrawal.

If the physician orders nicotine replacement therapy, record the instructions you provided concerning nicotine patches, gum, or spray and the adverse effects of nicotine replacement therapy. Document that you taught the patient which signs and symptoms to report and that you reviewed the dangers of smoking during nicotine replacement therapy. Finally, record the names of smoking-cessation programs and support groups to which you referred her.

WHEN YOUR PATIENT HAS CONTRABAND

A patient with an unlicensed weapon, street drugs, or other illegal or prohibited items poses a danger to himself, staff members, and other patients. Alcohol is usually considered contraband unless the physician prescribes it for the patient's medical use.

Unless the contraband is in plain view or the patient tells you he has it, stop and think before you search his person or belongings. Remember that you have no authority, right, or responsibility to conduct such a search without his permission—unless you believe that he might use the contraband to harm himself.

How to Respond

Review your facility's policy on contraband possession. If your facility has no policy, speak to the appropriate nurse administrator and risk manager about developing one. All personnel should use a consistent approach so that patients know that contraband is forbidden under all circumstances.

If you work on a unit in which some patients are more likely to have contraband, such as a psychiatric or drug rehabilitation unit, explain the rules about contraband on admission, and state exactly which items are forbidden. If your patient is allowed to leave the facility on a pass, remind him of the unit's rules each time he leaves and returns. That way, he's more likely to hand over the contraband to you.

Dealing with Street Drugs and Alcohol. If you discover street drugs or alcohol, tell your patient that the substance isn't permitted in the facility and must be disposed of or sent home. Don't try to take it from him because he may become violent if he feels threatened by your actions.

If the patient refuses to dispose of or hand over the contraband, notify the physician, your nurse administrator, and the facility's security department. They'll reinforce what you've told the patient and offer him the choice of handing over the contraband or leaving the facility.

Dealing with Weapons. If you believe that your patient has a weapon, notify the security department immediately. If you've established a rapport with the patient, accompany the security guard when he talks with the patient. Otherwise, stay away and allow the guard to handle the matter.

The security guard may confiscate the weapon. If the patient or a family member can produce a weapon permit, the guard may give the weapon to the family member to take home. Otherwise, the police should be contacted and the weapon turned over to them. (See *Preserving the chain of custody*.) If your patient refuses to relinquish the weapon, an appropriate staff member, such as the physician or a security guard, should tell him to leave the facility.

What to Document

Document that your patient received instructions about the facility's contraband policy on admission or at another appropriate time. If your facility asks patients to sign a form acknowledging awareness of these rules, place a copy of the signed form in the patient's medical record.

If you find a substance that you suspect to be contraband on your patient or in his room, fully document the situation, including the circumstances of your discovery. If the item was in a closed drawer or under his clothing, explain how you found it. If you searched your patient's belongings because you suspected that he might harm himself, document this action and the rationale for your suspicion.

Describe the substance objectively. For instance, write "loose white powder" or "clear, brown liquid" rather than "cocaine" or "Scotch." Remember—you don't know for sure what the

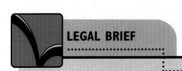

LEGAL BRIEF

PRESERVING THE CHAIN OF CUSTODY

If you've notified the police that your patient has contraband, you'll need to maintain the chain of custody—proper possession of the evidence—in case it becomes legal evidence. To show that evidence hasn't been lost or tainted, the police must indicate the chain of custody from the time the evidence is discovered until the defendant's trial. A break in the chain could cause the court to rule that the evidence has been tampered with and can't be used against the defendant.

To preserve the chain of custody, note everything that occurs to the contraband. Record the names of all people who have had contact with it from its discovery until the police arrive to inspect it. If anyone handles it, record this action and the time. Also document the name of the police officer who removes the contraband from the health care facility.

substance is until it's been tested. If the patient tells you what it is, state in your notes that he has named it.

Record your conversation with him about the contraband, using direct quotes to document his words. If he let you dispose of it, document the measures you took, including the name of the staff member who witnessed the disposal. Record the full names of security guards involved and explain their roles. Also document your communications with your nurse administrator and the physician. Record their names, the times and content of your discussions, their instructions, and your actions.

Then complete an incident report as indicated by facility policy. If the police were involved, attach a copy of the police report to the patient's medical record.

WHEN YOUR PATIENT TAMPERS WITH MEDICAL EQUIPMENT

Whether accidental or deliberate, tampering with medical equipment can cause a catastrophe. For example, a patient who alters her IV pump settings may stop receiving a prescribed drug or experience a lethal overdose. One who manipulates the stopcocks on a pulmonary artery catheter or twists a central line's IV tubing connection may experience an air embolism or exsanguination. A patient who disconnects the suction tubing from a drain may develop an infection, a hematoma, or internal fluid accumulation.

Patients tamper with medical equipment for various reasons and are seldom aware of the possible consequences. A child may play with equipment out of curiosity, especially if it blinks or beeps. An adult may tinker with a medical device to see how it works. A confused patient may tamper with equipment if it bothers her or if she thinks that manipulating it will somehow adjust the room temperature, change the lighting, or call the nurse.

A patient who suffers an injury because of altered equipment performance may claim negligence by health care workers, even though her actions contributed to the injury. In many states, however, the doctrine of contributory negligence applies, and the patient doesn't recover damages. (See *Understanding contributory and comparative negligence*, page 268.) Your documentation must show that you took steps to correct the problem, prevent patient injury, and avoid a recurrence.

How to Respond

Before your patient has a chance to tamper with medical equipment, teach her about the equipment's purpose and stress the importance of not touching it. Whenever possible, place the equipment out of her reach, especially if she's a child or confused.

If you discover that your patient has tampered with the equipment, assess her for changes and correct the equipment problem. If necessary, notify the physician immediately, and prepare to carry out urgent treatment instructions. For instance, if your patient received a higher-than-prescribed dose of potassium, the physician may order blood tests immediately and prescribe a drug to lower her serum potassium level.

Then discuss the incident with the patient. Reinforce the importance of not touching the equipment. If you suspect that she intended to harm herself, notify the physician and request a psychiatric consultation. Reposition the equipment to limit her access. If possible, place a shield over the display buttons or dials so she can't change the settings.

If your patient is confused, your instructions probably won't prevent a recurrence. Depending on the potential danger and the equipment's location, you may need to restrain her. Before doing so, obtain a physician's order. When applying restraints, be sure to follow facility policy. (See *When your patient must be restrained,* pages 244-251.)

With a pediatric patient, try simple diversion by offering an age-appropriate electronic game, a toy that beeps or blinks, a coloring book and crayons, or a TV program.

What to Document

No matter how minor the incident, always document equipment tampering in case complications arise or the incident becomes part of a behavior pattern. Document exactly how you discovered the tampering. Record only your observations, not your assumptions. For instance, if you didn't see the patient change her IV pump settings, state that you discovered the settings were different from those recorded. If the patient admits she changed the settings or if you saw her touch the equipment, document this.

TIPS & ADVICE

CUSTOMIZING A FLOW SHEET

Besides tables for recording dates, times, and interventions, most flow sheets provide several blank lines for writing interventions specific to your patient's care. This lets you customize the flow sheet to address such problems as a patient's potential for tampering with medical equipment.

Simply write in the topic you want to address on the blank line. Depending on facility guidelines, you may insert a yes-or-no phrase that requires caregivers to place a checkmark next to the action carried out. For instance, they would check the box next to "IV pump out of reach" to verify that they took this action. Or you may insert a phrase that requires recording of specific information. For example, next to "Placement of IV pump," caregivers would record exactly where they placed the pump to prevent the patient from tampering with it. The sample below uses this format.

PATIENT: Amy Myerson			
DATE: March 23, 2006	**2300 - 0700**	**0700 - 1500**	**1500 - 2300**
IV THERAPY Tubing change	None. BW	None. KS	1900. RS
Dressing change	None. BW	None. KS	1900. RS
Site appearance	No edema or redness. 2330. BW	No drainage, no edema, no redness. 1300. KS	No redness, no edem 1900. RS
Placement of IV pump	Out of reach Ⓛ side bed. 2330. BW	Out of reach Ⓛ side bed. 1300. KS	Out of reach Ⓛ side bed. 1900. RS

Also record your assessment findings. If you notified the physician of changes in your patient's condition, document the physician's name, time of notification, instructions received, your interventions, and the patient's response.

Then document the measures you took to prevent a recurrence of tampering. As appropriate, note that you discussed tampering with the patient, repositioned equipment, and took other steps. Document the incident in the nursing plan of care to inform all staff members.

When recording your patient's routine care on a flow sheet, also document interventions to prevent equipment tampering. This reminds other nurses who care for the patient to address this potential problem. (See *Customizing a flow sheet.*) Finally, if your patient experienced an adverse outcome from equipment tampering, complete an incident report according to your facility's policy.

WHEN YOUR PATIENT HIDES HIS DRUGS

Your patient may hide his prescribed drug if he thinks that he doesn't need it or believes that it's doing more harm than good. If he's receiving a narcotic, he may hide daytime doses so that he can take a larger dose at bedtime to help him sleep. A depressed patient may stockpile drugs for a suicide attempt.

Whatever the reason, hiding drugs is a problem for you as well as your patient. Unless he has impaired cognition, it may indicate that you haven't communicated with him effectively about the importance of taking the drug as prescribed.

How to Respond

If you discover hidden drugs, broach the topic with your patient by stating that you've noticed he hasn't been taking his drugs as prescribed. Then ask whether he has a problem with the drugs, and tell him you'd like to help him solve it. As you speak with him, assess his cognitive status and evaluate his statements for logical progression. Document your discussion and assessment findings, placing quotation marks around the patient's words. Then notify the physician of the patient's behavior, and document the time of notification and the physician's instructions.

If Your Patient Is in Pain. If you suspect that your patient is saving narcotic doses for nighttime pain relief, discuss this with him or consult a pain-management nurse. If necessary, consult the physician about adjusting the drug schedule so that the patient receives additional doses at night.

If Your Patient Lacks Knowledge. If your patient says that he doesn't need the drug or thinks that he should take it only when he doesn't feel well, reinforce your teaching about the drug's purpose. If he's still reluctant to take it as scheduled, explore the issue further to elicit other fears or concerns.

If Your Patient Cites Scheduling Problems. If your patient says that the drug interferes with his daily schedule, consider strategies for adapting his dosing schedule to his lifestyle. For instance, if he doesn't want to take a second dose of a diuretic at 6 P.M. because it makes him urinate at night, talk to the physician about adjusting the timing of doses to avoid nocturia.

If Your Patient Fears Drug Effects. If your patient tells you that he's afraid to take a drug, determine whether his fear is reality-based. If he says his best friend got sick or died after taking the same drug, his fear is realistic. If he refuses to take the drug because he believes that the physician wants to poison him, his fear is unfounded.

If the patient has a realistic fear, provide teaching to help him overcome it, including statistical information on the drug's safety from clinical trials, if appropriate. Teach him the signs and symptoms of adverse effects and what to do if they occur.

If the patient's fear isn't realistic, discuss with the physician ways to ensure that he receives the correct dose. After administering each scheduled dose, ask him to open his mouth so that you can check under his tongue. If appropriate, ask the doctor to substitute a liquid drug form because it's easier to verify that the patient swallowed a liquid. Convey your plan to all caregivers involved in his drug therapy.

If You Suspect that Your Patient Is Suicidal. If you suspect that your patient is stockpiling drugs for a suicide attempt, take suicide precautions and notify the physician as soon as possible. (See *When your patient threatens suicide,* pages 254-259.) Stay with the patient until help arrives. If possible, keep him talking and listen empathetically.

When you leave his room, take the stockpiled drugs with you. Count the tablets or capsules and identify them. If you're not sure what they are, have the pharmacist identify them. Then store them or remove them from your unit according to your facility's policy. Don't recycle them for future doses. Tell the physician how many tablets or capsules the patient stockpiled so that the physician knows how many doses of which drugs the patient missed.

What to Document

If you find hidden drugs, document the situation in detail. Record the drug's name and the number of hidden tablets or capsules you found. Note the circumstances of your discovery. If the drugs were in a closed drawer or under clothing, explain how you found them to defend against possible charges that you invaded the patient's privacy or conducted an unreasonable search. (See *When your patient has contraband,* pages 269-272.) If you searched his belongings because you suspected that he might harm himself, state this in your documentation and provide supporting data.

Also record your discussion with the patient about the hidden drugs and his explanation for hiding them. Use direct quotes when recording his words. Document your assessment of his cognitive status. Record your teaching about the drugs and his response.

If you believe that the patient was stockpiling drugs for a suicide attempt, record the actions you took to ensure his safety. Also document that you notified the physician, and record the time of notification, the physician's instructions, and your interventions. Describe the incident in the nursing plan of care and flag the medication administration record to alert other caregivers who administer drugs to the patient.

WHEN YOUR PATIENT REMOVES HER ENDOTRACHEAL TUBE

An endotracheal (ET) tube is used to provide a means for mechanical ventilation or to prevent airway blockage caused by edema. A patient whose gas exchange depends on an ET tube may die immediately from respiratory compromise if she pulls out the tube. Or she may suffer severe laryngeal or vocal chord damage if she removes the tube with the cuff inflated. You must record this life-threatening emergency clearly and thoroughly to show that you took appropriate action to stabilize and treat the patient. (See *Doting on details*.)

How to Respond

If you discover your patient has pulled out her ET tube, call for help immediately and assess for signs of respiratory distress, such as wheezing, bilateral air exchange, cyanosis, use of accessory breathing muscles, decreased level of consciousness, and tachycardia. Record your findings as soon as time allows.

TIPS & ADVICE

DOTING ON DETAILS
Thorough, accurate documentation of a challenging patient situation may be your only protection against a finding of negligence. Sketchy documentation—especially when your patient's condition has deteriorated—can hurt you in court. The physician could claim that you didn't provide adequate details of an emergency or notify him in a timely manner to prevent irreversible complications.

If your patient pulls out her endotracheal tube, for instance, be sure to record every detail you reported to the physician initially. Depending on your assessment findings, you may need to document your patient's breathing difficulty as shown by use of accessory breathing muscles, a rapid respiratory rate, or a decreasing pulse oximetry reading. Also record the physician's name, the time you notified him, his instructions, and your actions.

If the patient is connected to a pulse oximeter, compare the current reading with previous readings. If her pulse oximetry level falls below 92%, notify the physician at once. As ordered, start supplemental oxygen by face mask at a liter flow comparable to what she was getting through the ET tube. Continue to assess her for respiratory distress, and compare her pulse rate with baseline.

If Your Patient Is in Severe Respiratory Distress. If the patient shows signs of severe respiratory distress, such as periods of apnea and cyanosis, manually ventilate her using a handheld resuscitation bag with a face mask and 100% oxygen. Extend her neck and deliver 12 breaths per minute (for an adult). Call for help and have someone notify the physician immediately. Monitor the patient's heart rate and note bradycardia, which may indicate severe hypoxia and can progress to cardiac arrest. Calmly tell her what you're doing, and explain that the physician will insert a new tube to help her breathe more easily.

Have a coworker bring emergency equipment to the room. When the physician arrives, help him position the patient for reintubation. After he inserts a new ET tube, inflate the cuff and auscultate breath sounds in both lungs. Note the centimeter marking where the ET tube meets the patient's lips (or her nose for nasal intubation), and then secure the tube with tape. Next, arrange for a chest x-ray to be taken at the bedside. If necessary, obtain a physician's order for wrist restraints. Following facility policy, apply the restraints so that the patient can't pull out the ET tube again.

If Your Patient Isn't in Respiratory Distress. If your patient displays no signs of respiratory distress, she may not need to be reintubated. Obtain an order for oxygen by face mask or nasal cannula. Make sure that the physician evaluates the patient. Then check her respiratory status every 15 minutes for the next few hours. Monitor her continuous pulse oximetry readings and review her arterial blood gas analysis results, as appropriate.

If the patient progresses to respiratory distress, notify the physician and prepare for reintubation. If her vital signs, pulse oximetry readings, and respiratory status remain stable, maintain supplemental oxygen as prescribed and monitor her respiratory status as appropriate.

What to Document

Record your assessment findings and interventions from the time you discovered that your patient removed her ET tube. Document how you learned of the incident, such as by hearing an alarm or witnessing the patient's action. Record your observations of her respiratory status and document her vital sign measurements and pulse oximetry readings. Also document that you called for help (noting the time of your call), initiated oxygen therapy, or provided manual ventilation.

If the patient is reintubated, record the following:

- name of the physician who performed the procedure
- size of the new ET tube
- centimeter marking where the ET tube meets the patient's lips (or nose for nasal intubation)
- method used to secure the tube
- oxygen administration through the ET tube, including the flow rate and delivery device
- patient's tolerance of the procedure
- time the chest x-ray was taken
- chest x-ray results and the name of the physician you reported them to
- use of restraints, if appropriate

WHEN YOUR PATIENT REMOVES HIS CHEST TUBE

A chest tube is usually inserted into the pleural cavity to remove air (from a pneumothorax) or blood (from a hemothorax). If your patient pulls out his chest tube, air or blood may enter the pleural space, leading to lung deflation that could cause fatal respiratory compromise. Also, tube removal at the wrong angle can damage underlying tissue.

To minimize patient injury during this life-threatening emergency, you must respond quickly and document the situation thoroughly. If your patient is injured, your documentation must show that you took every possible step to prevent a catastrophic outcome.

How to Respond

Call for help and notify the physician immediately. Apply pressure over the tube's insertion site with sterile petroleum gauze covered by a sterile gauze dressing. Securely tape the dressing in place. As ordered, administer oxygen.

Next, assess the patient for respiratory distress. Check for bilateral air exchange (because exchange on the side of a pneumothorax or hemothorax is poor) and for the use of accessory breathing muscles. If the patient is connected to a pulse oximeter, compare his current reading with previous readings. Also compare his pulse rate with the baseline measurements. In a calm, reassuring tone, explain to him everything you're doing.

If Your Patient Develops Respiratory Distress. If your patient is in respiratory distress—for example, if his pulse oximetry reading drops below 92%, his heart rate increases, and he becomes cyanotic—have someone call the physician right away. As ordered, administer oxygen. To prepare for chest tube reinsertion, ask another staff member to bring a chest tube tray and another sterile chest tube to the bedside. If a chest tube tray isn't available, have an assistant gather sterile drapes, sterile gloves, a local anesthetic with syringe, suture material, povidone-iodine sponges, and sterile dressing supplies, including petroleum gauze.

When the physician arrives, note the time and help him position the patient and establish the sterile field. Continue to talk to the patient calmly. The physician will clean the area, inject a local anesthetic, and reinsert the chest tube. As instructed, connect the tube to water-seal drainage or a water-seal suction device. Note the centimeter marking where the tube enters the skin. Apply a sterile dressing, and place the petroleum gauze under sterile gauze pads. Then apply nonporous tape over the insertion site to prevent air entry.

Next, arrange for a chest x-ray to be taken at the patient's bedside. Evaluate the need for wrist restraints to prevent him from removing the chest tube again. If indicated, obtain an order for restraints, and apply restraints according to facility policy.

If Your Patient Isn't in Respiratory Distress. If your patient displays no signs of respiratory distress, the chest tube may not need to be reinserted. The physician will order a chest x-ray to check lung expansion and to detect blood accumulation in the pleural space. When deciding whether or not to reinsert the chest tube, the physician considers the patient's respiratory status and x-ray findings. If the insertion site is painful, administer an analgesic, as prescribed.

What to Document

Record your assessment findings and interventions from the time you discovered that the chest tube was removed. Document how you learned of the incident, such as by finding the tube in the patient's bed or seeing him pull it out. Record your assessment of his respiratory status and document his vital sign measurements and pulse oximetry readings.

Describe other actions you took, including summoning help, applying an occlusive dressing, and initiating oxygen therapy. Be sure to note the time of each action. Also document the name of the physician you notified, the time of notification, and his instructions. If the chest tube was reinserted, document the following:
- name of the physician who reinserted it
- chest tube size
- centimeter marking where the tube meets the patient's skin
- use of a petroleum gauze dressing over the insertion site
- type of drainage or suction device in use
- patient's tolerance of the procedure
- time the chest x-ray was taken
- chest x-ray results and the name of the physician you reported them to
- use of restraints, if appropriate

After writing your notes, review them closely for misleading statements. (See *Did you write what you meant?*)

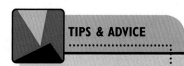

TIPS & ADVICE

DID YOU WRITE WHAT YOU MEANT?
When you write a nurse's note, your thoughts may get ahead of your pen—especially when you document an urgent situation. Before you start writing, gather your thoughts. If your thoughts run together, use several short sentences rather than a long one. After writing your notes, review them. Do they say what you want them to say? If not, they may mislead the reader. Here are examples of misleading notes:

Patient evaluated by physician at bedside, who was short of breath and using abdominal muscles to breathe.
This statement indicates that the physician, not the patient, was short of breath.

Physician inserted #22 Fr. chest tube after anesthetizing with lidocaine.
This note implies that the physician anesthetized the chest tube, not the patient.

Dressing applied with petroleum gauze and water-seal with 20-cm suction.
This statement indicates that the dressing was applied with water-seal suction.

WHEN YOUR PATIENT SPEAKS A DIFFERENT LANGUAGE

For a non-English-speaking patient, being hospitalized can be frightening. The patient knows that people are talking about her, but she can't understand what they're saying. They may touch her, give her drugs, or insert tubes into her, but she doesn't understand why. Worst of all, she can't ask them what they're doing or tell them if they're hurting her.

Caregivers are at a disadvantage too. The inability to speak a patient's language can impede every aspect of your care. You can't obtain her health history, elicit descriptions of symptoms, or receive feedback to evaluate treatment effectiveness. What's more, you can't teach her about her illness or self-care.

A language barrier can also prevent the physician from obtaining informed consent. To give consent, the patient must receive information about the proposed treatment or procedure in a language she understands.

How to Respond

If possible, arrange for an interpreter. If an accompanying family member speaks English, find out whether this person is willing to act as interpreter. Then, with this person present, make sure the patient agrees to having him act as interpreter. If your patient is alone or doesn't want to give sensitive health information to a family member, locate a staff member who speaks your patient's language by consulting your facility's list of employees fluent in other languages. (See *When an interpreter isn't available.*)

To communicate with a patient about commonly requested items, use a picture board or flash cards. Through the interpreter, explain to the patient what each picture on the board means, and instruct her to point to the picture that indicates her needs. For instance, tell her to point to the picture of a toilet if she needs to go to the bathroom or to the picture of the syringe if she needs an analgesic. If the board has a clock picture, change the position of the clock's hands to show what time a procedure or care activity will be done.

If you're using flash cards, write the English word or phrase on one side of the card and have the interpreter write the word or phrase in the patient's language on the other side. Then instruct the patient to use the appropriate card to indicate her needs.

Post notices in the patient's medical record and room identifying her language

••••••••••••••••••••••••••••••
DID YOU KNOW?

WHEN AN INTERPRETER ISN'T AVAILABLE

If an interpreter isn't available when you need one, your medical dictionary may come to the rescue. Some dictionaries, such as *Mosby's Medical, Nursing, and Allied Health Dictionary*, 6th ed., and *Taber's Cyclopedic Medical Dictionary*, 17th ed., contain a section that lists commonly used medical terms and phrases in English and other languages, such as French, German, Italian, and Spanish.

If your unit doesn't have such a dictionary, talk with the appropriate nurse administrator about buying one. Or if your unit cares for many patients who all speak the same non-English language, consider investing in a medical phrase book specifically for that language.

and the communication method she's using, such as a picture board or flash cards. This will help other health care team members communicate with her.

What to Document

In the patient's medical record, nursing plan of care, and your nurse's notes, indicate the language she speaks. Document in your notes the steps you took to arrange for an interpreter. Write the names of available interpreters and their telephone numbers on the front of the record. If you're using a picture board or flash cards, document instructions for using this communication method in the nursing plan of care.

If you used an interpreter to obtain the patient's consent, record the interpreter's name in your nurse's notes and on the consent form. If a family member acted as interpreter, document that the patient agreed to this.

WHEN YOUR PATIENT HAS A HEARING IMPAIRMENT

A hearing impairment can range from a slight hearing loss to profound deafness. Depending on the impairment's severity, your patient may be unable to communicate his needs, relate his health history, and describe his symptoms. Even if he can speak clearly, read lips, or use sign language, his hearing impairment calls for extra steps in your nursing care.

A hearing impairment also may interfere with informed consent. The health care team may need to give the patient extensive written information or use a sign language interpreter to convey the information he needs to consent to treatment.

How to Respond

First, determine the severity of your patient's hearing impairment, and find out whether he uses a hearing aid, reads lips, or knows sign language. If he's profoundly deaf, find out whether he's also mute.

Ask the patient's family what methods they use to communicate with him. Suggest that a family member act as interpreter, if the patient agrees. If the patient knows sign language, obtain a sign language interpreter.

Always enter your patient's room within his line of sight so that he knows you're there. If you can't position yourself where he can see you, gently tap him on the shoulder. Keep a pen and pad at his bedside so that you can communicate in writing, if necessary.

If Your Patient Reads Lips. When speaking, face a lip-reading patient directly, and avoid placing your hand or some other object in front of your mouth. Don't speak more slowly than usual because this changes your lip movements, making it harder for him to lip-read. If you're using an interpreter or other third party, face the patient even when talking to the other person so that the patient can understand what you're saying.

Tell the patient to make a note on the bedside pad when he doesn't understand you. Tell a mute patient to write answers to your questions on the pad.

If Your Patient Doesn't Read Lips. As appropriate, communicate with your patient in sign language or in writing if he doesn't read lips. If he has difficulty writing, consider using a picture board. Through an interpreter, tell him what each picture on the board means, and ask him to point to the appropriate picture to indicate his needs. For instance, tell him to point to the picture of a toilet if he needs to go to the bathroom or to the picture of the syringe if he needs an analgesic. If the board has a clock picture, change the position of the clock's hands to show what time a procedure or care activity will be done.

You may use flash cards with common terms instead of a picture board. Instruct the patient to indicate his needs by showing the appropriate card. Also consider trying an alphabet board so the patient can spell out his thoughts or requests.

If Your Patient Has a Hearing Aid. Make sure the patient wears his hearing aid when you teach him about his care. Then incorporate hearing aid care into routine care. (See *Where to document your patient's hearing aid*.) Check the hearing aid's batteries and obtain new ones, if necessary. Post signs at his bedside and on the door so other caregivers know he has a hearing aid.

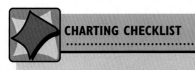

CHARTING CHECKLIST

WHERE TO DOCUMENT YOUR PATIENT'S HEARING AID
If your patient uses a hearing aid, document this on his medical record and on other appropriate forms your facility uses. The list below tells where to document each aspect of his hearing aid use.

❑ Health history
  • Duration of hearing aid use

❑ Initial assessment form
  • Hearing aid's location (left or right ear)
  • Patient's ability or inability to hear words at a normal volume when wearing the hearing aid

❑ Belongings list
  • Hearing aid's size, model, and type (such as over-the-ear or in-the-ear)

❑ Consent form
  • Patient's use of the hearing aid when the physician explained the procedure and obtained consent

❑ Preoperative checklist
  • Hearing aid removal before the patient entered the operating room
  • Hearing aid's location after removal

❑ Routine morning care (nurse's notes)
  • Offer of the hearing aid to the patient or your insertion of it for him

❑ Routine evening care (nurse's notes)
  • Removal of the hearing aid
  • Hearing aid's location after removal

❑ Patient teaching plan
  • Instruction to other caregivers to make sure the patient wears the hearing aid during teaching sessions

❑ Discharge notes
  • Patient's departure from the health care facility with hearing aid

Remember that many patients with a hearing aid also read lips, so be sure to face your patient when talking to him. Minimize extraneous noise because a hearing aid conveys all sounds equally. Machine noise or a nearby conversation may prevent him from hearing you.

What to Document

Document the patient's hearing impairment in his medical record, in the nursing plan of care, and in your nurse's notes. Record the steps you took to arrange for a sign language interpreter if appropriate. Write the names and telephone numbers of available interpreters on the front of his record. If the patient reads lips or uses a picture board or flash cards, document instructions for the chosen communication method in the nursing plan of care. When documenting patient teaching, record the method used to present the information. For example, you might write, "Used sign language interpreter provided by hospital when instructing patient."

If the patient uses a hearing aid, record its care and the times he usually wears it. Also document his hearing aid use on other forms your facility requires.

If the patient consented to treatment through an interpreter, record the interpreter's name in your nurse's notes and on the consent form. If a family member acted as interpreter, document that the patient agreed to this. If the patient wears a hearing aid, record that it was in place when the physician provided information for consent. If the patient received written information, place a copy of this information in his record.

WHEN YOUR PATIENT HAS A VISION IMPAIRMENT

A vision impairment can range from slight vision loss to blindness. Depending on the severity of your patient's vision impairment, the strange sounds, smells, and occurrences in a health care facility may seem nightmarish. Her vision impairment also places extra demands on caregivers. You'll need to be especially creative when teaching her about care activities, treatments, and drugs.

How to Respond

On admission, assess your patient's vision. Find out whether she can see shadows or faint objects in a limited area. If she sees well enough to recognize faces and read large print, test her visual acuity using a Snellen eye chart. If she can't read the chart, hold a few fingers in front of her face and ask how many fingers she sees. Also determine whether she uses devices to improve her vision or navigate the environment. (See *Documenting visual acuity*.)

TIPS & ADVICE

DOCUMENTING VISUAL ACUITY

To document your patient's visual acuity, record her best response to visual acuity testing while she wears eyeglasses, contact lenses, or other corrective vision device. Document her response as follows:

• Reads eye charts at 20′ and 14″
• Identifies the number of fingers held in front of her
• Sees a hand waving in front of her face
• Sees a penlight shining into her eyes

After you take the patient to her room, tell her how many steps she must take to reach the door, the bathroom, the chair, and other landmarks. Put her hand on the call button so that she knows where it is. Mention how many rooms are on the unit, and describe the location of the nurses' station relative to her room. If she can walk, help her to the bathroom and describe its layout. To orient her, place her hand on the toilet paper dispenser, soap dispenser, and paper towel dispenser.

Then help her stow her personal belongings—and never rearrange them without her permission. Remember that the routine tidying you do for other patients can confuse a vision-impaired patient, who finds items by touch and remembers exactly where she left them. Moving something even a few inches can frustrate her.

To maintain your patient's independence and dignity, announce yourself before you enter her room. Otherwise, your sudden presence at her side might startle her.

Obtaining Informed Consent. Make sure the patient receives a complete verbal explanation of the care she is being asked to consent to. Depending on the extent of her vision impairment and your facility's policy, she may need to sign a large-print or Braille consent form. Some facilities have a blank line on the standard consent form for a translator's or facilitator's signature. This person must read every word on the document to a vision-impaired patient but isn't responsible for answering questions about the proposed treatment or procedure. The physician should be present to answer questions and provide explanations.

Providing Routine Care. Explain everything you do when caring for a vision-impaired patient. If you must touch her, tell her precisely where you'll touch before she feels your hands. If she has eyeglasses or contact lenses, make sure she wears them during your care to increase her comfort with her surroundings and your care.

When serving food, describe where each food is located on the tray in terms of a clock face. For instance, you might tell the patient the meat is at 6 o'clock, the vegetables are at 10 o'clock, and the beverage is at 2 o'clock. Describe which foods are hot and which are cold. If necessary, help her open containers and remove lids.

Ensuring Safety. To help prevent injury, make sure the floor and furniture in the patient's room aren't highly polished. If possible, leave the door open completely so that she won't walk into it, and keep her path clear to keep her from tripping. Each time you enter and leave her room, check for and remove debris or liquid on the floor.

If your patient has some sight, provide adequate lighting. To reduce the glare of bright sunlight, close Venetian blinds or draw sheer curtains, as necessary. Keep night-lights on in the bedroom and bathroom at night.

If your patient is ambulatory, instruct her to ask for assistance when she wants to leave her room. Otherwise, she may get lost, even if her room and the elevators have Braille markings.

What to Document

Document the level of your patient's vision impairment and the devices she uses to improve her vision or navigate the environment. Also record that you provided orientation to her environment, including:

- room layout
- bathroom location and layout
- location of the nurses' station
- call button location
- safety measures

Document your explanations of your care. If appropriate, record that the patient wore eyeglasses or contact lenses when you provided care. Also document that a facilitator participated in obtaining the patient's consent, if appropriate.

In the nursing plan of care, record where the patient stores each personal belonging and document the safety measures you take. Indicate her vision impairment on her medical record, and direct other health care team members to the nursing plan of care so they can maintain consistent interventions. Post a sign on her door to inform staff and visitors of her vision impairment and to remind them to announce themselves before entering.

WHEN YOUR PATIENT IS OBESE

A major public health problem, obesity is a chief cause of such disorders as cardiovascular disease and type 2 diabetes mellitus. An obese patient may be *overweight*, with a body mass index (BMI) that falls between 25 and 29.9 kg/m²; *obese*, with a BMI of 30 to 35 kg/m²; or *morbidly obese*, with a BMI greater than 35 kg/m². Morbid obesity is especially likely to complicate your nursing care. So when documenting your physical examination findings and interventions, be sure to record how and why you adapted the patient's care.

How to Respond

First, obtain an accurate body weight for your patient and document it in the medical record. If you use a special scale to weigh him, note this too. Calculate and record the patient's BMI, noting whether he's overweight, obese, or morbidly obese.

Checking for Obesity-Related Health Problems.
Thoroughly investigate and record the patient's health history, but be sensitive to his feelings, especially when asking about his weight and eating habits. He's likely to be painfully aware that he's overweight and may have tried to lose weight numerous times. Also, he may know the health risks of obesity and feel guilty about endangering his health.

When interviewing the patient, ask about and document a history of obesity-related disorders, such as diabetes mellitus and hypertension. Also determine whether his serum cholesterol and triglyceride levels have been checked recently. If so, record the results and note whether he's being treated for high cholesterol or other abnormalities.

Review the patient's eating patterns, preferably with a 24-hour recall of his usual diet. Also assess his physical activity and exercise patterns, and any previous attempts at weight loss. Try to determine whether his obesity is long-standing or relatively recent. If it's recent, ask whether he knows what prompted the weight gain, such as recent use of a corticosteroid or other drug with weight gain as an adverse reaction. If the patient is female, also ask about recent pregnancies and changes in menstrual patterns. Document the patient's responses.

Also investigate whether your patient is depressed, bored, or less mobile as a result of an injury or disorder. These factors can provide clues to the cause of obesity and its possible treatments. Record all history findings, particularly noting possible causes and effects of the patient's obesity.

Modifying Care.
Whenever your patient is obese, record any modifications your must make to his care. Be sensitive to your patient's need for privacy and discretion. If a patient gown doesn't cover him fully, let him wear his own clothing, as appropriate.

Adapt your examination techniques as needed for your obese patient. In areas that he may not be able to reach, such as his skin-folds, feet, and toenails, carefully examine the skin for signs of disease or poor hygiene. If you have difficulty eliciting his deep tendon reflexes, try placing your fingers on the tendon and feeling for a response. To palpate abdominal organs through excess adipose tissue, try using bimanual palpation to trap or hook an organ. If you can't detect peripheral pulses by palpation, use a handheld Doppler ultrasound device. When excess adipose tissue impedes auscultation of the heart and lungs, reduce ambient noise by closing the door to the patient's room and turning off unnecessary equipment. Also turn the patient on his left side to bring the heart closer to his chest wall, which may improve heart sound auscultation. Make a note of the alternative examination techniques you used so that other health care team members can repeat them and have a context for your findings.

To ease the care of your obese patient, use special equipment (or adapt existing equipment) as needed and record its use. For example, use a large cuff to ensure accurate blood pressure measurement. If adipose tissue interferes with light penetration and prevents the oxygen saturation probe from working properly, place an adhesive probe on the bridge of his nose to obtain a more accurate reading. To enhance patient comfort and safety, plan to use a large-sized bed, commode, and wheelchair and a large-capacity scale, if possible.

Before discharge, teach the patient about the importance of nutrition, exercise, and weight loss to his health. If he's open to your discussion, suggest a consultation with the physician or a nutritionist to develop an individualized weight loss plan. Keep in mind, however, that the physician isn't likely to order caloric restrictions while the patient is critically ill. Be sure to record your teaching and referrals.

What to Document

In the medical record, record your obese patient's body weight, BMI, and degree of obesity. If his weight gain is recent, record the percentage over his usual body weight and possible reasons for the weight gain. Also record the following information:
- obesity-related disorders
- drugs used at home, especially those that can produce weight gain
- 24-hour dietary recall
- patient's usual physical activity level

- physical examination findings
- patient care modifications, including the availability and use of special equipment
- patient teaching about nutrition and weight loss
- the patient's motivation to lose weight
- results of discussions or consultations about a weight loss plan for the patient

WHEN YOUR PATIENT CAN'T GIVE INFORMED CONSENT

B efore a patient undergoes a treatment or procedure, she must give informed consent. Her signature on an informed consent form means that she has received, in terms she understands, all the information she needs to decide whether to consent to the proposed treatment or procedure. (See *Understanding informed consent.*) If she signs a consent form without understanding what the treatment or procedure involves, her consent isn't informed and therefore isn't valid.

Only an adult or emancipated minor of sound mind can give informed consent. The definitions of adult and emancipated minor differ among states. For example, in some states, a pregnant 16-year-old is considered an adult, and a married teenager is considered an emancipated minor. In some states, a mature minor also can give informed consent if she demonstrates that she understands the risks involved.

How to Respond

The physician is responsible for obtaining informed consent. If you witness your patient sign an informed consent form, you could be asked to testify that she was able to give consent. Also, if you perform a treatment or procedure on a patient who won't or can't give informed consent, you could be charged with battery. If you believe that your patient can't give informed consent, don't

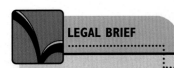

LEGAL BRIEF

UNDERSTANDING INFORMED CONSENT
Informed consent rests on the concept that every adult of sound mind has the fundamental right to decide whether to allow violation of her body's integrity. Consent can be expressed or implied.

Expressed consent, which can be given orally or in writing, specifies the actions to which the patient is consenting. Obtaining consent in writing is a way to prove that consent was given. *Implied* consent is conveyed by the patient's actions or circumstances. For instance, a patient who sees a physician for a physical examination gives implied consent to having her blood pressure taken and her lungs auscultated. If she signs a consent form allowing blood to be drawn for human immunodeficiency virus testing, she's giving expressed consent for that procedure.

Consent Requirements
For informed consent to occur, the patient must receive:
- a description of the proposed treatment or procedure
- names and qualifications of the people who will perform it
- an explanation of the risks of death, serious harm, or adverse effects from the treatment or procedure
- an explanation of alternative treatments or procedures
- a description of the possible consequences of not having the treatment or procedure
- an explanation that she can refuse the treatment or procedure without having other care or support withdrawn
- an explanation that she can withdraw her consent after giving it

participate in obtaining her consent or performing the treatment or procedure. Instead, notify the appropriate nurse administrator of your belief and provide supporting data.

If Your Patient Is Incompetent. A mentally incompetent patient can't give informed consent. All adults are presumed to be legally competent unless judged incompetent in a formal court proceeding. A patient who is legally competent may be clinically incompetent—that is, unable to understand the full extent or implications of a proposed treatment or procedure. In most cases, the physician determines clinical competency based on whether the patient:

- understands the information presented
- engages in rational decision making
- can make a definitive and reasonable decision regarding the proposed treatment or procedure

Except in an emergency, a clinically incompetent patient can't receive treatment until consent is obtained from her legal guardian. The physician usually consults the patient's spouse, adult child, or other family member about treatment decisions. Many states recognize the family's right to make decisions for a loved one, provided they act in good faith. If the patient has a durable power of attorney that designates her surrogate health care decision maker, that person must be consulted as the legal decision maker when the patient is incompetent.

If family members or other legally appointed decision makers disagree on a treatment plan or if you question their motives or ability to make health care decisions, notify the appropriate nurse administrator and your facility's risk manager. Your facility may want to start guardianship proceedings.

Before witnessing a consent signed by the surrogate decision maker for your legally or clinically incompetent patient, ensure that the health care team has followed your facility's policy to identify the legal decision maker. If the patient has given someone durable or health care power of attorney, this person should make treatment decisions. Otherwise, consult the appropriate nurse administrator and, if needed, the facility's legal counsel to determine the appropriate decision maker, such as the spouse, the oldest adult child, another adult child, a parent, or a sibling.

If Your Patient Is a Minor. The custodial parent must give informed consent for a minor. Remember, though, that the parent who brought the child to the health care facility may not have full custody, so be sure to determine who is legally responsible for the child. Unless the parents are separated or divorced, assume that the natural parent has legal responsibility. Keep in mind that most states will abide by the decision of the parent who admits the child, whether he or she is the custodial parent.

In other circumstances, consult your facility's risk manager to determine the legal decision maker. Keep in mind that grandparents, aunts, uncles, and siblings can't give informed consent for a minor unless they've been appointed legal guardian or have legally valid *in loco parentis* (in place of the parent) status.

If Your Patient Is an Emancipated Minor. States define *emancipated minor* differently. Generally, an emancipated minor is a child age 14 to 17 who no longer depends on her parents for support or isn't subject to parental control. Nearly all states that recognize emancipated minors stipulate that the minor be self-supporting and not live in the parents' home. Married minors are usually considered emancipated. In some states, minors in the military or in college also are considered emancipated.

Depending on the state, an emancipated minor may have the right to consent to nonemergency treatment without parental approval. Twenty-three states now recognize an emancipated minor's right to make medical decisions for herself.

If you're not sure whether your patient is an emancipated minor, delay the planned treatment or procedure until you've consulted your facility's risk manager about the patient's status. If the patient is deemed emancipated, she can give consent as long as she understands the consequences.

If Your Patient Is a Mature Minor. Four states recognize mature minors—children age 15 or older who make their own decisions on daily affairs, are independent financially, and can understand the risks and benefits of a proposed treatment or procedure. Usually, the court makes this determination when the best interests of the child are met by excluding parental consent—and when the minor shows that she can give informed consent. A child can be deemed a mature minor based on her age, abilities, experience, education, degree of maturity, soundness of judgment, conduct, and demeanor. Also she must demonstrate the capacity to understand the risks and consequences of a procedure.

What to Document

Your documentation must show that you assessed the patient's mental status and decision-making ability and took steps to safeguard her right to informed consent. Record her orientation and ability to understand simple explanations, such as how to operate a bed control or use a call button. Document her understanding of the terms used in the informed consent form. To show whether her decision was firm or vacillating, record her statements about it, placing quotation marks around her words.

To document the patient's thought process, record her stated reason for her consent decision. If she says that she wants to undergo surgery so that she can recover and return to work, she's demonstrating rational thought. If she agrees to surgery because she says Doug Ross or Marcus Welby will make house calls afterward, she's demonstrating irrational thought.

If you believe that your patient is clinically incompetent, document the name of the person you notified, the supporting evidence you presented, and the person's response. As appropriate, note the method used to identify the patient's surrogate decision maker. If the patient has a durable or health care power of attorney, place a copy of that document in her medical record. If a family member made the decision to consent, record this person's name and the reason he has decision-making power. Also record the names of family members who didn't participate in the decision. This information identifies the people who were available at the time consent was given in case a family member claims he was passed over unjustly.

For a minor, document the family situation, the name of her decision maker, and the reason this person is considered the decision maker. If the minor is emancipated or mature, record the reason for her legal status. Also document the data your facility used to determine that she was emancipated or mature, including the name of the lawyer or risk manager involved. If the minor has a court-appointed guardian or is in an adult's legal custody, include a copy of the court document in her record.

Also, this information must be provided in terms the patient understands, and the patient must consent voluntarily. Know that obtaining informed consent doesn't mean that health care providers can't be sued for negligence if substandard care is rendered. A patient never consents to substandard care.

WHEN YOUR PATIENT DOESN'T UNDERSTAND THE PROCEDURE HE'S ABOUT TO UNDERGO

Unless your patient understands the information he has received about a proposed treatment or procedure and its effects on his health and lifestyle, he can't give informed consent. Although the physician is responsible for providing the information, you must make sure your patient understands it. (See *How much information is enough?*) As a nurse, you also have an ethical duty to answer your patient's questions truthfully.

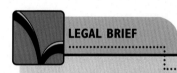

LEGAL BRIEF

HOW MUCH INFORMATION IS ENOUGH?
For years, the courts have wrestled with the question of how much information a physician must disclose to obtain a patient's informed consent. In some cases, courts have measured disclosure in terms of good medical practice. In others, they've applied the standard of what a reasonable practitioner would provide in the same circumstances or what medical practice in a given community demands. In many states, the law requires the physician to disclose what a reasonable patient would need to know before making an informed choice.

In *Canterbury v. Spence*,[1] a landmark informed consent case, the U.S. Court of Appeals held that a patient can exercise the right to self-decision only if he has enough information to form an intelligent decision. Although the court acknowledged that physicians sometimes may have to speculate about what information the patient considers significant, it stated that their medical experience and training provides a basis for deciding how much information an average, reasonable person of the patient's background and condition needs.

[1]*Canterbury v. Spence, 464 F.2d 772 (D.C. App., 1971).*

How to Respond

If your patient asks you about a planned treatment or procedure, answer his questions to the best of your ability. Then, determine his understanding by evaluating his response to your clarification. If you believe that he still doesn't understand the treatment or procedure, advise him not to sign the consent form. Immediately contact the appropriate nurse administrator and the physician, and ask the physician to speak with the patient. He'll probably appreciate your observation. If he doesn't, prepare to go up the chain of command to uphold the patient's right to informed consent.

Try to attend when the physician clarifies the procedure with the patient. If he doesn't elicit the patient's feedback, ask him to explain what the physician just told him in his own words to assess his understanding. Find out whether he understands the procedure's full intent and possible implications. For example, does he believe that he's only having a breast lump removed even though the physician is asking him to consent to breast removal? Does he realize he'll have a colostomy after proposed bowel surgery? If he doesn't consent to the entire procedure, it shouldn't be performed.

What to Document

Document the conversation that led you to believe that your patient didn't understand the proposed treatment or procedure. Record the patient's exact words, placing quotation marks around them.

Then document your actions. If you conveyed your belief to the physician, document your conversation with the physician, the time it occurred, and the physician's response. If the physician provided additional information to the patient, document what he said and the patient's response. Record the entire question-and-answer session and the patient's return explanation of the proposed procedure to help determine whether he received and understood the information needed to give informed consent.

WHEN YOUR PATIENT'S EQUIPMENT FAILS

M edical equipment failure can range from a minor incon-
venience to a life-threatening event. Caring for a patient
with life-sustaining medical equipment poses a challenge even
when everything works properly. When her equipment fails, the
challenges multiply. Thorough documentation of your actions and
the patient's responses may protect you if an adverse outcome
leads to a lawsuit.

How to Respond

Remain calm and assess the situation objectively. First, assess for
changes in your patient's condition. If she's in immediate danger,
such as from mechanical ventilator or intra-aortic balloon pump
failure, call for assistance and start emergency interventions immediately. Have someone notify the physician.

If the equipment failure doesn't pose an immediate threat,
assess your patient, notify the physician of the incident and your
assessment findings, and then implement the physician's instructions. Next, try to troubleshoot the equipment and correct the
problem. If you can't correct it quickly, ask a colleague to obtain
replacement equipment and then replace the faulty item. Tell the
patient that the equipment isn't working properly and that you're
replacing it.

Remove the equipment from the patient's room. In large
letters, attach a note stating "REPAIR NEEDED" along with a
brief description of the equipment's performance. Report the
malfunction to the appropriate nurse administrator, who then will
have the faulty equipment transported to the biomedical equipment department or other appropriate area.

To reduce the patient's anxiety, assure her that you'll take
special measures to make sure the new equipment works properly. Explain the alarm settings and review the schedule you'll use

to evaluate her condition and the equipment's performance. Then follow this schedule diligently.

What to Document

In your nurse's notes, describe how you discovered the equipment failure. Record your assessment of the patient's condition and the steps you took to prevent injury. Also describe your actions in troubleshooting the problem or note that you replaced the equipment, as appropriate.

Document the brand name, model, and serial number of the faulty equipment. Record the name of the nurse administrator and physician you notified, times of notification, their instructions, your interventions, and the patient's response. Also document your conversations with the patient about the faulty equipment.

Indicate that you tagged the equipment for repair and attached a description of the problem. Also record the actions you took to check the new equipment's performance. (See *Documenting follow-through actions*.)

If the patient developed adverse effects from the equipment failure, complete an incident report according to your facility's policy (but don't mention the incident report in your nurse's

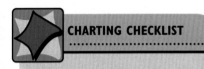

CHARTING CHECKLIST

DOCUMENTING FOLLOW-THROUGH ACTIONS
When you document an equipment failure or other problem, you must show that you followed through on it by taking appropriate corrective action. For each problem you record, document:
- ❑ your description of the problem
- ❑ your actions to safeguard the patient
- ❑ how and when you notified the physician
- ❑ the physician's instructions and the time you implemented them
- ❑ the patient's response to interventions
- ❑ your reassessment of the patient

If a colleague will reassess the patient, document this person's name and the times when reassessment should occur.

notes). If your unit has an equipment problem log, record the malfunction there, and describe the location of the malfunctioning equipment. Also, speak to your nurse administrator about filing a report with the Food and Drug Administration (FDA). (See *Reporting medical device failure to the FDA*, pages 303-304.)

TIPS & ADVICE

REPORTING MEDICAL DEVICE FAILURE TO THE FDA
The Food and Drug Administration (FDA) Safety Information and Adverse Event Reporting Program, also known as MedWatch, allows health care providers and consumers to report adverse events related to defective medical devices. This voluntary program supplements mandatory reporting requirements for manufacturers. Through MedWatch, a facility or individual can file form 3500 with the FDA to report events that result in death, life-threatening illness, hospitalization, disability, or congenital anomaly or that require medical or surgical intervention to prevent permanent impairment.

In some facilities, a member of the risk management team or biomedical engineering department fills out form 3500. However, if you must complete the form yourself, be prepared to provide data about the patient and yourself, as well as the following information:

Adverse Event and Product Problem (Brief)
- Brief description of the adverse event
- Brief description of the product problem, which may involve contamination, defective components, therapeutic failure, or product confusion caused by name, labeling, design, or packaging
- Outcome caused by the adverse event—including death, life-threatening illness or impairment, hospitalization, congenital anomaly (if device failure with a pregnant woman affected the fetus)—and required intervention to prevent permanent impairment
- Date of the event
- Date the report was filled out
- Brief description of the adverse event or product problem

Adverse Event (Detailed)
- Detailed description of the event
- Relevant clinical information, including diagnostic tests and any preexisting medical conditions
- Copies of the patient's medical record with all identifying information deleted.

Continued

TIPS & ADVICE
....

REPORTING MEDICAL DEVICE FAILURE TO THE FDA—cont'd
Product Problem (Detailed)
• Brand name
• Type of device
• Manufacturer's name and address
• Product identification numbers, including model number, catalog number, serial number, lot number, and expiration date
• Operator of device
• Implantation and explanation dates
• Name and address of company the reprocessed or refurbished the device
• Availability of device for evaluation
• Use of concomitant medical products

WHEN YOUR PATIENT'S BELONGINGS ARE MISSING

M ost patients bring some personal belongings when they enter a health care facility. If your patient loses any of his belongings during his stay, he may grow mistrustful of you and other caregivers. What's more, he may wonder how staff members can manage his medical care if they can't even keep track of his belongings.

The health care facility may be found liable for a patient's missing belongings. Individual employees are seldom held accountable unless evidence suggests that they were involved in the item's disappearance. If the patient takes legal action, documentation of your attempts to locate the missing item helps show that the staff didn't treat the incident lightly.

How to Respond

When your patient is admitted, inform him of the facility's policy about personal belongings. If he later sues over a missing item, your thorough documentation of these instructions can aid your facility's defense. Encourage the patient to send valuables home or lock them in the facility's safe. According to your facility's policy, inventory his belongings. (See *Eliminating belongings lists*.)

If your patient reports a missing item, show your concern. Check the belongings inventory (if one exists), and question family members to make sure they didn't take the item home with them. Then help the patient search his room. (If you're too busy to search right away, explain that you'll return later to search.) Find out when and where he last saw the item. Ask other staff members if they remember seeing it. If your facility has a lost-and-found department, check for the missing item there.

DID YOU KNOW?

ELIMINATING BELONGINGS LISTS

Some acute care facilities have stopped taking inventories of patients' clothing and all other belongings on admission. Instead, they encourage patients to send items home, document the valuables sent home, and ask patients to sign a statement that clothing and valuables are the patient's responsibility.

If your search turns up nothing, notify the security department and the appropriate nurse administrator. (In most cases, you don't need to notify the police.) Tell the security guard what steps you took to locate the item and help him complete his report.

What to Document

On admission, document a complete list of your patient's belongings, if required in your facility. Describe each item objectively, without guessing at its value or composition. For instance, describe a patient's ring as "a yellow metal ring with a clear stone" rather than "a diamond ring with a gold band."

When documenting a missing item, include the following:
- date and time you learned of its disappearance
- its description
- time and place it was last seen
- name of the person who last saw it
- names of family members, staff members, and others you questioned
- areas searched, including the lost-and-found department

- names of the security guard and nurse administrator you notified, and times of notification
- actions taken by the security guard and nurse administrator
- patient's response to the incident

Depending on facility policy, you may also need to complete an incident report.

Eliminating belongings lists can lighten the paperwork burden. To implement this policy at your facility, talk with the appropriate nurse administrator and your facility's risk manager.

WHEN YOUR PATIENT'S FAMILY QUESTIONS THE QUALITY OF CARE

Answering patients' and family members' questions is a basic nursing responsibility. If a patient's family members question the quality of the care their loved one is receiving, you may become uncomfortable. If handled incorrectly, such questions may provoke anger and hostility in the family and dissension and feelings of rejection among the staff. A hasty response may fuel a lawsuit.

How to Respond

Take all quality-of-care questions seriously and respond sincerely. Never dismiss or ignore such questions. Acknowledge family members' concerns and have them explain why they believe that the patient is receiving poor care. Clarify their response with them to make sure you understand their concerns.

Handling Questions About Nursing Care. If family members question the patient's nursing care, answer honestly. If their concerns are based on a misunderstanding, provide appropriate teaching or clarification. For instance, if they ask why the patient's IV site has the same clear plastic dressing as the previous day, explain that facility policy specifies that transparent dressings be changed every other day. If necessary, tell them you'll ask the physician to discuss the issue with them.

Keep the lines of communication open. Don't be afraid to say, "I don't know the answer, but I'll have the physician (or my supervisor) discuss it with you." Within the limits of confidentiality, keep family members updated on the patient's treatment and condition.

If family members seem upset, don't argue or try to defend yourself or a colleague. A defensive posture may escalate the conflict and make them suspect that you're trying to cover up a problem. Instead, notify the appropriate nurse administrator as soon as possible. She may speak with them herself or have another administrator do so. She'll probably bring you back into the discussion once she's investigated the complaint.

Dealing with Questions About Medical Care. If the complaint goes beyond the scope of nursing practice, describe to family members the care the physician has prescribed. Then tell them you'll have the physician discuss the treatment plan with them, if the patient agrees to this. Notify the physician of the family's concerns, and tell the family members when he'll be available to talk with them.

Also refer questions about the patient's declining health status to the physician. If family members are reluctant to talk with him, have them speak with the facility's risk manager and patient advocate. After the family speaks with the physician or risk manager and patient advocate, talk to family members to make sure their questions were answered. Keep them informed about the patient's care and the reasons for changes in her condition.

What to Document

Document the family's questions and concerns and your responses. Record the names of family members present during your discussions. Document the names of the physician, the nurse administrator, and others you notified, along with times of notification.

Document what you, the physician, and other staff members told the family. Also record your conversations with the nurse administrator and the physician. Keep your documentation objective, and use direct quotes whenever possible. Record the name of the risk management staff member and patient advocate assigned to interact with the family and the instructions they gave you.

If a quality-of-care lapse occurred, you may need to file an incident report. Check your facility's policy.

WHEN YOU SUSPECT THAT YOUR PATIENT HAS BEEN ABUSED

A serious problem that crosses all age, gender, racial, and socio-economic boundaries, abuse is a harmful action committed knowingly by one individual against another. More specifically, the U.S. Department of Health and Human Services defines *abuse* as the "willful infliction of injury, unreasonable confinement, intimidation, or punishment with resulting physical harm or pain or mental anguish, or deprivation."

If you suspect that your patient has been abused, you have a professional duty to intervene on his behalf and a legal duty to report the crime—whether the patient is a minor or an adult. Keep in mind that your report of suspected spousal abuse is a privileged communication that doesn't subject you to legal action.

The federal Child Abuse Prevention and Treatment Act of 1973 made failure to report suspected abuse or neglect of a minor a crime. A physician or nurse who fails to report suspected abuse or neglect of a minor may be prosecuted for criminal liability and sued for malpractice.

Nearly every state also has mechanisms to protect victims of elder and spousal abuse. Most states permit such victims to obtain a civil injunction or restraining order against the abuser. Some have provisions and funds for removing the victim from the home temporarily. (See *Protecting long-term-care facility residents.*)

Most states also have good faith reporting laws, which protect health care workers against liability in lawsuits brought by people falsely accused of abuse. The health care worker must prove he or she had reasonable cause to believe that the patient's injuries weren't accidental.

How to Respond

Review your state's laws on reporting suspected abuse, and learn which public agencies deal with abuse. Also check your facility's policy and protocol for reporting abuse.

Because many victims hesitate to admit their abuse out of shame or fear of reprisal, watch for psychogenic and physical signs of abuse, such as fractures, bruises, welts, GI disorders, acute back pain, choking sensations, and constant headache. If you detect such signs in your patient, determine whether he's in immediate danger. If you believe that he is, notify his physician and the appropriate nurse administrator of your suspicion of abuse and your actions, and try to arrange for his removal from the abusive situation. If he has severe physical injuries, his admission to the health care facility will accomplish this goal. For an elderly patient or child, the appropriate state agency can make arrangements for temporary custody or housing as needed.

If the patient is already hospitalized or isn't in immediate danger, notify the appropriate agency of the suspected abuse. In some facilities, a team of professionals counsels and follows up on abuse victims. If your facility doesn't have such a team, consult the social services department about assigning a social worker to your patient's case.

Offer the patient support and understanding and refrain from judging him. Remember that he may be embarrassed by his situation. Ask open-ended questions and explore available support resources, such as friends and family members. As needed, help him make alternative living arrangements or contact legal authorities to remove him from an abusive home. If he's been admitted to your facility, offer the option of visitor restriction to limit contact with his abuser. (See *Enforcing visitor restrictions.*)

What to Document

If your facility has a special form for recording suspected abuse, complete it and send it to the appropriate administrator. Place a copy in the patient's medical record.

If your facility doesn't have a special form, document the situation in your nurse's notes. Include the following information:
- patient's demographic data, such as name, address, and number and ages of children
- type of abuse suspected
- name and address of the suspected abuser
- information reported by the patient, such as his reason for seeking medical care and his explanation of the cause of his bruises, fractures, or other physical signs of abuse

CHARTING CHECKLIST

ENFORCING VISITOR RESTRICTIONS
If your patient doesn't want to see certain visitors, ask whether he'd like to restrict them from visiting. Activating a visitor restriction takes coordination and cooperation among several departments. To cover all the bases, make sure to document the restriction as follows:

❑ *Nurse's notes.* Document your discussion with the patient about visitor restrictions, the names of people he wants to restrict from visiting, and his reason. In the nursing plan of care, record the names of restricted visitors and describe the steps to take if they try to gain access to the patient.

❑ *Nursing unit.* Inform the appropriate nurse administrator of the visitor restrictions. She should document the restrictions on her report sheet for the duration of the patient's stay on the unit.

❑ *Security department.* Send a memo to the security department detailing the visitor restriction and the possible need for intervention by security guards.

❑ *Information desk.* Send a memo to the information desk instructing them to request identification from anyone who asks to visit the patient and outlining the steps to take if a restricted visitor tries to see the patient.

- your assessment findings, including observations of the patient's body language and mental status
- names of facility staff members contacted
- names of people contacted at state and law enforcement agencies
- other related actions taken, such as imposing visitor restrictions and intervening for physical injuries

WHEN YOUR PATIENT'S VISITORS WON'T LEAVE

F amily members and other visitors can provide emotional support to a loved one in a health care facility, possibly helping to shorten her stay and promote her recovery. However, sometimes visitors interfere with patient care activities and may tire or upset the patient.

Most facilities have guidelines governing visiting hours and special visiting circumstances. If your patient's visitors won't observe these guidelines, dealing with them can be a challenge.

How to Respond

To prevent visitor problems, review your unit's visiting policy with your patient and her family when she's admitted. If possible, provide written guidelines so that they'll know who may visit and when. If visiting hours differ for certain types of visitors (such as extended spousal visits in a maternity unit), review the information that applies.

If your patient's visitors refuse to leave, avoid confrontation whenever possible. Find out why they want to stay. Evaluate them for anxiety, and acknowledge and explore their concerns. Are they afraid the patient's condition will change for the worse after they leave? Do they think she'll become anxious if left alone?

Provide information, as appropriate, to address visitors' concerns. To reduce their anxiety, describe the patient's condition and care. If they need additional reassurance, ask the appropriate nurse administrator and the physician to talk with them.

Then determine whether special circumstances may apply. If your patient's condition is unstable, for instance, and close family members can't visit at other times, consult your nurse administrator about making special arrangements, such as allowing them to arrive at 8 P.M. and leave by 9 P.M., even though visiting hours officially end at 8 P.M. Be sure to include limits in the special arrangement.

If visitors refuse to leave despite your interventions, notify the appropriate nurse administrator and ask her help in getting them to leave. As a last resort, call the security department to escort the visitors off the unit. If your patient doesn't want to see certain visitors, consider obtaining visitor restrictions. (See *Enforcing visitor restrictions*, page 310.)

What to Document

On admission, document that you informed the patient and her family of visiting hours. If you gave them a written summary of the visiting policy, note that too.

If the patient's visitors refuse to leave, document their behavior and your assessments and actions in your nurse's notes. Include each visitor's name and relationship to the patient. Record your conversations with them, including the time you notified them that visiting hours were over. Document their responses and explanations for not wanting to leave. Describe the methods you used to elicit this information. Also document your explanations to them to reduce their fears about the patient's condition. If the physician or a nurse administrator spoke with them, record what this person said and the visitors' responses.

Document the final outcome and the time the visitors left. If the security department was involved, record the security guard's name and actions and the patient's response to the incident.

If you've made special visiting arrangements, document the reason for the arrangement, the name of the person who permitted it, the visitors' names, and the specifics of the agreement, including the time the visitors are expected to leave. Also record this information on the nursing plan of care to inform other caregivers. Notify the security department of the visitors' names, the times when they're permitted to arrive, and their required departure times.

WHEN YOUR PATIENT IS SERIOUSLY ILL

A patient with an acute illness or serious injury, such as cerebrovascular accident or head trauma, may not be able to communicate fully because of his condition or the use of mechanical ventilation or heavy sedation. This inability to respond can pose problems, especially if you need the patient to supply information for his care and the medical record. Yet good communication skills, sensitive nursing care, and careful documentation can help you surmount these problems.

How to Respond

First, assess and record the patient's level of consciousness and orientation to person, place, and time. Also note his vital signs; stability of his airway, breathing, and circulation; and other pertinent physical data.

If your seriously ill patient can't provide extensive information and a family member isn't available, obtain and document vital data only, such as his level of pain. Then tell him you'll ask more questions later. That way, he won't feel rushed or taxed and will be more likely to answer your questions as completely as he can.

For a patient who is conscious but can't speak because of mechanical ventilation or another barrier, establish a communication method that lets him respond nonverbally to simple questions. To obtain basic information including his level of pain and anxiety, identify gestures he can use to indicate his responses to questions. For example, tell him to squeeze your hand once for "no" and twice for "yes."

Before recording the patient's answers, test to make sure he understands the gestures and uses them appropriately. For example, ask a question that has a known answer, such as, "Is your name Joseph?" He should respond correctly by squeezing your hand the proper number of times. In your notes, document the communication method you established as well as the patient's demonstrated ability to use it.

Providing Comfort Measures. Immobility, pain, discomfort, anxiety, or depression can interfere with a seriously ill patient's ability to focus on questions or instructions. So after establishing a communication system, evaluate these factors in your patient. Ask how he's feeling. Determine whether he can talk at length or whether he needs to keep his responses short because of immobility, pain, or discomfort. Before proceeding with the interview—or any nursing care—address the patient's immediate discomfort. For example, help him into a more comfortable position or offer a cool beverage, if permitted. If he's in pain, give the prescribed analgesic; then wait for it to take effect before performing non-urgent care.

To further ease the patient's pain or discomfort, try guiding him through progressive muscle relaxation. Instruct him to perform this 10- to 30-minute exercise by progressively tightening and then relaxing one muscle group at a time until his whole body is relaxed.

Or try guided imagery, which is more effective for some patients. To do this, gently instruct the patient to imagine he's in one of his favorite places, coaching him to mentally experience it through all of his senses. This should have a relaxing effect and enable you to proceed with the interview. (See *Collecting information from a patient in severe pain.*) In your notes, document all measures you take to make the patient more comfortable as well as his responses to them.

Caring for an Unresponsive Patient. If your patient becomes unconscious or comatose, don't assume he can't hear you. Instead, speak to him while you perform nursing care and provide explanations as if he were awake. Before cardiac auscultation, for example, you might say, "Now I'm going to listen to your heart." He may be able to hear your voice and find your words soothing. Also, remember not to discuss other patients' private information in his presence.

What to Document

Caring for a seriously ill patient can challenge your clinical skills—and your communication skills. Yet the information you gather from the patient or his family can be critical in guiding his care. So it's vitally important to obtain accurate information

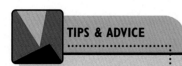

COLLECTING INFORMATION FROM A PATIENT IN SEVERE PAIN

When gathering information from a patient in severe pain or discomfort, plan to use your best interview skills. Then document his answers thoroughly to help avoid him having him repeat himself to other caregivers. To make the interview go as smoothly as possible, follow these suggestions.

Get Off to a Good Start
- If your patient feels well enough to talk at length, start by asking open-ended questions. This should help him feel more comfortable with you. Also use natural pauses in the conversation to ask closed-ended questions and obtain more details.
- Keep the conversation flowing so that the patient stays focused on your questions rather than his discomfort or the surroundings. Also, occasionally nod your head or make brief remarks to show you're listening closely to his responses.

Deal with the Patient's Fears
- If your patient asks whether he's going to die or be permanently disabled or disfigured, answer him honestly. Remember—most patients don't ask such questions unless they already suspect the answers or are ready to hear them, regardless of whether the news is good or bad.
- Prepare for this situation by doing some soul-searching. Before you can deal with the patient's fears, you need to examine your own attitudes toward illness, disability, disfigurement, and death. Consider whether you can talk openly about these topics without being overwhelmed by your anxieties.
- If you decide that you're not up to the task, ask whether the patient would like to speak with a counselor, religious leader, or other person who feels comfortable discussing these matters.

Accept the Patient's Tears
- If bad news about the patient's health brings him to tears, resist the urge to cut short his crying.
- Stay with the patient, but don't rush to say something you hope will make him feel better. Instead, quietly offer a box of tissues or touch him on the arm to show your acceptance of his feelings and willingness to listen.
- Even if you feel uncomfortable with his tears, avoid talking. If you feel you must speak, offer a few sympathetic words about how hard it must be for him to go through such an ordeal. Try to accept his crying for what it is: coming to terms with painful emotions. Your acceptance can help him realize it's normal to feel the way he does.

and carefully note it in the medical record. When documenting information about a seriously ill patient—and your method for obtaining it—be sure to record the following:

- patient's level of consciousness and orientation to person, place, and time
- description of his medical condition and stability, including vital signs, airway patency, breathing, and circulation
- severity of pain, rated on a 0-to-10 scale, with 0 representing no pain and 10 representing the most severe pain
- communication system established, such as squeezing your hand, and its effectiveness
- comfort measures taken, such as administering an analgesic
- patient's response to comfort measures
- patient's emotional state and any emotional support you provided
- source of patient information, which may be the patient himself or a family member. If someone other than the patient supplied data for the medical record, document that person's name and relationship to the patient

WHEN YOUR PATIENT ASKS YOU TO WITNESS HER LAST WILL AND TESTAMENT

Your patient may ask you to witness her last will and testament, especially if she thinks that she's facing death. Or she may request that you witness her oral statement about how she wants her property distributed after death. Some patients may even ask you to prepare a written will for them.

Before responding to such a request, make sure you understand the legal implications and know how to document the situation. The last will and testament is an important legal document that declares a person's wishes about property distribution after death. It also indicates who should administer the person's estate and may name the guardians of minor children.

State laws specify how a will must be drawn up. If certain statutory requirements aren't met, the will may be invalid. To ensure that the person's intentions are carried out after death, a competent, qualified lawyer should draw up the will.

How to Respond

In most states, you can witness a patient's signature on a will or can witness her oral statement unless you're named as a beneficiary. Although witnessing a patient's will may contribute to her peace of mind, you have no legal or ethical obligation to do so.

What Your Signature Means. Usually, when you sign your name as a witness on a patient's will, you're simply verifying that you saw her sign it. You're not verifying that she's mentally competent, signing of her own free will, or making wise choices about property disposition. (See *Execution of wills: Judging mental capacity*, pages 318-319.)

In some states, your signature on a will also indicates you heard the patient state that the document she's signing is her last will and testament and that the person who drew up the will and the other witnesses were present at the signing. (Most states require at least two witnesses.) If in doubt as to what your signature means, ask your facility's legal counsel for clarification.

How to Sign. Be sure to verify that the document you're signing really is your patient's last will and testament. Carefully read the information above and below your signature line to make sure it indicates you're signing as a witness. When signing, write your full legal name legibly. You don't have to include your credentials and title but doing so may explain to lawyers and others why you were present at the time of signing.

If You Want to Decline. If you decide not to be a witness, decline politely. Offer to arrange for a patient representative or other staff member to serve as a witness.

If you suspect that your patient is mentally incompetent or acting under duress, don't sign as a witness. Instead, notify the appropriate nurse administrator or the patient's physician. If you knowingly witness an illegal signing, you may be charged with a crime.

If your patient asks you to prepare her will, explain that you're not legally qualified to prepare a will. Offer to contact your facility's

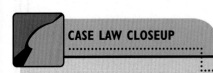

EXECUTION OF WILLS: JUDGING MENTAL CAPACITY
By witnessing a patient's will, you make no claims about his mental capacity to make a will, which the courts call his testamentary capacity. However, your nurse's notes may speak volume about the patient's mental capacity—and protect his legal right to dispose of his property according to his last wishes.

Understanding the Case
Pollard v. Hastings[1] addressed the issue of mental capacity to execute a will by Mr. Pollard, a nursing home resident with bouts of confusion, agitation, and acting out. While in the nursing home, Mr. Pollard was visited regularly by certain family members. About 16 months before his death, he executed and signed a will leaving his entire estate to a nephew and the nephew's wife. This nephew and Mr. Pollard's long-time friend had arranged for a lawyer to draft the will. The long-time friend witnessed the signing of the final document.

Mr. Pollard died at age 90, survived by a brother and many nieces and nephews. After Mr. Pollard's death, his brother filed a lawsuit, declaring that the will was void because Mr. Pollard didn't have the mental capacity to execute a valid will. His motive in filing the suit was that he—and not the nephew—would have inherited the entire estate if Mr. Pollard had died without a valid will.

At the trial, Mr. Pollard's physician and the nursing home psychiatrist testified that, although Mr. Pollard had lapses in mental capacity, he was generally competent. In their opinion, he had the mental capacity to sign a valid will. The brother's lawyers hired a physician as an expert witness. This expert testified that Mr. Pollard had long periods of dementia and was not mentally competent. As the source of his information, the expert used entries from the patient's chart, including physician's and nurse's notes.

How the Court Ruled
The court noted that a person has the mental capacity to execute a will if, at the time of the execution, he has sufficient mind and memory to understand that he's making a will, understands the property he owns and wishes to leave in the will, knows and recalls the people he wishes to leave his property to, and has plans for dividing the estate. The key legal factor isn't the person's overall mental status, but the mental capacity he possessed at the time the will was signed.

---

[1]*Pollard v. Hastings, 862 A. 2d 770 (Rhode Island, 2004).*

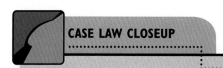

CASE LAW CLOSEUP

EXECUTION OF WILLS: JUDGING MENTAL CAPACITY—cont'd
The court also noted that any expert witness can rely on observations charted by caregivers in formulating an expert opinion about a patient. However, it faulted the expert in this case for highlighting Mr. Pollard's isolated episodes of confusion, agitation, and acting out (which suggested dementia), without relating them to the exact date and time that Mr. Pollard made and signed the will. During the patient's stay in the nursing home, medical and nursing staff members had made multiple references in progress notes about his mental agility and appropriate comprehension. Thus, without exact data to show that Mr. Pollard was incompetent *at the time of signing the will,* the court couldn't determine whether the will was valid and remanded the case for a new trial.

The Lesson Learned
Although no nurses testified in this case, their careful, accurate nursing documentation of the patient's mental status was a critical factor in the court's decision. The law has long recognized that patients may have the mental capacity to execute wills, sign informed consent forms, or refuse consent for selected procedures even if they have bouts of confusion or dementia. For such a patient, accurate and thorough nursing documentation may be the court's only means of validating whether or not the patient was mentally able to make decisions for himself at the time.

legal department, which can send someone to prepare her will. (See *Giving advice about a will: Your legal limitations,* page 320.)

What to Document

Document that you saw the patient sign her will and that you signed it as a witness. Record the names of other witnesses and anyone else present at the signing.

Also document the patient's physical and mental status at the time. Note whether she'd recently received a narcotic or other drug, and record the drug's name, dosage, and time of the last dose before she signed the will. Also describe significant changes in her condition just before she signed, such as deteriorating vital signs or hemodynamic status. Record her level of consciousness, including her degree of alertness and orientation to time, place,

LEGAL BRIEF

GIVING ADVICE ABOUT A WILL: YOUR LEGAL LIMITATIONS
Unless you're a properly qualified lawyer, you could be accused of practicing
law without a license if you give your patient advice about her will, tell her how
to phrase it, or comment on its contents. If she asks you to write her will, tell
her that you're not qualified to do so. Advise her to discuss these matters with
a lawyer or a trusted family member or friend. If she doesn't have a lawyer,
offer to contact your facility's legal department or patient representative.

Documenting the Patient's Request
In the patient's medical record, document her request, your response, and the
steps you took to arrange for will preparation.

and person. Document whether her speech was clear and articulate, and describe her emotional status, noting whether she was anxious, fearful, angry, or unusually docile.

If you witnessed your patient's dying declaration or oral will, record her statement verbatim in the medical record and a memorandum. If other people heard her statement, document their names and relationships to the patient. Note the patient's mental and physical condition at the time of her statement. Then give the appropriate nurse administrator a copy of your memorandum. The administrator should tell the patient's family that this memorandum exists.

WHEN A PATIENT DIES

When your patient dies, you must perform postmortem care for the body, provide emotional support to family members, and return the patient's belongings to his family. Thoroughly documenting such care may prove crucial if his family claims his body was mishandled or his belongings were lost.

How to Respond

Postmortem care depends on the circumstances of the patient's death. In most states, a patient who dies within 24 hours of admission or surgery or who wasn't under a physician's care when he died must be referred to the medical examiner.

If the Body Will Be Sent to the Medical Examiner. If your patient's body will be referred to the medical examiner, preserve evidence of invasive procedures and treatment measures. Provide the usual postmortem care as described below—but keep tubes, IV lines, and internal monitoring devices in place. Cap an IV catheter or tie a knot in the tubing. Then cut the tubing, loop it on top of the dressing, and cover it with a clean dressing. Hide medical equipment to the extent possible by covering it with clothing or dressings. For more information on preparing the patient's body for the medical examiner, review your facility's policy and your state's laws.

Before taking family members into the patient's room, prepare them for what they'll see. Explain that tubes and devices must be left in place until the medical examiner reviews the patient's case. When they're ready to enter, take them to the room, answer their questions, and then excuse yourself to give them privacy.

If the Body Won't Be Sent to the Medical Examiner. Prepare the body for family viewing. If the patient had a roommate, take him to another room or a lounge until the patient's body is removed. Have family members step outside while you prepare the body. Offer to have the chaplain see them. If they want to call anyone, show them to a telephone.

If no family members were present when the patient died, ask the physician to call the family to inform them of the patient's death and ask whether they want to see his body.

After you've cleared the room, bathe the patient and remove visible medical devices, such as an endotracheal tube, IV catheter, or indwelling urinary catheter. Cover wound and puncture sites with clean dressings. Provide mouth care and change the bed linens and the patient's gown. Close the patient's eyes and place a rolled washcloth under his chin to keep his mouth closed. Tidy the room, remove unused equipment, and empty the trash can.

Then escort the family into the room. Provide chairs and tissues. Answer their questions and arrange for the physician to talk with them, if they want him to do so. Tell them where you'll be and how to contact you when they're ready to leave. Then excuse yourself to give them privacy.

Caring for the Patient's Belongings. Gather the patient's belongings and check off each item on the admission inventory (if used in your facility). If additional items are present, note them on the list. Give the belongings to a family member, and have this person sign the list to acknowledge receipt.

Check the patient's body for jewelry, and give jewelry to a family member. Record this person's name and relationship to the patient. If you can't remove a ring, place a piece of tape over it so that it won't fall off during transport or embalming.

If no family member is present, copy the belongings list and place it in a bag with the patient's belongings. Prepare the body for transport to the morgue according to facility policy. Then deliver the belongings to the security department, and have the security guard sign the belongings list to acknowledge receipt. The patient's belongings will be held for the family.

What to Document

Your documentation should reflect the care you provided for the patient and family and indicate the disposition of the body and the patient's belongings. Record the time and manner of the patient's death. Document the circumstances of his death, including treatment he was receiving at the time. If resuscitation was in progress, indicate when it started and ended, its outcome, and the location of resuscitation documentation (for instance, on the code sheet). If the death wasn't witnessed and resuscitation wasn't attempted, note that the time you've recorded is the time the patient's body was found, not when his heart stopped beating.

Also document the name of the person who verified the patient's death. Some states permit nurses to verify death. Be sure to follow your facility's policy. Make sure your documentation also includes:

- names of family members present at the time of death
- whether the case was referred to the medical examiner
- postmortem physical care you performed

- medical devices removed or left in place
- staff members who interacted with the family and the type of interaction
- family members who viewed the body
- belongings removed from the room and those left on the patient's body
- disposition of the patient's belongings
- presence of gold fillings or bridges
- body's disposition
- name of the funeral home notified to retrieve the body from the morgue, if appropriate

WHEN YOUR PATIENT DONATES AN ORGAN

A patient's heart, kidneys, corneas, skin, and bone marrow can be transplanted or her blood can be transfused into another patient. The Uniform Anatomical Gift Act permits organ harvesting from a deceased person who completed and signed an organ donor card. (However, some states also require permission from the next of kin for organ donation, even if the patient completed an organ donor card.) If a card wasn't signed, the Act also permits the deceased patient's family to consent to donation of her organs. Most facilities require that the next of kin sign a separate consent form witnessed by two people. The donor or her next of kin also must sign a separate consent form to allow human immunodeficiency virus testing.

Make sure you're familiar with your facility's organ donation policy. (See *Understanding required referral*, page 324.) The policy should address which patients can donate an organ, the consent form required, and which people must be notified of the planned donation.

How to Respond

A patient or the family of a patient who decides to donate an organ needs your emotional support and nursing skills. Provide information as appropriate. Thoroughly document the patient's

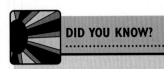

DID YOU KNOW?

UNDERSTANDING REQUIRED REFERRAL
For hospitals to qualify for Medicare and Medicaid reimbursement, the Health Care Financing Administration (HCFA) requires hospitals to report all cardio-vascular and brain deaths to the local organ procurement organization (OPO). This reporting (or referral) not only allows reimbursement, but also identifies more potential organ donors, which helps to reduce the donor organ shortage.

To promote compliance, local and federal branches of the HCFA examine hospital records to ensure that staff members report all deaths and ask the patient's family about consenting to organ donation. To help ensure that your records meet HCFA requirements, obtain forms that list the required infor-mation from your hospital or local OPO. In general, you'll need to document the following:
• time and date of the patient's death
• name of the person you notified at the local OPO
• organs' suitability for transplantation

condition, the circumstances of the decision to donate, and the names of people involved in the decision.

If the Patient Has Died. For a deceased patient, contact your local organ procurement organization (OPO), which will obtain the family's consent. If you don't know the name of your local organization, contact the United Network for Organ Sharing (UNOS). This national agency can direct you to your local organ-ization, which will review the patient's case and tell you which physical care measures to perform. For instance, if your patient is a candidate for cornea donation, you'll be instructed to place saline-soaked gauze over her eyes to prevent corneal drying. As needed, obtain physician's orders to implement required care. Also make sure the necessary consent forms have been signed and placed in the medical record.

If the Patient Is Brain-Dead. The local OPO can help you and the physician discuss organ donation with the family of a "brain-dead" patient. (See *Teaching about brain death*.) After reviewing the case, the organization will consult the physician about medical

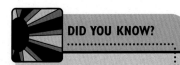

treatment or drug therapy required to maintain the patient's organs for donation.

Implement care as prescribed. As appropriate, reinforce teaching with the family and answer their questions. Emphasize that organ donation is a gift of life.

Providing Care During Organ Harvesting. Before organ harvesting begins, answer family members' questions and provide emotional support. Reassure them that organ harvesting isn't disfiguring and won't prevent an open-casket funeral, if desired. As appropriate, call the chaplain or social services department to provide additional support.

Depending on the organ involved, harvesting may take place in the patient's room or in an operating suite. Corneal harvesting usually takes place at the bedside. To prepare for corneal harvesting, gather needed equipment and escort family members out of the room. If the family wants to see the patient after the procedure, close the patient's eyes and cover them with a dressing.

Major organs are harvested in an operating suite. Verify that consent has been obtained, and complete your notes before the patient's body leaves the unit. In most cases, the body goes directly from the operating room to the morgue.

Caring for a Living Donor. If your patient decides to donate an organ, provide the usual preoperative care. Make sure she has signed a consent form and has undergone necessary laboratory work.

Also provide emotional support. Remember that the patient who donates an organ faces a loss and a body image change. Arrange for a chaplain or social worker to talk to her, if necessary, to provide additional counseling. If the organ recipient is a family member, keep the patient informed of the recipient's condition.

After organ harvesting, check the incision site frequently. Provide routine postoperative care and monitor affected body functions. For example, if the patient donated a kidney, record her fluid intake and output and monitor her blood urea nitrogen and creatinine levels. Teach her how to perform self-care at home to promote health and avoid complications. Explain the importance of follow-up care after discharge.

What to Document

Document the circumstances of the decision to donate an organ. Record the times of your and the physician's discussions with the patient and family. Write down what family members were told about the patient's prognosis before they decided to donate their loved one's organ. If the patient had an organ donation card, copy it for the medical record. If the organ donation team will use the consent form required by your facility, place a copy in the medical record.

Document the names of organ procurement team members who met with the family, and record the meeting date and time. Document the name of the physician who harvested the organ, and record the date and time of the procedure. If the procedure took place at the bedside, document the condition of the patient's body afterward and the family's response to the procedure.

For a living donor, document preoperative and postoperative care and your patient's response to the procedure. Record your referrals to the chaplain or social services department, along with the reason for referral. Also document patient and family teaching and the patient's and family's understanding of your instructions.

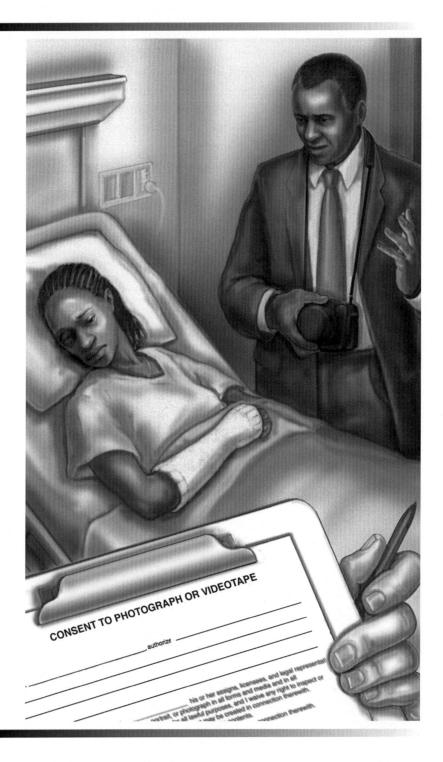

CONSENT TO PHOTOGRAPH OR VIDEOTAPE

_____, authorize _____

_____ his or her assigns, licensees, and legal representat
_____ ortrait, or photograph in all forms and media and in all
_____ all lawful purposes, and I waive any right to inspect or
_____ ___ may be created in connection therewith.
_____ _____ contents, _____ connection therewith.

PART 3

Handling Difficult Professional Problems

The physician orders a drug you believe will harm your patient. A coworker performs a clinical procedure incompetently. You suspect that a colleague has tampered with the nurse's notes. Are you sure of your responsibilities in these dilemmas? Do you know how to document properly to reduce your legal risk?

As you've probably discovered, working with other health care professionals makes you vulnerable to many legal dangers. Part Three explores your legal responsibilities when a health care team member's actions put you in a precarious position, violate professional standards, or break the law. It helps you recognize your legal obligations, avoid potential conflicts, choose an appropriate course of action, and document defensively to protect yourself legally.

Besides clarifying the situations described above, this section explores your legal accountability and documentation responsibilities when taking a telephone or verbal order from a physician, handling a physician's illegible order, documenting a colleague's care, and dealing with criticism in the patient record. It also explains legally safe actions to take—and sound documentation to write—when facility practices put you at legal risk. For instance, it outlines your options if your employer expects you to cosign colleagues' notes, document care given by unlicensed assistive personnel, or work in an understaffed unit. It also tells how to document your actions in these situations.

To be prepared for an on-the-job dilemma, you need to learn everything you can so that you can act wisely when the situation arises. Of course, being prepared also means being familiar with your facility's policies and procedures, including those on record retention. (See *Telephone triage logs: Ruling on record retention*.) For instructions on how to act in a specific situation, you'll need to consult your facility's risk manager or legal counsel.

CASE LAW CLOSEUP

TELEPHONE TRIAGE LOGS: RULING ON RECORD RETENTION

If you're like most nurses, you may wonder how long to keep patient records, hesitate to destroy old records in the course of business, and worry about needing them in court *after* they've been destroyed. Fortunately, case law can help you understand your legal obligations—and reduce your fears.

Understanding the case

Thornton v. Shah[1] demonstrates the importance of properly timed record retention and destruction. In this case, Mrs. Shah experienced multiple complications of pregnancy. For advice and appointments, she frequently telephoned the health maintenance organization (HMO) through which she had medical insurance coverage. After the pregnancy ended with the stillbirth of a previously viable fetus, she filed a lawsuit against the HMO's physician for negligence of her prenatal care.

During the trial, Mrs. Shah's attorney tried to show that she was diligent in alerting the HMO about changes in her condition and that the stillbirth directly resulted from a lack of care by the HMO's attending physician. Her attorney requested copies of all patient call logs in order to show how often she had called the HMO.

Upon receiving the request the triage log books, the HMO informed the patient's attorney that they had been destroyed in the ordinary course of business 6 months after they were created. The attorney then changed his motion to include spoliation of (interference with) evidence by the HMO.

---

[1] *Thornton v. Shah,* 202 WL 1822126 (Ill. App., August 8, 2002).

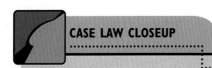

CASE LAW CLOSEUP

TELEPHONE TRIAGE LOGS: RULING ON RECORD RETENTION—cont'd
How the Court Ruled
The court stated that spoliation of evidence wasn't a valid motion in this case because it wasn't relevant to the litigation. From the court's perspective, the HMO didn't have a legal obligation to preserve the nurses' telephone triage logs longer than the logs had medical relevance to suits that may be brought by HMO members against physicians or nurses. Because there were no allegations of professional misconduct against the HMO's nursing staff, the records were destroyed as part of the usual business routine. The court noted that businesses are free to create policies about data preservation and can destroy such data in the ordinary course of business. It also saw no indication that the logs would have proven negligence by the attending physician. For these reasons, the court ruled that there was no intent to prevent or interfere with a later lawsuit.

The Lesson Learned
State laws generally stipulate the amount of time required for retaining actual patient records. However, they don't cover telephone triage records. That leaves businesses free to determine when and how to destroy such ancillary records.
   So whenever you must document in ancillary records, do so accurately. Then when the time comes, destroy these records according to facility policy. Most important, don't worry needlessly about not having them in the facility's files as a defense against later lawsuits.

Keeping the Medical Record Relevant

To protect yourself, your colleagues, and your facility against undue legal risk, make sure that the information you write in the patient's medical record belongs there. Don't use the record to document complaints about understaffing, instances of substandard nursing care, or conflicts with a colleague. Instead, address these concerns with the appropriate nurse administrator or the colleague you're having trouble with. If your facility's policy requires you to document such concerns, use the appropriate form—for instance, an unusual occurrence form or risk management form.

WHEN A PHYSICIAN OR COLLEAGUE ILLEGALLY ALTERS THE MEDICAL RECORD

A health care professional who tampers with (illegally alters) a patient's medical record places herself, her colleagues, and, possibly, her employer at legal risk. In court, an altered medical record has no credibility.

The person who tampers with the record can be charged with fraud, which carries a longer statute of limitations than malpractice. Using sophisticated ultraviolet and infrared techniques, expert document examiners can determine handwriting age and detect late additions.

Defining Tampering. Actions that constitute tampering include:

- improperly adding to a colleague's notes
- destroying all or part of a patient's medical record
- rewriting all or part of the record
- omitting significant facts
- deliberately documenting inaccurate information
- falsifying an entry date or time or adding to an entry later without indicating that the addition was late

Reasons for Tampering. Most commonly, a health care professional tampers with a medical record to cover up improper or ineffective care. Imagine, for instance, the following scenario: Your patient has severe hypertension and heart failure. At 0200, you call the admitting physician to report that the patient's blood pressure keeps rising despite antihypertensive drug therapy. The physician tells you to continue observing the patient, further restrict his fluids, and obtain blood in the morning for electrolyte, blood urea nitrogen, and creatinine measurements. You document these telephone orders and note that you've initiated them. In the nurse's notes, you record the information you reported to the physician, the instructions she gave, and the time.

At 0430, the patient's blood pressure remains extremely high, especially the diastolic value. When you report this to the physician, she prescribes a different oral antihypertensive drug to be given immediately. You suggest that perhaps the patient needs a nitroprusside drip. The physician ignores your suggestion and repeats her prescription for an oral antihypertensive drug.

You give the drug, but it barely affects the patient's diastolic pressure. You document your earlier conversation with the physician, her orders, the time she gave them, and the patient's response to the drug. When giving a report to the day shift at 0700, you mention your telephone conversations with the physician.

When you arrive for work the next night, you find that the physician has written an order, timed at 0300, for a nitroprusside drip titrated to keep the patient's systolic pressure below 140 mm Hg and diastolic pressure below 90 mm Hg. The nurse giving you report asks why you didn't initiate the order. You realize that the physician must have falsified the time of her nitroprusside order when she realized that the oral antihypertensive drug she prescribed at 0430 was ineffective.

How to Respond

If you discover that someone has altered your patient's medical record, notify the appropriate nurse administrator or your risk manager right away. Don't try to correct or add to the altered entry. In the scenario above, for instance, your nurse's notes would indicate that you received the physician's order for a different oral antihypertensive drug (rather than a nitroprusside drip) at 0430—even though she wrote on the order sheet that she prescribed the nitroprusside drip at 0300.

What should you do if a physician or nurse colleague asks you to change your nurse's notes because they conflict with hers or cast hers in a bad light? Say no—or risk placing all your documentation in question and exposing yourself to extensive legal liability.

What to Document

If a coworker alters a medical record or asks you to alter your notes, continue to document truthfully and objectively. Trust that your notes will support your documentation.

The appropriate nurse administrator or risk manager should photocopy your notes and the altered portion of the medical record. If required by your facility, complete an incident report describing your conversations with the coworker who altered the record or asked you to do so. In the report, note the times you made documentation entries in the medical record.

Making a Legal Alteration. Most nurses occasionally make honest mistakes in a patient's record, such as misidentifying which of the patient's arms has an IV line. To correct a simple error like this, draw a single line through the mistaken entry, write "Mistaken entry" above or next to it, specify the reason for the alteration, record the date and time, and then initial the correction. This shows that you've taken ownership of the mistake and aren't hiding anything. (See *Correcting a mistaken entry.*)

TIPS & ADVICE

CORRECTING A MISTAKEN ENTRY
When correcting a patient's medical record, follow the general guidelines below, as well as your facility's policies and procedures.

Do
- *Do* draw a single line through the mistaken entry so that your original words remain visible.
- *Do* write "Mistaken entry" above or next to your original words to explain why you drew a line through them.
- *Do* write your initials and the date and time next to the words "Mistaken entry."
- *Do* follow the proper procedure for making a late entry if you must add information.

Don't
- *Don't* try to squeeze corrected information around the original entry.
- *Don't* use correction fluid, draw a thick line through the mistaken entry, or otherwise make the original words unreadable.
- *Don't* write "Error." Juries tend to associate this word with a clinical error that led to patient injury.
- *Don't* try to hide your mistake. If the jury suspects that you're hiding something, it's likely to rule against you even if you did nothing wrong.

If you've made a more serious mistake, such as writing another patient's laboratory test results on your patient's record, you may need to take additional steps—especially if other caregivers have based their interventions on the incorrect results. In most cases, an explanation of the reason for the correction will suffice. For example, if you discover that you've documented in the wrong patient chart, write "Data entered in wrong chart." For specific instructions, however, consult your facility's risk manager. Also inform health care team members of the error so that they can reevaluate the patient's treatment plan as needed.

WHEN A COLLEAGUE CRITICIZES YOUR CARE IN THE MEDICAL RECORD

You're caring for an 80-year-old patient who's undergoing her third round of cancer chemotherapy. When reviewing her record, you see that a nurse on the shift after yours has written, "On assessment, noted that patient was left with infiltrated IV line by previous nurse."

Chances are, you'd take exception to this nurse's using the patient's medical record to criticize your care. Blaming a colleague—especially in the medical record—casts all nurses on the unit in a bad light and indicates lack of effective team work. (See *Collegiality: A nursing standard*, page 336.)

It's also bound to raise suspicions of incompetent care in the minds of judges and juries. If the patient in the scenario above sued for malpractice, her attorney could construe the written criticism as evidence that you provided poor care. Your employer would probably settle out of court to avoid more extensive questions about the quality of patient care in the facility.

How to Respond

Disagreements among staff members don't belong in the patient record. If a colleague writes a comment that criticizes your care, notify the appropriate nurse administrator. Don't respond to the

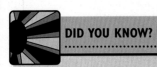

COLLEGIALITY: A NURSING STANDARD
If you're concerned about the quality of a colleague's care, don't air your concerns in the medical record. Instead, address them in a constructive, nonthreatening way, as directed by the American Nurses Association's Standard IV.

Titled "Collegiality," this standard states that the nurse should contribute to the "professional development of peers, colleagues, and others." To meet the criteria for collegiality, you must:
- give peers constructive feedback about their practice
- share your knowledge and skills with colleagues and others
- contribute to an environment that promotes clinical education of nursing students, as appropriate

criticism in writing, alter the record, delete the note, or add to your original note to refute the criticism. These acts may constitute tampering and bring serious repercussions. (See *When a physician or colleague illegally alters the medical record,* pages 332-335.)

Instead, speak with the critical colleague and try to resolve the matter privately. Request that she complete an incident or unusual occurrence (variance) report, and offer to help her write it. As she writes the report, make sure she keeps her documentation objective, describing only what she found without blaming you.

If you're uncomfortable making this request, speak with the appropriate nurse administrator, who may be able to address the issue more effectively. Consider suggesting that your administrator call a unit meeting to discuss the correct use of nurse's notes and to improve working relationships.

What to Document

If you believe that a colleague's actions have jeopardized your patient, don't record your suspicions or criticisms in the record. Instead, complete an incident or unusual occurrence report to document your beliefs. Don't cast blame in the report. Stick to facts and observations. Simply state what you saw, heard, smelled, or felt and describe your interventions. (For detailed information, see *How to complete an incident report,* pages 383–386.)

WHEN YOU FIND AN INAPPROPRIATE COMMENT IN THE MEDICAL RECORD

You've been assigned to care for a patient who's recovering from a cerebrovascular accident on your rehabilitation unit. When reviewing the nurse's notes, you see that the nurse on the previous shift has written, "While walking in hallway, patient's legs gave out and he fell to the floor. Patient has done this before on purpose. This nurse refuses to ambulate him again." A little further on you read, "Patient refuses medications and A.M. care. Patient is crazy and needs a psychiatrist."

Such attacks against patients don't belong in the medical record. The attorney for an injured patient could claim that the record proves the patient received incompetent care.

What's more, documenting critical comments about a patient may interfere with patient care and reflects poorly on the responsible nurse, the unit, and the nursing profession. Instead of criticizing the patient, the medical record should identify the patient's behavior, list medical and nursing interventions performed, describe the patient's response to interventions, and identify consultations obtained for supportive therapy, such as physical therapy or psychiatry.

If the patient fails to adhere to or accept prescribed interventions, the record shouldn't fault him. It should simply describe his actions, your response, and staff members' actions to ensure delivery of competent care.

How to Respond

If you discover an inappropriate comment in your patient's medical record, don't refute or address it in the record. Instead, notify the appropriate nurse administrator, who will investigate why the note was written and take steps to ensure the continuity

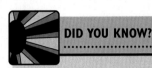

DID YOU KNOW?

HOW A NURSE ADMINISTRATOR CORRECTS THE RECORD
Don't be surprised if a nurse administrator *legally* alters a medical record after reading an inappropriate comment. Her alteration provides legal protection, showing that she took steps to ensure the quality of patient care and promote cooperation among employees. The administrator should also explain her actions to the staff member who made the comment.

Making the Change
To indicate that the inappropriate comment doesn't belong in the medical record, the nurse administrator crosses out the comment with a single line, writes the date and time, and initials the original note. Then she asks the staff member who wrote the inappropriate comment to initial her alteration.

of competent care. (See *How a nurse administrator corrects the record.*) For the colleague who wrote the inappropriate comment, the administrator should explain the proper channels and methods for addressing patient noncompliance.

What to Document

According to your facility's policies and procedures, file an unusual occurrence (variance) form, an incident report, or a quality management report. If appropriate, also send a memo to the nurse administrator. She can submit a written request to the continuing education department suggesting teaching sessions on documentation for all staff members. On the report or form you file, document that you made this recommendation, if appropriate.

WHEN A PHYSICIAN ASKS TO REMOVE A MEDICAL RECORD FROM THE FACILITY

The patient's medical record is a legal document that belongs to the health care facility or agency. Although health care professionals may request a copy of the record for valid purposes, they don't own or have exclusive control of it and they can't remove the original record from the facility. (See *How the courts rule on lost medical records,* pages 339-340.)

How to Respond

If the physician says she's removing a patient's medical record from the facility, politely remind her that she's not permitted to remove the original. Offer to copy the portion she needs, and record the names and dates of the sections you copy. If the physician needs

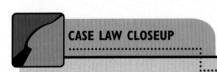

CASE LAW CLOSEUP

HOW THE COURTS RULE ON LOST MEDICAL RECORDS
Loss of a patient's record not only complicates his care and creates extra work for the health care team, but also may expose you, your colleagues, and your facility to legal risks, as the case below illustrates.

Understanding the Case
Phillips v. Covenant Clinic[1] concerns the unintentional loss of medical records for Mr. Phillips, age 80, who came to the clinic with flulike symptoms and chest pain. A physician's assistant (PA) took his history, examined him, and made extensive notes in his clinic record. The PA informed the clinic physician of the patient's history of congestive heart failure and current report of chest pain. The physician ordered an electrocardiogram (ECG) and chest x-ray.

After obtaining an ECG tracing, the PA allowed the patient to walk to the hospital nearby for the chest x-ray. On the way to the hospital, the patient collapsed. When the hospital informed the clinic of the patient's status, a second clinic physician grabbed the patient's record—including the PA's notes and the ECG tracing—and rushed them to the intensive care unit (ICU) where Mr. Phillips had been admitted. Despite a full resuscitative attempt, Mr. Phillips died shortly after admission.

Mr. Phillips' family filed a lawsuit against the clinic and both clinic physicians. Their attorney demanded to see the patient's clinic record, which the clinic no longer possessed and had no way to locate. Without the record, the family's attorney had no facts to prove negligence in the clinic's care of Mr. Phillips.

The court was going to dismiss the case, but the family's attorney argued that the missing record caused *spoliation* of (interference with) the evidence and that the clinic was indeed negligent.

[1] *Phillips v. Covenant Clinic, 625 N. E. 2d 714 (Iowa, 2001).*

Continued

CASE LAW CLOSEUP

HOW THE COURTS RULE ON LOST MEDICAL RECORDS—cont'd
How the Court Ruled
The Supreme Court of Iowa acknowledged that spoliation of evidence is a valid legal concept but stated that the concept didn't apply to this case. The clinic couldn't have intentionally altered, destroyed, or lost the record because it couldn't have known in advance that the patient would die in the ICU and that the clinic would be sued. According to the court, common sense would hold that someone who destroyed or lost a document relevant to litigation must have felt threatened by its contents. Spoliation of evidence can't occur and no assumptions can be made when evidence is destroyed unintentionally or during routine destruction of old files. The court concluded that the record was lost in the ICU by unit personnel with no intent to protect the clinic.

The Lesson Learned
The case illustrates to need for nurses and other personnel to diligently preserve records. This particular record may have been lost because the code or Mr. Phillips' rapid admission and discharge may have created a chaotic environment. Nevertheless, nurses have a duty to preserve patient records and track their location.

Furthermore, the case shows that the courts will view alterations or destruction of patient records after notice of impending litigation as intentional spoliation of evidence. This ruling serves as a warning not to lose, destroy, or add information to a patient's record after a legal action is filed or even contemplated. If you must make a late entry in a patient's chart, do it promptly and according to facility policy. And remember *never* to remove or allow others to remove portions of the patient record.

the patient's most recent laboratory or radiology reports, keep in mind that most facilities provide additional copies of such data to physicians or can transmit computerized data to the physician's office directly.

If the physician insists on removing the medical record from the facility, page the appropriate nurse administrator immediately. Remind the physician that the patient's record is the facility's official business record and can't be removed from the premises. Hold onto the record physically if necessary. By the time you've finished your explanation, the nurse administrator may have arrived to reinforce your explanation. (See *Preventing medical record destruction.*)

If the physician is determined to take the record and you can't stop her without risking physical harm, let her take it. Then inform the risk manager or legal counsel of the physician's actions and follow that person's recommendations. Take other appropriate steps your facility requires, such as completing special forms.

If the physician says that she needs the medical record to dictate notes or write new prescriptions, suggest that she take it to the facility's dictating area. Before she does this, remove the portions you're currently using so that you can continue to document patient care while the record is unavailable.

What to Document

In the patient's medical record, document the physician's statement that she intends to remove the record from the facility. Record her name, the date and time of her statement, and your response. Also document the names of witnesses and the nurse administrator you notified.

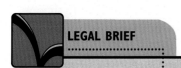

LEGAL BRIEF

PREVENTING MEDICAL RECORD DESTRUCTION

The most serious form of tampering, destruction of a patient's medical record is legal suicide. The health care provider who destroys the record—and possibly her employer—stands virtually no chance of prevailing in court if a patient sues for malpractice. The jury will assume that the record was destroyed because it contained extremely damaging information.

Taking Precautions

If you suspect that your colleague is planning to destroy all or part of a patient's medical record, alert the appropriate nurse administrator immediately. If needed, ask her to help you copy the record. Then give the copy to the medical records department for safekeeping.

If the physician leaves the facility with the patient's record despite your interventions, start a second record and label it "Temporary record." Write a note explaining why you created the temporary record, and thoroughly document the events leading to the physician's removal of the record.

If you must reconstruct part of the original record, document the date and time of reconstruction and identify the source of the original information. Then obtain copies of prescriptions from the pharmacy and copies of other important documents from appropriate departments. (For more information, see *When your patient's medical record isn't available,* pages 208-212.)

As required, complete an unusual occurrence (variance) or incident report. (If your facility uses a nurse administrator's report for this type of incident, complete a separate unusual occurrence report if the administrator's report isn't a permanent record.) Document the name of the risk manager or legal counsel you spoke to, that person's recommendations, and your actions.

When the physician returns with the patient's record, the nurse who's most familiar with the patient's care should review the record for alterations and deletions and should document such changes on an unusual occurrence report. Notify the admitting and consulting physicians of the changes this nurse detects so that they can rewrite orders or review the treatment plan as needed. In the nurse's notes, document the time the physicians were notified, their responses, and other measures taken to safeguard the patient.

HOW TO HANDLE A PHYSICIAN'S QUESTIONABLE ORDER

Although you have a duty to implement a physician's orders as written, your primary duty is to protect your patient's well-being. At some time, you may need to question a physician's inappropriate or potentially harmful order—or even refuse to carry it out. Increasingly, courts are ruling that nurses must speak out on their patients' behalf and document their concerns about questionable orders. If you implement a questionable order, you may be held liable for subsequent patient injury if a lawyer shows that you had the last clear, direct chance to prevent the injury.

How to Respond

Never countermand a physician's questionable order, for instance, by altering it. (See *Question, don't countermand*.) Instead, if you believe that carrying out the physician's order will harm your patient—or if the physician fails to order a test or treatment that you believe your patient needs—try to get a second opinion from a trusted colleague. Then discuss your concerns with the physician and document the discussion in the record. If the physician insists that you administer the questionable treatment, you have a duty to refuse and to document your refusal and rationale. These duties also apply if the physician's order goes beyond the scope of your practice or directly violates your state's nurse practice act, facility policies and procedures, or professional standards.

Also, review your facility's policy to determine which steps to take if a physician places a patient in jeopardy or fails to meet the standards of medical care. For example, the policy may require you to discuss your concerns with the appropriate nurse administrator and to write a memo to that person and higher-level managers. At some point, the chief of staff or medical director may need to become involved too.

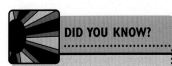

DID YOU KNOW?

QUESTION, DON'T COUNTERMAND
Although you're obligated to question a physician's potentially harmful or inappropriate order, you have no right to countermand or alter it. Countermanding or altering an order is a violation of the nurse practice act and exposes you to charges of insubordination and practicing medicine without a license.

If you believe that you could harm the patient if you carried out the questionable order, try to delay implementation until the issue has been resolved. If you can't resolve the issue by speaking directly with the physician who gave the order, talk with the appropriate nurse administrator and, if necessary, a higher-level administrator.

What to Document

To support your belief that the physician's order is questionable, record patient assessment findings and other pertinent information. Then document your discussions with the physician about the patient's treatment. If you've refused to carry out a prescribed treatment, document your refusal, the rationale, and the names of the physician and nurse administrator you notified. Record their responses and note the times.

Then, in a memo or letter, inform the nurse administrator of your concerns. Describe the facts objectively, including the patient's condition, your discussion with the physician, and your rationale for refusing to implement his order.

Some facilities may require you to use a special form for this information. If necessary, consult your facility's risk manager or legal counsel to make sure you've filled out the form correctly. Keep copies of the form for your files.

WHEN YOU TAKE A TELEPHONE OR VERBAL ORDER

Telephone and verbal orders are easily misunderstood. Many facilities specify the circumstances under which physicians may give such orders and require them to cosign the orders within 24 hours. These policies help ensure that a physician corrects a miscommunicated or misunderstood order promptly and that orders aren't implemented too late or for longer than intended.

How to Respond

Don't accept a telephone or verbal order unless the physician has a valid reason for giving one. For instance, if your patient develops hypotension after her physician has scrubbed for the operating room, the physician must give telephone orders to treat the patient's acute situation. Because many facilities have a policy against accepting verbal orders when the physician is in the nursing unit, ask the physician to write the order if he's present.

When you receive a telephone or verbal order, repeat it back to the physician using his exact words. If the order seems ambiguous or incomplete, ask him to clarify it. If possible, have a colleague verify the telephone order by listening on a second extension and then cosigning the order on the physician's order sheet.

Before the physician hangs up, review your notes to make sure he has given all the required components, such as the administration route for a prescribed drug or the duration of a prescribed infusion. If you have questions, ask him to clarify. If you're not sure you heard the drug name correctly or if several other drugs have similar names, ask him to spell the drug name.

What to Document

Write the order on the physician's order sheet—not scratch paper—as soon as possible, while it's fresh in your memory. Record the date and time you received the order, and note whether it was a telephone order (t.o.) or verbal order (v.o.). Write your name and full credentials, and have the colleague who verified the order write her name after yours. Then transcribe the order as you would any other.

If the physician gave his order in response to assessment findings that you reported, document in the nurse's notes your reason for notifying him and the assessment data you conveyed. Then record that you implemented the order, and document the patient's response. (See *Telephone orders: What the courts look for,* pages 346-347.) For instance, if the physician instructs you to assess the patient for an additional hour, make sure your notes indicate that you carried out this order and called the physician later to report the new assessment data. Also record the additional hour of patient observation on the physician's order sheet. A sample order sheet entry might read:

3/29/06, 0400. Observe patient for signs and symptoms of heart failure. Notify me immediately if systolic blood pressure falls below 90 mm Hg, heart rate exceeds 150 beats/minute, urine output drops below 30 ml in a 2-hour period, or patient becomes confused or restless. t.o. Dr. Dennison/M. Rowell, RN/K. Somer, RN (witness).

If your facility allows you to accept orders from an intermediary, such as a physician's assistant, record the intermediary's

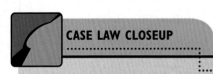

CASE LAW CLOSEUP

TELEPHONE ORDERS: WHAT THE COURTS LOOK FOR
Implementing telephone orders correctly can help you and your employer in court—especially if you can also show that you performed competent patient assessment and promptly reported your findings to the physician. In the following case, the nurses' careful documentation and prompt implementation of the physician's telephone orders helped tip the outcome of a lawsuit.

Understanding the Case
In *Pugh v. Mayeaux*,[1] Mrs. Pugh, a full-term obstetric patient, was admitted with intermittent labor contractions and slight cervical dilation. Shortly after her admission, the nurse noted that Mrs. Pugh showed signs of possible pancreatitis. When she called the physician to report these findings, the physician gave verbal orders based on the provisional diagnoses of pregnancy at term and, possibly, gastroenteritis. These orders included continuous monitoring for signs of fetal distress, such as a decelerated heart beat, and notification that a cesarean section would be done if indicated.

According to the medical record, nurses assessed Mrs. Pugh 10 times between 1500 and 2315. At 1615, the physician called to prescribe an antiemetic in response to a nurse's report that Mrs. Pugh continued to have mild nausea and emesis. At 2315, the nurse telephoned the physician to report that the patient had abdominal distention and diffuse abdominal pain, was vomiting dark green emesis, and had a temperature of 99.3° F. The physician ordered a STAT amylase level measurement and insertion of a nasogastric tube connected to continuous low suction. The nurse implemented these orders.

When the laboratory results showed an above-normal amylase level, suggesting pancreatitis, the nurse called the physician again. He decided not to perform an immediate cesarean section because the pancreatitis didn't threaten the fetus. He also ordered continuous fetal monitoring and instructed the nurse to contact him immediately if she detected signs of fetal distress.

At 0445 the next day, the nurse telephoned the physician to report that Mrs. Pugh had continuing abdominal distress and distention. She was taken to the intensive care unit. Later that morning, when the fetal heart rate dropped, the nurse notified the physician immediately and prepared the patient for a cesarean section.

When signs of fetal distress developed, an emergency cesarean section was performed—but not soon enough to prevent damage. The neonate suffered permanent complications from hypoxic neurologic damage. The parents sued the physician, hospital, and nurses for negligence in not performing the cesarean section sooner.

---

[1]*Pugh v. Mayeaux, 702 S. 2d 988 (La.App. 1998).*

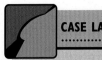

TELEPHONE ORDERS: WHAT THE COURTS LOOK FOR—cont'd
How the Court Ruled
The court exonerated the defendants. It found that the nurses had provided high-quality care and documented their care thoroughly, as shown by their notes describing comprehensive assessment, prompt physician notification of assessment data, and immediate implementation of the physician's orders.

The Lesson Learned
This case underscores the importance of nurses reporting significant findings immediately, physicians giving telephone or verbal orders promptly in response to nurses' reports, and nurses implementing telephone orders as soon as possible. It also shows that just documenting a telephone or verbal order isn't enough. You must also record the reason for notifying the physician, the patient's signs and symptoms, and your prompt implementation of the physician's orders.

name on the order sheet, and transcribe the order as a standard telephone or verbal order. For instance, write, "J. Ortiz, PA, called in the order for Dr. Dennison." Then, in your nurse's notes, document that J. Ortiz, PA, called the unit for Dr. Dennison and note that the order was implemented. No matter who places the verbal or telephone order, flag the chart to signal the prescriber to authenticate and cosign the order.

WHEN A PHYSICIAN'S ORDER IS ILLEGIBLE

Physicians have a duty to write complete, legible, medically sound orders. If you're not sure what a physician's order says or if you believe that it's incomplete, don't implement it based on your best guess. If you guess wrong, you could give the wrong

....
TIPS & ADVICE

WHAT TO DO IF YOU CAN'T REACH THE PHYSICIAN

If you can't reach the physician to clarify his order, notify the appropriate nurse administrator. In an emergency or urgent situation, she may consult the chief of staff or medical officer about the patient's care. Or she may ask the physician's medical partner to clarify the order.

If the physician is busy treating a patient who's in more critical condition than yours, document that you contacted him and expect him to respond in person as quickly as possible. This notation protects you and the physician in case your patient later sues.

drug, prepare the wrong dosage, or use the wrong administration route. If your guess leads to patient injury, you may find little sympathy from jurors.

How to Respond

Clarify an illegible order with the physician at once. Then ask him to rewrite his order to eliminate uncertainty about its content. If the physician has left the unit and you can't reach him, notify the appropriate nurse administrator. (See *What to do if you can't reach the physician.*)

Also tell other nurses on the unit that you're having trouble reading the order. A colleague who's more familiar with the physician's handwriting may be able to interpret the order.

Above all, don't let the situation cloud your thinking or force you into implementing an illegible or incomplete order—even in an emergency. The risk for error and consequent patient harm is too great.

Suggesting Routine Order Reviews. As a long-term measure, consider writing a memo to the appropriate nurse administrator documenting the need for that physician to review orders with the nurse or unit secretary before he leaves the unit. Or ask the physician to review his orders with you routinely before he leaves the unit. Emphasize that you don't want to delay implementing his orders but that you need to make sure you carry them out exactly as he intended.

What to Document

Document your attempts to contact the physician to clarify his order. Record the method of contact, such as telephone or pager, and the time of each attempt.

Once the physician clarifies the order, transcribe it on the physician's order sheet, marking your entry as a clarification of an earlier order. A clarified entry might read:

3/25/06, 1500. Clarification of orders for 3/25/06, 1430: Ampicillin 250 mg
P.O. g 6 hr.t.o. Dr. Johnson/J. Martinez, RN, BSN

Then document in your nurse's notes that the orders have been rewritten. Other health care team members will then see that the order was clarified.

If a colleague has interpreted the order for you, ask her to print the questionable word or words above the physician's original writing and then sign and date her notation.

WHEN A COLLEAGUE ASKS YOU TO DOCUMENT HER CARE

Like most nurses, you've probably documented procedures and treatments performed by physicians, recorded the events of a code or surgical procedure, or documented routine care provided by physical therapists and other health care professionals. These and certain other types of indirect documentation are legally acceptable. (See *Documenting monthly summaries*, page 350.)

Delegated documentation, as when you record care provided outside your presence, subjects you to legal risk. If you document a colleague's care that you didn't witness or participate in, you can be held liable for her errors. The courts regard delegated documentation as secondhand information with little credibility. What's more, delegated documentation fails to meet the standards of care that a reasonable and prudent nurse would provide.

How to Respond

Refuse to document care that you didn't witness or participate in. Tell your colleague that agreeing to her request would place you both in a legally indefensible position. If possible, offer to help her complete other patient care tasks so that she has more time for documentation.

If you notice the same colleague asking other nurses to document for her, notify the appropriate nurse administrator. The administrator should speak to your colleague directly and may want to hold an in-service session by a nurse-attorney to review the legal aspects of documentation.

Taking Telephone Reports from Colleagues. If a colleague calls the unit after her shift ends to report information she forgot to document, you're legally permitted to record this information. Just be sure to label it as a telephone report from the previous nurse, note the date and time of the entry, and record your colleague's name. In this situation, your entry might read:

> *2/28/06, 2020. K. Collins, RN, telephoned to report that patient voided 300 ml of clear, yellow urine immediately after admission to Room 382B. Patient had no difficulty voiding, and palpation showed no evidence of retained urine.—G. Gonzalez, RN*

If a colleague calls with routine information that she can easily document on her next shift, suggest that she record the information as a late entry. If the information is crucial to the patient's care or could affect care during the subsequent shift, document it right away, noting that it was reported to you. If required by your facility, use a special form to record telephoned information instead of recording it in the nurse's notes.

LEGAL BRIEF

DOCUMENTING MONTHLY SUMMARIES
Most long-term care facilities require nurses to write a monthly summary of each resident's general condition. Although this practice requires you to document care and observations that you didn't give or witness, it's legal as long as you label the report "Monthly summary of the medical record."

In this situation, your signature indicates only that you've read and summarized the notes from all nursing shifts. It doesn't indicate that you're personally attesting to the information. On the other hand, if you document the observations and care in the note as your own, you *could* be held responsible for the information.

WHEN A COWORKER GIVES YOUR PATIENT DRUGS IN YOUR ABSENCE

You've probably administered prescribed drugs to a coworker's patients or asked colleagues to administer drugs to your patients. If you work on a busy unit, this situation may arise more often than you'd prefer. During an emergency, sharing tasks with colleagues helps ensure that all patients on the unit receive necessary care on time. However, you're at risk for committing a medication error if you administer a drug that another nurse has poured, removed from the unit-dose package or bottle, or predrawn into an unmarked syringe.

How to Respond

Unit-dose packaging has decreased the drug administration problems described above. If you discover that a colleague has given your patient a drug while you were off the unit, thank her and make sure she has completed all the necessary documentation. For instance, if she gave the drug in response to a patient's symptom, such as pain, she should record her assessment findings, intervention, and the patient's response in the nurse's notes. Also have her document and sign the medication administration record.

What to Document

The nurse who administers a drug must complete all related documentation, including patient assessment, physician notification of significant findings, and patient response to the drug. If a colleague gave your patient a prescribed drug, make sure she documents it as described above. Then complete your documentation, including patient assessment findings you gathered when you returned to the unit. If your colleague initiated an infusion that wasn't completed when you returned, document the time the infusion ended and record the care you provided at the IV site when you discontinued the infusion.

WHEN YOU SUSPECT THAT A COLLEAGUE IS NEGLIGENT

All state nurse practice acts and professional standards of care emphasize the nurse's duty to protect patients from harm. The American Nurses Association Code for Nurses requires that nurses report a colleague's negligence or unsafe practice.

The doctrine of qualified privilege legally protects the nurse who reports a negligent colleague. (See *Understanding qualified privilege.*) However, reporting a colleague can lead to retaliation. Some health care workers who have reported colleagues have been harassed, fired, demoted, denied job-related requests, and forced into retirement.

How to Respond

If you suspect a colleague of professional negligence, first make sure you're seeing the whole picture. Gather all the facts that you can—from the patient, witnesses, the medical record, and other documents. What appears to be negligence may be an acceptable alternative method of providing care.

If your review of the data convinces you of your colleague's negligence, report your belief through the appropriate channels.

LEGAL BRIEF

UNDERSTANDING QUALIFIED PRIVILEGE
Normally, someone who impugns a person's professional reputation or capacity can be sued for defamation. However, nurses and others with a legal obligation to report honestly on colleagues' performance are protected by *qualified privilege.* This doctrine gives you immunity against charges of libel (written defamation) and slander (oral defamation) because the overriding public interest—patients' well-being—takes precedence over a person's professional reputation.

Keep in mind, though, that qualified privilege applies only to statements made to protect patients. It doesn't apply to idle gossip that reflects on a colleague's professional capabilities or motives, even if those statements are true.

In most facilities, you must notify the appropriate nurse administrator first. Expect her to request details, and don't be surprised if she asks you to discuss the issue with the colleague you've reported.

If your administrator won't pursue the issue, be prepared to stand your ground. Notify the next person in the chain of command, as dictated by your facility's reporting channels. You may need to contact top-level administrators and the board of directors or, if all else fails, outside agencies, such as the appropriate licensing board.

What to Document

According to facility policy, complete an incident or unusual occurrence (variance) report. Keep your language factual and objective. Without casting blame, describe the events that concern you and cite specific patient or witness statements. Record the names and titles of people who provided information about the incident and of those you notified. Also describe your actions to prevent further patient harm. Then give the report to the appropriate nurse administrator. Notify the patient's physician that you've filed the report, even if he's the one you're reporting. In the nurse's notes, document the care you provided to prevent or minimize patient harm. Don't note that you filed an incident report.

HOW TO DOCUMENT CARE GIVEN BY UNLICENSED ASSISTIVE PERSONNEL

Like other nurses, you may routinely document coworkers' care, such as treatments that physicians perform, portable x-rays that radiology technicians obtain, and blood samples that laboratory technicians draw. The physician's progress notes and laboratory and radiology reports can verify your documentation.

Care provided by unlicensed assistive personnel (UAP) may not be verifiable because it's typically not cross-referenced in other records. To address this problem, some facilities require UAP to fill out checklists that indicate the tasks or procedures they've performed. Most checklists involve routine and daily care, such as baths, linen changes, back rubs, meal service, and measurement of fluid intake and output and vital signs.

Some facilities also have a separate permanent form on which UAP record patients' vital sign measurements. Licensed nurses review the UAP's documentation and follow up on the data as necessary. Usually, the unit secretary transfers the information from the checklist to individual medical records.

Documenting Nonroutine Care. If you document nonroutine tasks performed by a UAP, such as assessing a patient's response to treatment, you could be in legal jeopardy unless you personally witnessed or verified the assessment findings or other care. Remember—your name appears on the patient's medical record. You will be the first person questioned if the patient files a lawsuit that alleges negligent nursing care.

How to Respond

Review the facility's policies on documenting care given by UAP. Find out whether your documentation means that you personally witnessed or can verify the care they provided or only that such care was reported to you.

If your documentation means that you witnessed or can verify the UAP's care, try to substantiate what the UAP reports by conducting interviews and spot checks. For instance, if she reports that the patient has been ambulating in the hall and ate all his meals today, ask the patient if this is true and try to recall whether you saw him walking in the hall. Elicit the patient's evaluation and perception of the care he received. Find out how much of his meals he ate and how much liquid he drank. Also inspect his skin, dressings, and general appearance.

Check the patient's room for clues too. If the UAP reports that the patient sat up in a chair for an hour, check for a chair in the room. If you don't see one, this could mean that the patient hasn't been out of bed all day, making the UAP's report incorrect. If the bed sheet has the same stain you saw yesterday, assume that the linens weren't changed, even if the UAP reported changing them.

If the patient can't speak or is confused, ask family members about the care he received, and assess him carefully before documenting the UAP's care. Then record only what the UAP and the patient or his family can verify. (See *Corroborating reports from unlicensed assistive personnel.*)

Reducing Your Legal Liability. If you must document nonroutine care provided by UAP, urge administrators to develop reasonable work assignments, documentation policies, and appropriate forms that don't require you to document findings or care you didn't witness or participate in.

What to Document

In the nurse's notes, record the name of the UAP who provided the care you're documenting. Clearly distinguish what was reported

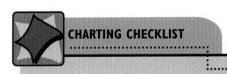

CHARTING CHECKLIST

CORROBORATING REPORTS FROM UNLICENSED ASSISTIVE PERSONNEL
Before you document care performed by unlicensed assistive personnel (UAP), try to corroborate the UAP's report and the patient's response. Usually, you can corroborate routine care by:
❑ asking the patient what happened during the day
❑ noting whether his bed linens have been changed and a chair is in his room
❑ asking the patient what he had for lunch or dinner and how much of each meal he ate
❑ asking family members about the patient's care if they visited that day
❑ recalling your observations. For instance, did you see the patient ambulating in the hall, as the UAP reported?
   If you doubt the accuracy of the UAP's information, investigate further before recording and signing the entry.

to you from what you've verified. For instance, you might document as follows:

> *4/13/06, 1100. Maureen Powers, UAP, reported that the patient was bathed, ambulated 50' in hall, and ate 50% of her sandwich for lunch. This nurse observed patient freshly shaved and ambulating with assistance of UAP in hall. Patient reports he received full bath from UAP. This nurse observed that patient's room was tidy with fresh linens on bed, and saw half of sandwich on lunch tray.—Cathy Stevens, RN, BSN*

If the UAP filled out a flow sheet that will become a permanent part of the medical record, refer to this in your notes. When documenting vital signs that the UAP measured, be sure to record the UAP's name.

WHEN YOU'RE ASKED TO COUNTERSIGN A COLLEAGUE'S NOTES

Countersigning a colleague's notes means that you're attesting to their veracity. Depending on your facility's policy, countersigning may or may not imply that you performed or witnessed the care documented in the entry. It always indicates that you reviewed the entry and agree with the information. Despite the legal issues that countersigning raises, many health care administrators view it as a quality management tool that helps maintain patient care standards and promotes legible, effective documentation.

How to Respond

Never countersign notes that you haven't read. Remember—if the medical record suggests or indicates a potential patient problem, you could share liability for patient injury.

Review your facility's policy on countersigning. If it states that countersigning means that you witnessed the care described or that the care was performed in your presence, don't countersign unless you actually witnessed the care.

If countersigning in your facility means that you've verified that the documented information is true, don't countersign until you've investigated the information. For instance, quickly assess the patient and ask her about the care she received during your shift. If necessary, have your colleague notify you when she starts a task that you'll need to countersign. Then stop by to make sure she's providing the care you'll be countersigning.

After verifying that the documented care was provided, read your colleague's entry carefully for accuracy, logic, and misspelled or misused words. Correct confusing or illogical entries. If necessary, make comments or corrections to ensure clarity and accuracy, or insist that your colleague do this. Make sure the entry clearly identifies who performed the procedure and exactly what was done. Check for all required data, such as the patient's response to treatments or drugs. If the entry suggests or describes a problem that requires follow-up action, make sure the action has

TIPS & ADVICE

WRITING A DISCLAIMER
Depending on your facility's policy, you may want to add a disclaimer in front of your countersignature. Keep in mind that a disclaimer doesn't extend to subsequent signatures. You must write a new one each time you countersign.

Types of Disclaimers
If your countersignature means only that you've reviewed your colleague's note according to facility policy, your disclaimer may read:
Linda Schmidt, SN/Entry reviewed by Mary Harper, RN

If you've verified the information in the entry, you may write:
Linda Schmidt, SN/Entry verified by Mary Harper, RN

If you can't verify the information in the entry, write a disclaimer such as:
Signed in accordance with policy. Signature does not indicate personal knowledge of the information above charted by student nurse. Mary Harper, RN

If you participated in the care, you don't need a disclaimer. You can countersign as follows:
Linda Schmidt, SN/Mary Harper, RN

been taken. If necessary, perform the action yourself, and then document the appropriate entry and countersign the entire patient record for that day or shift. You may need to add a separate entry to the record to ensure that your colleague's documentation accurately depicts nursing assessment and interventions.

If your countersigned signature means that you observed all the care and findings described in the entry, considering adding a disclaimer before your signature. (See *Writing a disclaimer*, page 357.) Work with the appropriate nurse administrator to have your facility's policy changed so that you don't have to observe the care you countersign for.

WHEN YOU MUST WORK ON AN UNDERSTAFFED UNIT

Health care facilities have a duty to ensure adequate staffing. On the other hand, floating staff members to understaffed units can increase the facility's liability risk if the floating nurses have less expertise in caring for patients on the new unit. A patient may win a lawsuit by showing that he was injured because of understaffing or improper floating. (See *Legislation for safe staffing*.)

If you work on or are floated to an understaffed unit, you're at increased risk for being sued. To reduce your liability, you'll need to prioritize and delegate tasks appropriately and document the situation carefully.

How to Respond

If you've been asked to float to a unit that's understaffed or has extremely high patient acuity, you may be tempted to refuse the assignment. Such a refusal could be considered insubordination and grounds for immediate termination. However, if you accept an assignment and then leave, you could be guilty of abandonment, a form of nursing negligence. (If you're part of a collective bargaining unit, your contract may address your right to refuse an assignment.)

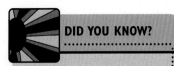

DID YOU KNOW?

LEGISLATION FOR SAFE STAFFING
In 2005, the U.S. House of Representatives introduced the Quality Nursing Care Act (H.R. 1372). The bill aims to ensure adequate registered nurse (RN) staffing in health care facilities and protect RNs who report patient care issues, including inadequate levels of nurse staffing.

Instead of mandating specific nurse-to-patient ratios, the act requires the development of a system to ensure adequate staffing for patient care on each shift and in each unit of the facility. The staffing system must:
• Be designed by direct-care RNs or their designated representative
• Account for the number of patients, the level and intensity of care required, the environment's architecture and geography, and the available technology
• Reflect the level of education and experience of those providing care
• Incorporate staffing levels recommended by specialty nursing organizations
• Prohibit RNs from being pulled to another nursing unit without appropriate training and orientation

Some states have already enacted similar legislation regarding safe staffing. To determine whether your state has such laws, contact your state nurses association or your state.

Instead of refusing the assignment, try to negotiate a compromise with the appropriate nurse administrator if you're uncomfortable with your responsibilities, for instance, if you've been floated to an understaffed unit in a specialty area other than your own. For instance, ask whether you can perform tasks other than drug administration. Medication errors are among the most common causes of patient harm and subsequent lawsuits stemming from floating. Or ask to work with a buddy—a nurse colleague who's familiar with the unit and can provide help and guidance during your shift. Also request basic nursing tasks, such as monitoring vital signs, documenting fluid intake and output measurements, and providing simple wound or personal care.

Prioritizing Care. To reduce your legal liability when floating, give high priority to tasks that could harm the patient if not done, such as administering drugs and measuring vital signs.

Assign lower priority to less important tasks. Depending on your workload, you may have to leave the less important tasks undone.

Delegating Care Appropriately. Delegating tasks also promotes adequate patient care on an understaffed unit. Make sure to delegate care only to staff members who can legally perform such tasks. For instance, don't delegate a tube feeding to an unlicensed assistive worker or a family member.

What to Document

If your unit is understaffed, document the situation by writing an incident report or memo. This shows that you recognized and reported a potentially dangerous situation to those responsible for resolving it. Keep one copy of the report or memo for yourself and give copies to managers at each level, including the appropriate nurse administrator and the facility's administrator or risk manager.

Some nursing associations and collective bargaining organizations have developed protest-of-assignment forms, which serve the same purpose as the incident report or memo. If these forms are available, complete one to document the circumstances and staffing shortage during your shift. Remember to keep one copy for your records.

WHEN YOUR PATIENT OR HER FAMILY ASKS YOU FOR MEDICAL ADVICE

Sooner or later, a patient or one of her family members is bound to ask your opinion of a recommended treatment or a physician's abilities. Perhaps you'll feel obligated to answer because you believe that your role as patient advocate demands it. (See *Patient advocacy: Your role and its risks.*)

Before you answer, think twice. If your response crosses the line to medical advice, you could be charged with practicing medicine without a license—even if your advice concerns something as trivial as a cough remedy. And if you state your opinion

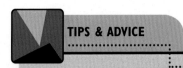

PATIENT ADVOCACY: YOUR ROLE AND ITS RISKS

Can you define your exact responsibilities as patient advocate? If you can't, you're not alone. Even experts debate the nurse's role as patient advocate. Some believe that a patient advocate's primary role is to mediate conflicts between the patient and health care providers. Others maintain that it is to protect the patient's right to self-determination.

In its *Code of Ethics for Nurses* (2001), the American Nurses Association (ANA) focuses on the nurse's responsibility to safeguard the patient's interests.

The nurse's primary commitment is to the health, welfare, and safety of the patient across the life span and in all settings in which health care needs are addressed. As an advocate for the patient, the nurse must be alert to and take appropriate action regarding any instances of incompetent, unethical, illegal, or impaired practice by any member of the health care team or the health care system or any action on the part of others that places the rights or best interests of the patient in jeopardy. To function effectively in this role, nurses must be knowledgeable about the *Code of Ethics,* standards of practice of the profession, relevant federal, state, and local laws and regulations, and the employing organization's policies and procedures.

Understanding the Risks

A patient advocate must walk a fine line between promoting patient self-determination and giving medical advice or defaming a colleague. Doing the latter could cause legal problems.

Be aware, too, that the road to advocacy may be paved with retribution. Some nurses have lost their jobs and licenses when promoting patient self-determination.

Taking Precautions

To protect yourself in your role as patient advocate, follow these guidelines:
- Always check the facts before giving your opinion about a recommended treatment or a physician's abilities.
- Present information about options rather than giving advice.
- Follow the chain of command as needed to ensure your patient's safety. For example, promptly alert the appropriate nurse administrator to patient care concerns so she can discuss them with other administrators or the medical chief of staff before a crisis occurs.
- Document your observations and actions.
- Record the names of the people you spoke with about patient concerns. For instance, if you consulted the diabetes educator about a patient's questions, document the educator's name and the time of the consultation.

of a physician's abilities, you could be charged with defamation of character, slander, and interfering with the physician-patient relationship.

How to Respond

If your patient or a family member asks about treatment options, provide objective information, not advice. Even if your patient is seeking reassurance about her medical care, your best approach is to teach her the rationale for each treatment rather than recommending one over another.

Determine what the patient knows about each treatment option. Ask what the physician has told her and what she has heard. Listen for clues to her underlying concerns about treatment. For instance, perhaps the physician has prescribed a certain drug that the patient's brother says will keep her awake all night.

After you've determined the patient's knowledge base and elicited her concerns, formulate an appropriate answer. To alleviate her fears, explain how the treatment works to relieve or cure her condition. If she still has concerns, advise her to consult her physician. Then inform the physician of the patient's concerns, relate the information you provided, and suggest that he speak with her.

Fielding Questions About a Physician's Abilities. Responding to questions about a physician's skills or expertise can be far more challenging. Try to find out why the patient has asked the question. Has she heard something negative about the physician? Has she had a bad experience with him?

As you respond, don't defame the physician, even if you have doubts about his abilities. If the patient seems doubtful of the physician's abilities or the treatment he has recommended, advise her to seek a second opinion. Most physicians expect patients to seek a second opinion, and some routinely advise them to do so.

What to Document

In your nurse's notes, document the patient's or family member's questions and your responses. If your responses included teaching, record the information taught and the patient's or family member's understanding. If you told the patient that you would speak with the physician about her concerns, document this. Also record your conversation with the physician, his response, and your follow-up discussions with the patient.

If your patient asks for advice when you can't speak to the physician promptly, such as during the night shift or on a weekend, record what you stated about the patient's questions when you gave report to the nurse on the next shift. Also document the name of the person responsible for speaking with the physician about the patient's concerns.

WHEN THE PHYSICIAN AND FAMILY DECIDE TO TERMINATE THE PATIENT'S LIFE SUPPORT

The decision to terminate a patient's life support has wide-ranging legal and ethical implications. Most states have right-to-die laws, which recognize the patient's right to refuse extraordinary treatment when he has no hope of recovery. Most states also permit the patient's next of kin to decide whether or not to discontinue life support if the patient can't make that decision. Health care facilities typically honor the family's request, rather than insisting on a court order.

If the patient is competent, health care providers should honor his right to refuse extraordinary treatment. If he's incompetent or unconscious, his next of kin may express his desires. A written statement of the patient's wishes provides the best evidence of what treatment he would consent to if he could communicate. The Patient Self-Determination Act (PSDA) requires health care facilities to ask the patient on admission if he has an advance directive (a statement of his wishes if he should become unable to make decisions for himself). An advance directive may include a living will, which takes effect when the patient can't make decisions, and a durable power of attorney for health care, which names a surrogate decision maker. (See *Understanding advance directives*, page 364.)

UNDERSTANDING ADVANCE DIRECTIVES

An advance directive is a written document that specifies how the patient wants medical decisions to be made for him if he can't make them himself. Although not required by law, an advance directive is recommended for everyone age 18 or older. It should be reviewed every year to make sure it still reflects the patient's wishes. If the patient revises the document, he should give a copy of the new directive to his physician, family, close friends, and lawyer.

Types of Advance Directives

The two main types of advance directives are the living will and the durable power of attorney for health care.

Living Will.   Also called a treatment directive or a natural death act, a living will describes the types of medical treatment the patient does and does not want to receive. It usually gives specific instructions about individual treatments, such as cardiopulmonary resuscitation, drugs, blood transfusions, mechanical ventilation, tube feedings, and dialysis. The patient can choose to receive all, some, or none of the measures listed.

He can also give different instructions for different situations. For instance, he can state that he wants to receive tube feedings if he's comatose but not if he has end-stage cancer.

Be aware that although a living will lets the individual make specific treatment decisions, giving clear instructions in a written document can be difficult. Also, the patient may not anticipate every conceivable situation, and general instructions may be too vague for real-life situations.

Durable Power of Attorney.   Also called a proxy directive, a durable power of attorney for health care is a document that designates another person to make medical decisions when the patient can't make them himself. The designee, referred to as an agent, proxy, or surrogate decision maker, has the authority to accept or refuse treatment for the patient. Most people choose a spouse, parent, adult child, or close friend as their designee. Before signing the document, the patient should discuss with the designee the types of treatment he does or doesn't want.

A durable power of attorney for health care has an advantage over a living will: it allows the designee to make decisions for the patient even if the situation doesn't exactly match the instructions the patient has given. Because of the designee's power, it is especially important that the patient choose someone he can trust to follow his instructions.

The PSDA also mandates that the patient receive written information regarding his right to make decisions about his medical care.

How to Respond

If the physician and family want to terminate life support for an incompetent or unconscious patient, try to determine the patient's wishes by checking his record for an advance directive. If you can't find one, ask the physician whether she or a family member has a copy.

If you find an advance directive, review it with the facility's risk manager or legal counsel to determine the patient's instructions on withholding treatment and the name of the person he designated as his decision maker. The risk manager or legal counsel must verify that the advance directive meets state and facility legal standards. (Ideally, this review should take place when the document first enters the medical record so that the patient can revise the directive, if necessary.) Also check your facility's policy on life-support termination, and make certain the necessary consent forms have been signed and placed in the medical record. If the patient's condition or the proposed life-support termination doesn't match his wishes as stated in the directive, notify the appropriate nurse administrator as well as your facility's legal counsel or risk manager.

If your patient doesn't have an advance directive, notify the appropriate nurse administrator and risk manager. The risk manager will evaluate the situation in light of applicable state laws, including those addressing family consent. Depending on circumstances, a court hearing may be required before life support can be terminated.

Providing Care After the Decision. Offer family members the counseling services of the social work department or chaplain. Arrange for them to spend some time alone with the patient to say good-bye, and ask whether they would like to be present when life support is discontinued.

The patient's physician should attend when life support is terminated. In fact, some facilities require that she personally discontinue the ventilator and extubate the patient. After the equipment is turned off, remove it from the room and clean secretions or tape residue from the patient's face.

Then provide privacy for the family and patient. Stay in the room if family members ask you to. Be aware that the patient may not die right away. If appropriate, administer prescribed drugs to promote his comfort and ease the work of breathing.

What to Document

Document the presence or absence of an advance directive in the patient's record. If indicated, note that you read the directive and had it reviewed by your facility's legal counsel or risk manager. If your facility requires a separate consent to terminate life support, document that this form has been signed and placed in the record.

Document the names of people you notified of the decision to terminate life support, notification times, and their responses. Record your conversations with family members and your offer of counseling.

Describe your physical care for the patient just before and after life-support termination. Document the time of termination, the name of the person who turned off the life-support equipment, and the names of others present. Record the patient's vital sign measurements and respiratory effort after extubation, and document the time he stopped breathing and was pronounced dead. Finally, document the family's response, and describe your interventions for them and the patient after his death.

WHEN THE PHYSICIAN WRITES A "DO NOT RESUSCITATE" ORDER

In all health care facilities, the standard of care calls for immediate resuscitation of a patient in cardiac arrest—unless her medical record contains a valid "Do not resuscitate" (DNR) order. Most patients with DNR orders have terminal diagnoses or other reasons for refusing extraordinary measures to prolong life.

DNR orders are fairly common in acute care and long-term care facilities. However, the meaning of DNR may differ among facilities. Also, some facilities have different DNR levels. Here's an example:

- Level 1 may prohibit endotracheal intubation and chest compressions but permit the use of bag-mouth ventilation and resuscitative drugs.
- Level 2 may prohibit endotracheal intubation and chest compressions but allow the use of drugs.
- Level 3 may prohibit all measures.

Your facility's policy specifies who can write a DNR order, what the order must say, how long the order can stay in effect, and what other documentation must exist. Some facilities also require that a second physician and the patient (or her designee) countersign the DNR order.

How to Respond

If your patient has a DNR order in her record, review your facility's definition of and policies on DNR orders. Learn who is permitted to write the order and who can give consent if the patient can't. Also find out when the DNR order must be renewed. Be aware that the physician who is primarily responsible for the patient's care should sign the DNR order.

Check the physician's progress notes and orders to make sure they comply with facility policies. If your facility doesn't require the patient or her designee to countersign the DNR order, make certain the physician's notes indicate that the designee or family agrees with the DNR decision. If the physician's notes conflict with the DNR order, ask the physician to document the name of the family member who consented to the order.

Finally, report the patient's DNR status to all staff members involved in her care. This helps ensure that no one takes unwanted resuscitative measures if her heartbeat or breathing stops.

Providing Care. Continue to assess and care for the patient as you would any other patient. Unless the DNR order specifically prohibits other treatments, such as antibiotics or IV vasopressors, continue to implement nonresuscitative measures, as ordered. Be aware that the patient may remain a candidate for surgery to relieve pain or prevent further deterioration.

Remember, too, that the DNR order doesn't mean that nursing care should stop. In fact, the patient's nursing needs typically increase. Be prepared to provide all-encompassing physical care, take steps to prevent complications, implement aggressive measures to promote comfort, and offer extra teaching and support to the family.

What to Document

Make sure the patient's record contains all necessary signatures, statements, and forms and specifies the DNR order's renewal date. (See *DNR orders: What the record should show.*) Document your conversations with the patient or family about her DNR status. If you were present when the physician spoke with them about withholding extraordinary measures, record what each person said.

Then, according to your facility's policy, write "DNR" clearly on the front of the patient's medical record, in the nursing plan

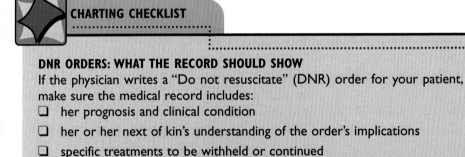

CHARTING CHECKLIST

DNR ORDERS: WHAT THE RECORD SHOULD SHOW
If the physician writes a "Do not resuscitate" (DNR) order for your patient, make sure the medical record includes:
- ❑ her prognosis and clinical condition
- ❑ her or her next of kin's understanding of the order's implications
- ❑ specific treatments to be withheld or continued
- ❑ the name of the person who made the DNR decision if the patient didn't make it herself

Make sure the medical record *doesn't* include:
- ❑ a verbal or telephone DNR order (unless your facility's policy allows it) because this can lead to errors
- ❑ an order for a "slow code," which directs staff members to walk slowly with the emergency cart or to call the physician before initiating resuscitation. "Slow code" orders are unethical and may expose the health care provider to legal action for malpractice and failure to provide an acceptable standard of care.

of care, and in the medication administration record. Or use a special DNR sticker for this purpose if your facility has one. Depending on facility policy, you may also need to place a special identification bracelet on the patient or add a label to her admission bracelet so that caregivers who respond in an emergency can instantly identify her DNR status.

WHEN YOU WITHHOLD A PRESCRIBED DRUG OR OTHER PATIENT CARE

To fulfill your role as patient advocate, you must exercise independent judgment when deciding whether to implement the physician's orders. If you believe that the prescribed treatment or drug could harm the patient, you must withhold it. (See *To give or not to give?*) Depending on facility policy, you may also have the authority to decide whether to give the entire dose of a prescribed drug.

What to Do
If you decide to withhold a prescribed drug or to halt an ordered treatment, inform the prescribing physician of your action and

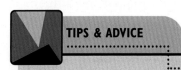

TIPS & ADVICE

TO GIVE OR NOT TO GIVE?
As a patient advocate, you're obligated to evaluate the potential consequences of administering or withholding a prescribed drug or other treatment. If you're considering withholding care, ask yourself how your decision could affect your patient's well-being. As a rule of thumb, if no contraindications exist, you should probably administer the treatment.

If you decide to withhold treatment, notify the physician immediately, if appropriate, and take steps to ensure the patient's safety if his status has changed significantly. Continue to monitor and document his status. Notify other health care providers as needed to ensure patient safety and continuing care.

its rationale. Depending on the circumstances, you may not have to notify her immediately. As a rule of thumb, the more serious the potential consequences to the patient, the sooner you should inform the physician.

For instance, if you withhold a drug prescribed for sleeping because you find the patient asleep when you go to his room to administer it, you don't need to tell the physician immediately. You can simply leave a note for her in the medical record. On the other hand, if you decide to withhold a prescribed digoxin dose because the patient's heart rate is 49 beats per minute, you should notify the physician right away.

What to Document

Follow your facility's policy on documenting that you've withheld a prescribed treatment or drug. If necessary, circle your initials on the medication administration record or nursing plan of care and fill in the correct code to indicate your reason for withholding care.

Also document withholding of treatment in the nurse's notes. Record the date and time the prescribed treatment or drug dose was due, your assessment findings, and your reason for withholding care. Document the physician's name, the time you notified her of your decision to withhold care, and her response. If she gave additional orders, record them and document when and how you implemented them. Also document other measures you took to protect the patient, noting the times you implemented them.

WHEN SOMEONE ASKS TO PHOTOGRAPH OR VIDEOTAPE YOUR PATIENT

The law protects all citizens against unreasonable and unwarranted interference with solitude. This right to privacy extends to your patient's name and picture. Using a patient's picture without consent violates the right to privacy and can result in legal action. Cases that involve unautho-rized publication of patients' photographs have led to large monetary awards against health care facilities.

To minimize the risk for lawsuits, most facilities require patients to sign a consent form before allowing them to be photographed or videotaped. As with consent for a medical procedure, such consent is valid only if it's informed and the patient is of legal age. With respect to photographs or videotaping, informed consent means that the patient is told why the photo or tape will be taken and where and how it will be used. If the photo or tape is later used for a differ-ent purpose, the patient may bring—and win—a lawsuit against the health care provider or facility. (See *Disputing disguised identity*.)

DID YOU KNOW?

DISPUTING DISGUISED IDENTITY

A patient may consent to being photographed or videotaped on the condition that her identity be disguised. But obtaining con-sent with this stipulation can be a no-win situation for everyone. Some health care facilities in New York and California have lost lawsuits brought by patients who requested disguised identi-ties but later learned that they could be identified. To avoid these problems, encourage patients who don't want their identities known not to consent to photo-graphing or videotaping under any circumstances.

How to Respond

Before your patient consents to a photograph or videotape, make sure your facility approves of the project. Don't let a researcher or journalist approach your patient unless this person has authoriza-tion from your facility.

Also, don't involve yourself in the request. Otherwise, your patient may feel pressured to consent because she wants to please you or fears mistreatment. Instead, have someone from the public information office or the person in charge of the project explain the request to the patient and ask for her consent. Make sure that all the patient's questions are answered and that she receives all the information she needs to make an informed decision.

What to Document

Most facilities have a special consent form for photography and videography. This form should specify how and when the photo-graph or videotape will be used and give the patient's full name, address, and telephone number. Place one copy of the signed consent form in the patient's medical record and give one to the patient and another to the photographer or videographer.

In your nurse's notes, document the name of the person who spoke to the patient about the project. Summarize the content of the discussion, its outcome, and the patient's response. If the patient changes her mind about consenting to a photograph or videotape, document her decision along with the time and date. Also document the names of the people you notified that the patient has withdrawn consent.

WHEN A MEMBER OF THE MEDIA ASKS FOR PATIENT INFORMATION

P rotecting your patient's privacy and confidentiality means keeping all information about him—even his admission to the health care facility—confidential. Disclosing patient information could constitute grounds for a lawsuit. (See *Disclosing patient information: The ANA's view*.) The right to privacy means that:
- your patient's name and photograph can't be used without his authorization
- his seclusion can't be violated
- health care providers can't publicly disclose medical information about him or make statements that place him in a false light

Understanding the Exceptions. The law requires health care providers to report communicable diseases to the state health department, positive human immunodeficiency virus test results to the Centers for Disease Control and Prevention, and suspected child abuse to local officials. Also, in some cases, the public's right to know may override the patient's right to privacy. If your patient is a public figure whose medical care and condition are newsworthy, disclosing medical information about him may be warranted.

How to Respond
Review and follow your facility's policy on disclosing patient information. Chances are, the policy will direct you to deny all

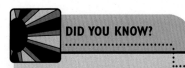

DID YOU KNOW?

DISCLOSING PATIENT INFORMATION: THE ANA'S VIEW
The *Code of Ethics for Nurses* (American Nurses Association, 2001) outlines your legal and ethical responsibilities in protecting your patient's confidentiality. It emphasizes that you must consider your patient's rights, well-being, and safety when deciding whether to disclose confidential information about him. It stresses that when disclosing patient information to other health care team members, you should include only the data that's pertinent to the patient's treatment and welfare.

The *Code* also addresses how to document the patient information required for peer review, third-party payment, and other quality management purposes. It states that you should disclose such data only according to written policies, mandates, or protocols—and make sure to maintain the patient's rights, well-being, and safety when doing so.

requests for patient information. Refer the journalist or other requester to the public affairs office or other department that deals with the media. Then notify the appropriate nurse administrator of the request, and tell other health care team members about the incident so they'll be on guard.

Keep in mind that a journalist may use deception to try to get you to answer questions. Don't be afraid to say "No comment" or to repeatedly direct him to the public affairs office. If he enters your unit, you may need to ask a security guard to escort him out.

What to Document

Document the name of the person who requested the patient information, his organization, and his specific request. Record your response and the name of the nurse administrator you notified.

If you saw the journalist in your unit or called a security guard to escort him out, document your action, the guard's actions, and the time of the incident. Record the names of staff members you informed of the incident. Also, if indicated, document further attempts the journalist makes to obtain information during your shift.

WHEN YOUR PATIENT IS TRANSFERRED OR DISCHARGED

When a patient is transferred to another unit or discharged from the facility, your primary goal is to ensure the continuity of her care. To achieve this goal, you must inform her new caregivers of her medical history, her current condition, and her treatment in a clear, organized manner.

Most facilities have special forms for communicating patient data to the receiving unit, facility, or home health care agency. On some forms, you can summarize your patient teaching, providing a reference the patient can use if she'll manage her care at home.

You must also protect your patient's confidentiality during her transfer or discharge. Usually, the general consent form that the patient signs on admission allows the facility to reveal her medical information to others involved in her care. This consent extends to home health care agencies, skilled nursing facilities, and other acute-care facilities.

How to Respond

Check your patient's medical record to see whether the physician has written a transfer or discharge order. If the order isn't in the record, verify that the physician wants the patient to be transferred or discharged.

Before the transfer or discharge, conduct a patient assessment to obtain baseline information for her new caregivers. Also make sure all teaching outcomes have been achieved. If necessary, reinforce weak teaching areas.

If the patient is being transferred to another unit or facility or to a home health care agency, give an oral report to the receiving nurse. Include the patient's name, age, medical history, social history (such as marital status and living situation), and the reason she was admitted to your unit. Summarize her treatment on your unit, her response, and her most recent assessment findings. Provide the name and telephone number of the attending physician. Also describe her treatment and drug regimens, and note the times of her last treatments or drug doses.

If your patient is being discharged to home, provide discharge instructions to her and her family. Include the names, purpose, doses, and administration times and routes of all prescribed drugs. Reinforce instructions about diet and activity, and review the treatments she must receive at home, such as wound care or colostomy irrigation. Also provide the physician's name and telephone number. Tell the patient which signs and symptoms to report, and remind her of the date, time, and location of her next medical appointment. Then give her a written copy of this information. Make sure she has prescriptions for each prescribed drug and the supplies she needs for at-home treatments, as appropriate.

Place relevant documents from the nursing plan of care and medication administration record with your patient's medical record. If she's transferring to another unit in the facility, send the original medical record with her. If she's transferring to a different facility, send a copy of the record with her. If she's going home, give the record to the unit secretary or put it in the appropriate bin for forwarding to the medical records department.

Ensure that all aspects of the transfer or discharge order are performed, such as discontinuing IV lines and reinforcing the physical therapist's instructions about using crutches. If the patient has valuables in your facility, arrange for their return and have her sign a form acknowledging receipt, according to facility policy.

Follow your facility's policy to arrange for transportation and to escort the patient from the facility. For insurance reasons, most facilities require that the patient leave on a stretcher or in a wheelchair.

What to Document

Record all appropriate data. (See *Documenting your patient's discharge or transfer*, page 376.) Document discharge assessment findings in your nurse's notes. Include vital sign measurements and measurements of wounds, incisions, and other skin markings. Document tubes left in place, such as an indwelling urinary catheter or a tracheostomy tube.

Also record the name of the receiving nurse who will assume care for the patient in the new unit or facility. If you speak with this nurse, document the time of your conversation and the information conveyed. If you use the facility's discharge-transfer

CHARTING CHECKLIST

DOCUMENTING YOUR PATIENT'S DISCHARGE OR TRANSFER
When your patient leaves your facility or unit, gathering all the necessary documents can be a daunting task. To make sure you cover all the bases, use the checklist below:

❑ discharge or transfer order (placed in the medical record)

❑ discharge-transfer summary (one copy in the record, one sent with the patient)

❑ discharge assessment notes (including vital sign measurements), written no more than 1 hour before transfer or discharge

❑ discharge or transfer instructions (one copy for the patient, one placed in the record)

❑ signed personal property form (if one was used) acknowledging the patient's or family's receipt of belongings (placed in the medical record)

❑ nurse's notes stating that report was given, transportation arranged, discharge instructions provided, and the documentation above checked. Also note the name of the person who will assume the patient's care in the new unit or facility

summary for your report, document that the information on this form was reviewed and record the name of the person who reviewed it. Also note that it accompanied the patient to the new unit or facility.

If your facility requires a narrative note instead of a discharge-transfer summary, make sure the note includes:

- patient's name, birth date, address, telephone number, identification (ID) number, insurance carrier, and insurance ID number
- patient's medical history
- history of current illness
- patient's status on admission
- significant events during patient's stay (including procedures and episodes of decline or improvement)
- resolved and unresolved patient problems
- patient's status on discharge
- discharge orders for treatments, drugs, nutrition, and activity

- facility name
- names of people involved in patient's care
- names and telephone numbers of people who patient should contact in an emergency
- physician's name and telephone number
- patient and family teaching provided
- times of follow-up medical appointments

If your patient is being discharged to home, document that you reviewed discharge instructions with her. Give her a copy of these instructions and ask her to sign a form acknowledging receipt. Place a second copy of the instructions in her record. Follow your facility's policy for distributing the remaining copies. Then document that you reviewed the discharge instructions with the patient and her family, as appropriate, and record their understanding of the instructions. If applicable, document that the patient or family received her valuables and other property.

Finally, document how the patient will be transported to her next destination and the name of the person who will assume responsibility for her, such as the receiving nurse on the next unit, an ambulance attendant, or the family member who drives her home.

HOW TO MAKE A LATE ENTRY

As you know, you should record your patient's care as promptly as possible. Occasionally you may need to postpone documentation while you attend to a critically ill patient. Or you may inadvertently omit important information from your notes. In these cases, you'll need to make a late entry. (See *Explaining your late entry*, page 378.)

No rules prohibit documenting out of chronological order. A late entry is better than no entry, and recording all pertinent information is more important than preserving the chronological order of entries. Be aware, though, that if your patient pursues legal action against your facility, an unusually long interval between

TIPS & ADVICE

EXPLAINING YOUR LATE ENTRY

How you explain and format your late entry depends on the circumstances. The samples below show how to write a late entry for several common situations.

The Patient's Record Was Unavailable When You Provided Care:

6/5/06   1000   *Late entry—record in medical records department being photo-copied for patient's transfer to the Heart Center_____*
6/5/06. 0900. Patient stated he had chest pain of 8 on 1-10 scale, with no radiation to jaw, back, or arm. Patient said it felt like his usual angina. BP 140/82 mm Hg. 12-lead ECG obtained. NSR, rate of 80. No ectopy. Paged Dr. Nobel; SL NTG 1/150; given as prescribed. Patient described pain as 3/10 1 minute after receiving NTG and 0/10 2 minutes after._____
0905. Dr. Nobel at patient's bedside. No further complaints of chest pain. No orders received from Dr. Nobel._____
_____ *Janice Brown, RN*

You Remember Important Information to Add to a Previous Note:

6/5/06   2100   *Late entry—additional information for earlier note_____*
6/5/06. 1730. Dr. Chu saw patient, removed L arm dressing. Wound clean and dry with pink edges. Minimal amount of serous drainage on old dressing. Dr. Chu applied dry, sterile dressing. Patient states wound and dressing change are "not painful."____ Mary Abel, RN

You Forgot to Write an Entry in Your Patient's Record:

6/5/06   0200   *Late entry—documentation inadvertently skipped_____*
6/4/06. 2330. On rounds, observed patient sleeping, with regular respirations, urine drainage bag with 100 ml clear, yellow urine.___
_____
6/5/06. 0130. Patient awake and asking for pain medication for ® shoulder pain. Gave 75 mg meperidine and 25 mg hydroxyzine IM as prescribed. _____
6/5/06. 0200. On rounds, observed patient sleeping. _____
_____ *J. Mara, RN*

patient care and its documentation could raise the suspicion that you made the late entry to hide a problem. (See *Taking a dim view of late entries,* pages 379-380.) So be especially careful to avoid making late entries.

What to Do

If you forget to document important information during your shift, call the unit and ask the nurse who's currently caring for your patient to write a note acknowledging that she spoke to you and to record the information you should have documented. When you arrive at work the next day, countersign her note. (See *When a colleague asks you to document her care,* pages 349-350.)

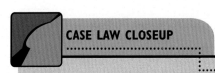

CASE LAW CLOSEUP

TAKING A DIM VIEW OF LATE ENTRIES
When a suit relies on your documentation, it had better be truthful, accurate, and *timely.* Otherwise, instead of saving you in court, late entries could sink you. The following case shows how.

Understanding the Case
Rothstein v. Orange Grove Center, Inc.[1] concerns the fraudulent charting of care for Ms. Rothstein, age 35, who was developmentally disabled. She lived in a group home, where she died from what was thought to be a seizure. Immediately before her death, she was placed alone in a darkened room, at the on-call nurse's direction, to try to calm her agitation and reduce her breathing difficulties.

Because death from a seizure made her a candidate for organ donation, the local organ bank contacted Ms. Rothstein's physician. He informed the organ bank that the patient had had viral cold symptoms and an elevated white blood cell (WBC) count, but then had a normal WBC count just before her death. Ms. Rothstein's autopsy revealed that she had died from bacterial meningitis caused by *Streptococcus pneumoniae.*

The patient's parents sued the group home and attending physician, claiming that they should have discovered the patient's illness was a serious (but treatable) bacterial infection—not a viral infection.

[1]*Rothstein v. Orange Grove Center, Inc.,* 60 S. W. 3d 807 (Tennessee, 2001).

Continued

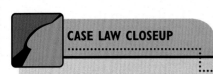

CASE LAW CLOSEUP

TAKING A DIM VIEW OF LATE ENTRIES—cont'd

How the Court Ruled
For the group home, two questions were key: When and how thoroughly were Ms. Rothstein's signs and symptoms reported to the attending physician? And what exactly happened to the WBC count the physician had ordered?

At the trial, the group home's attorney presented numerous phone message logs from nurses and other staff members, informing the physician of the severity and progression of the patient's illness. However, a handwriting expert testified that some phone messages and some patient record entries were created after the fact. Specifically, the expert noted that entries on the same page made different impressions because they were written with different materials under the page. In other words, the entries weren't made on the dates indicated. They were made later. The conclusion was that staff members were trying to create the false impression that they had fully advised the physician of the WBC count, which had either been mislaid or simply unappreciated for their importance.

The court awarded the family $275,000 with 20% apportioned to the group home and 80% to the physician.

The Lesson Learned
The obvious lesson is this: Never alter records to try to avoid liability. Aside from the fact that it's illegal and unethical, record alteration or creation after the fact is easily detected by technology. Plus, computerized documentation systems make it difficult or impossible to do. Instead, follow the rules for documentation, especially concerning late entries. And always seek advice from your facility's attorney or risk manager when you have questions about late entries.

What to Document

Follow your facility's policy on making late entries. Here are some general guidelines:

- Start your entry with the date and time you're writing it. In the body of the note, record the time of the event you're describing.
- Don't insert information in the margin or on top of an existing note. Instead, start your late entry on the next available line.
- Label your entry "Late entry."

- Document the reason you're writing the note out of sequence. Then note the date and time you should have written the entry.
- Make your entry as legible as possible.

HOW TO USE ABBREVIATIONS SAFELY

To save time and space, most health care professionals abbreviate certain words and terms when documenting patient care. But using abbreviations can lead to problems. An illegible or ambiguous abbreviation can be misread or misinterpreted, resulting in patient injury. (See *Avoiding ambiguous abbreviations*, page 382.)

Suppose, for example, that your patient is admitted for a left arm fracture. To indicate that she has no function of her left arm, you write "no fx L arm." The physician, however, might think you're documenting x-ray results and assume that "fx" means "fracture" rather than "function." If he then tries to move the patient's arm, she'll experience severe pain.

How you punctuate an abbreviation can make a difference too. For instance, if the physician uses periods when writing the abbreviation *qd* on a prescription, you may mistake *q.d.* for *qid* and incorrectly give a once-daily drug four times daily.

To prevent such misunderstandings, most facilities have an official list of approved abbreviations and discourage staff members from using others. If a staff member wants to add an abbreviation to the official list, the committee governing medical record procedures must approve the proposed addition. If your facility doesn't have its own abbreviation list, use the abbreviations recognized by the Joint Commission on Accreditation of Healthcare Organizations (JCAHO) in its National Safety Goals.

What to Do

Post a copy of your facility's approved abbreviation list at the nurses' station and other places where you and your colleagues typically

TIPS & ADVICE

AVOIDING AMBIGUOUS ABBREVIATIONS

To avoid problems caused by ambiguous abbreviations, use only the abbreviations approved by your facility or recognized by the JCAHO. Otherwise, you could jeopardize your patient's health.

Consider, for instance, the following note written for a postoperative thoracotomy patient with a chest tube.

1700. Pt returned from OR. Vital signs stable. ® anterior chest tube patent, attached to Pleur-evac suction system, 20 cm suction. BS diminished. Head of bed elevated 45 degrees. _____

Should you assume that BS stands for breath sounds or bowel sounds? Diminished bowel sounds may be an expected postoperative finding, whereas diminished breath sounds could signal a problem. What's more, BS isn't a JCAHO-recognized abbreviation and probably isn't on your facility's approved abbreviation list. Avoid using it.

In the next example, the nurse has written a confusing note for a patient with an infected knee replacement.

1800. Case reviewed with Dr. Summit. He will order PT for later today. _____

If you saw this note, would you look for an order for physical therapy or for a prothrombin time? Although PT is a JCAHO-recognized abbreviation for prothrombin time, the physician is just as likely to order physical therapy for this patient. In this case, spell out exactly what you mean to avoid confusion.

write in the medical record. If you consistently see unapproved abbreviations in documentation, inform the appropriate nurse administrator, who may address the topic at a staff meeting or ask the quality management committee to explore the issue.

What to Document

Use only approved abbreviations in the patient's record. Make sure your writing is legible so that others will understand your abbreviations. If you're not sure whether a particular abbreviation is approved or correct, don't use it. Instead, write out the complete word or words. Remember—the goal of using abbreviations is to communicate the patient's health care and response to treatment as succinctly as possible, but *only* if the abbreviation also communicates this correctly and clearly. When in doubt, don't abbreviate. Write out the full term instead.

HOW TO COMPLETE AN INCIDENT REPORT

A vital part of a facility's risk management or quality management program, incident reports can improve the quality of patient care. In fact, the JCAHO mandates incident reports, viewing them as a means for reporting and reviewing patient care.

Besides identifying areas that warrant further education, incident reports alert administrators to potential problems and help decrease the risk for similar incidents. (See *Incident reports: When follow-up fails*, pages 384-385.) A thorough review of a facility's incident reports can help identify an emerging pattern from events that may seem isolated to the caregivers who report them.

When to Complete an Incident Report. Prepare an incident report for any event that's out of the ordinary—not just when a patient is injured or has a high risk for injury. Examples of events that may warrant an incident report include:

- equipment malfunction, even if the equipment isn't used directly by the patient
- unexpected cardiac arrest
- unexpected patient death
- a patient's fall
- a medication error
- the wrong patient's name on a food tray or test report
- slow response time by another department
- documentation that's filed in the wrong medical record
- loss of a patient's belongings

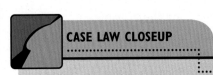

CASE LAW CLOSEUP

INCIDENT REPORTS: WHEN FOLLOW-UP FAILS

Incident reports can reveal quality management problems or even criminal conduct by health care providers. As the following case shows, patients may be harmed if caregivers fail to complete incident reports promptly or if the quality management department fails to follow up on the reports.

Understanding the Case

Gess v. United States[1] concerns a medical technician on duty in a hospital nursery when numerous adverse events occurred. According to nurses' documentation, several neonates developed severe breathing difficulties immediately after the technician transported them from the delivery area to the nursery. Incident reports showed that the technician was commonly the first one to arrive and to initiate resuscitation on the neonates.

A criminal investigation found that the technician had injected 1 new mother and 11 neonates with lidocaine or a similar drug. The woman and the families of the 11 infants filed suit against the facility and its staff for the patient harm and additional hospitalization resulting from the unauthorized injections.

How the Court Ruled

The U.S. District Court for the Middle District of Alabama held the hospital liable for negligence because the medical technician's criminal misconduct continued to harm patients—despite incident reports that provided a clear basis for investigation and intervention. The court found an obvious pattern to the suspicious events that should have been identified and corrected before so many patients were injured.

As the court saw it, a facility's quality management program must identify suspicious patterns in patient care episodes so that intentional criminal misconduct can be eliminated. Furthermore, the court said, the quality management program has a mission and a legal duty to identify patient care problems and take steps to prevent recurrences. The court emphasized that incident reports should be completed promptly to document nonroutine events and routed immediately to the quality management or risk management department. A further report should be prepared by the hospital employee designated to follow up on all incident reports to document the subsequent investigation, its findings, and actions taken to prevent recurrences.

---

[1]*Gess v. United States, 952 F.Supp. 1529 (M.D.Alza., 1996).*

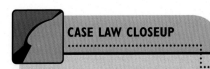

CASE LAW CLOSEUP

INCIDENT REPORTS: WHEN FOLLOW-UP FAILS—cont'd
The Lesson Learned
This case illustrates the need to complete incident reports promptly and investigate them thoroughly to detect patterns of adverse outcomes. If an incident report had been filed when the new mother reported she had received an injection from the medical technician, the quality management supervisor or risk manager might have realized that the technician was providing unorthodox care. And if all caregivers had completed incident reports when the first neonates required resuscitation, an astute quality management supervisor or risk manager might have suspected a developing pattern. A subsequent investigation might have revealed that the same medical technician was involved in every case, and administrators could have taken appropriate action before so many patients were harmed.

What to Do

Review your facility's policy to learn when and how to complete an incident report. Typically, the policy will direct you to complete an incident report whenever a nonroutine event occurs. Be aware that incident reports may go by a different name in your facility.

For example, in some health care facilities, the incident report may be called one of the following:
- variance report
- quality assurance report
- unusual occurrence report
- situation report

Remember that all parties in a potential lawsuit may read your incident report, so complete it properly. Avoid assigning blame or stating your opinion. Keep your language objective, and describe only what you saw, heard, felt, or smelled. Don't include nonessential information, such as a similar incident that happened the previous week.

After completing the incident report, forward it to the appropriate department in your facility. If another person witnessed the incident or related events, urge this person to cosign your report or complete a separate incident report.

What to Document

If the incident involved a patient, notify the physician as appropriate and describe the incident fully and objectively in your nurse's notes. Record the names of the physician and nurse administrator you notified, and document their responses. Also record the measures you took to prevent patient injury or treat an adverse outcome, and describe the patient's response.

In the medical record, don't mention that you completed an incident report. Also, don't place a copy of the report in the record. If appropriate, discuss ways to avoid recurrences with the appropriate nurse administrator verbally or in a separate memo.

HOW TO AVOID THE PITFALLS
OF COMPUTER DOCUMENTATION

Like traditional medical records, computerized records detail the patient's medical history, clinical status, diagnostic test results, treatments, response to treatments, and course of events during hospitalization. Unlike traditional records, computerized records are filed and stored electronically. Also, computerized documentation techniques are constantly being upgraded. (See *Advances in computerized documentation.*)

With most computerized systems, the user must log on to enter or retrieve patient information. After typing in a password, she can view updated information, such as laboratory test data and new physician's orders, or write assessment data or notes. The system automatically records the user's name and the entry date and time.

Advantages. Using computers speeds documentation, improves accuracy and legibility, reduces reliance on memory, minimizes redundant documentation, and enhances information exchange among health care providers. Most computerized systems also aid standardization of care and documentation by providing structure, comprehensive formats for input, and mandatory reporting fields for assessment findings and other data. Some programs

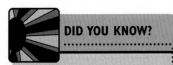

DID YOU KNOW?

ADVANCES IN COMPUTERIZED DOCUMENTATION

Computerized documentation is fast becoming the standard for records management in facilities across the nation. And with the introduction of so many technological innovations every year, even the most computer-savvy nurse can have trouble keeping up with the changes in patient care documentation. Here's a sample of some of the most recent advances in computer documentation:

- Computerized physician order entry (CPOE) systems let physicians prescribe drugs electronically. They also automatically produce medication administration records periodically. In addition, CPOE systems have built-in safeguards that warn nurses of potential medication errors (such as the wrong dose or a possible interaction) and abnormal laboratory test results.
- Bar code technology helps nurses administer drugs safely. It provides an identifying bar code on the nurse's badge, the patient's wristband, and the drug itself. When scanned, the bar codes provide an electronic record and prompt an alarm to signal when a medication error is about to occur.
- Wireless networking allows nurses and physicians to document patient information on a laptop computer at the bedside. This allows more immediate documentation and prevents health care providers from being tethered to a desktop monitor or network cable.

contain algorithms that help caregivers develop a plan of care, formulate patient goals, monitor patient progress, evaluate patient outcomes, and update prescriptions. Software that allows instant access to online discharge instructions and patient-teaching handouts can simplify and reinforce patient education. Other programs permit remote retrieval of such information as diagnostic test results, which allows physicians and other health care providers to prescribe treatment more quickly and efficiently.

Disadvantages. Health care providers who rely on computers may interact less with colleagues, reducing the collaboration and brainstorming that help refine plans of care and identify appropriate interventions. Also, computer-based record systems are expensive to design, implement, and maintain. Staff training adds to the cost.

What's more, computer malfunctions and routine maintenance can disrupt the flow of documentation and impede timely
information retrieval. Unless the system creates backup files, users
can't access information during down times.

Furthermore, computerized information isn't necessarily
secure. All computer systems are vulnerable to hackers (individuals who specialize in gaining unauthorized entry to computer
databases). They may also be accessed by hospital personnel who
aren't involved in the patient's care.

Protecting Patient Confidentiality

Confidentiality of computerized patient information remains a
challenge. Some patients may be reluctant to disclose information
if they know it will enter a computer database.

Also, once the user logs on to a terminal, many records may
remain open until the user manually logs off or until a time-out
feature kicks in, automatically closing the system after a specified
interval. If the user forgets to log off when she leaves the terminal, an unauthorized person could access patient records.

To protect your patient's privacy, make sure your password is
secure so that no one else can use it to enter or view medical
records. (See *Protecting your password*.) If possible, document with
the computer screen turned away from passersby. Also, don't leave
patient information displayed on the screen. When you complete
your request or entry, exit from the patient record. Then log off
the system before leaving the terminal.

What to Document

Document the same information you would enter in a traditional medical record. Before inputting data, make sure you've
retrieved the correct patient record. Then follow the user prompts
so that you won't omit important data fields or overlook conflict-
ing data.

After completing your entry, review what you've written
and run the computer's spelling check feature, if available. If you
must correct an entry, follow your facility's policy for making
corrections.

TIPS & ADVICE

PROTECTING YOUR PASSWORD

To keep patient information confidential, protect your computer password so that others can't use it to access patient files. Follow these suggestions when choosing and using your password:

- Select your own password rather than using an assigned one.
- If you must use an assigned password, such as when you first learn the computer system, change it as soon as possible to one that only you know.
- Don't choose a password that's easily associated with you—for example, your name, your birth date, your child's name, or your favorite color.
- Don't pick a password that you'll have trouble remembering.
- Don't write down your password.
- Change your password regularly in case someone has guessed it or has obtained it inadvertently.
- Enter your password only when no one else is observing you.
- If you suspect that someone else has been using your password, change it. Then report your suspicion to the appropriate nurse administrator in writing.
- Never let another person use your password or work at an active terminal where you're logged on. If a colleague needs to use the terminal, log off before you let the other person log on.

HOW TO PROTECT YOUR PATIENT'S PRIVACY WHEN FAXING MEDICAL RECORDS

Sending patient information by facsimile (fax) has become routine in many health care facilities. Because faxing speeds information transmission, it helps health care professionals make more informed patient care decisions quicker.

Without effective safeguards, however, faxing medical information can lead to violations of patient privacy and confidentiality.

To help protect your patient's privacy, learn when and how to fax medical information properly. (See *Keeping faxes confidential*.)

When to Fax Patient Information

Except in unusual circumstances, send or request patient information by fax only if you or a physician needs the data urgently. For instance, if a patient has been admitted with hypertensive crisis, the physician may need to review medical records held at a facility in another state before ordering treatments. In this urgent situation, it makes sense to request faxed copies of the patient's health history, laboratory test results, prescribed drugs, and physician's progress notes.

You also may fax information to a third-party payer to ensure payment certification. Suppose, for example, your patient has

TIPS & ADVICE

KEEPING FAXES CONFIDENTIAL
A facsimile (fax) machine that's used to send and receive patient information should be kept in a private area with restricted access. If possible, one person, such as the unit secretary, should monitor all fax transmissions. When a fax arrives, she should remove it immediately, count the pages to make sure she has received the entire fax, and review the material for legibility. If she finds a problem with the fax, she should call the sender to report the problem.

If the fax is complete and legible, the unit secretary should read the cover sheet for instructions on how to verify receipt. After verifying receipt, she should promptly notify the intended recipient, place the faxed document in an envelope, and seal and deliver the envelope. If the recipient isn't available, she should store the envelope in a secure area until it can be delivered.

Dealing with a Confidentiality Breach
To preserve your patient's privacy, take steps to prevent unauthorized or inappropriate people from reading or receiving faxed patient information. If you see a stranger reading a confidential fax, politely ask him to identify himself. If he's not involved in the patient's care, ask him to give you the fax. Then report the incident to the appropriate person—for instance, a member of the security staff, your nurse administrator, or the patient's physician. Document the event in an incident report.

coronary artery bypass graft surgery and then develops a postoperative complication, such as a cerebrovascular accident. To extend payment approval for his hospitalization, the insurer may require your facility to fax relevant medical information.

In some situations, automatic facsimile transmission (autofaxing) is acceptable. With autofaxing, a computer-generated report is faxed to selected people automatically. For example, a hospital laboratory may automatically fax a patient's laboratory test results directly to the hospital unit and the physician's office. Autofaxing systems should be tested routinely to make sure confidential information isn't faxed to the wrong person or site.

Important Safeguards. Before sending a fax, check the fax number twice to make sure you don't send the information to the wrong fax machine. To comply with the Health Insurance Portability and Accountability Act (HIPAA), remove identifying information, such as the patient's name and social security number. Always use a cover sheet that states the following:
- the date and time
- your facility's name, address, and telephone and fax numbers
- your name
- the recipient's name, address, and telephone and fax numbers
- the number of pages you're sending (including the cover sheet)
- the importance of keeping the faxed material confidential
- what to do if the fax is received by someone other than the intended party

Depending on facility procedures, you may also need to include instructions for verifying receipt of the fax.

If the intended recipient doesn't receive the fax, check your fax machine's logging system to determine where the fax was sent or whether a transmission error occurred. If the fax went to the wrong number, send another fax to that number explaining your mistake and requesting return of the material through the mail. Also, inform the appropriate nurse administrator and risk manager of the error. Then, fax the patient information to the correct number.

If a transmission error occurs during faxing, call the intended recipient, verify her fax number, and request that she check her fax machine for malfunction. Resend the material when she reports that her machine is working.

When Not to Fax Patient Information

Although few regulatory and accreditation agencies have specific guidelines on faxing patient information, some state laws address it. Several states prohibit faxing of information about a patient's psychiatric care or human immunodeficiency virus status. To prevent legal problems, review your state's laws.

Also, as a general rule, don't fax routine patient information to insurance companies or attorneys. Instead, send such information by regular mail.

What to Document

Typically, before you fax patient information, you must obtain the patient's written authorization. Certain exceptions apply. For instance, if a patient is comatose and his legal representative can't be found, your facility's legal counsel may permit you to fax medical information to a requesting health care provider.

After sending a fax, place the patient's signed authorization for faxing, the fax cover sheet, and the fax receipt in his medical record. Depending on your facility's policy, you may need to place a copy of the entire fax in the medical record. If not, be sure to document which information you faxed. Include the date, time, and your signature.

If you sent the fax to the wrong number, document the error and note that you re-sent the fax to the correct number. Record the name of the person who will mail the misdirected fax to your facility.

HOW TO PROTECT PATIENT CONFIDENTIALITY WHEN USING THE INTERNET

Many clinicians routinely use electronic mail (e-mail) to send and receive patient information, including laboratory test results, specialist referrals, hospital discharges, and prescriptions. Although this information could be sent by mail or facsimile, the ease and speed of Internet transmission make e-mail the preferred method in many facilities.

Despite the benefits of sending information instantly to remote locations, e-mail has certain disadvantages. For example, because e-mail messages are easy to forge or intercept, facilities must take steps to protect confidentiality. To help ensure that only the intended recipient reads e-mail messages, some e-mail systems use a unique key to encrypt, or code, messages. The receiver must have a key or the correct password to decode the message.

However, the efforts of some governments to control encryption could compromise transmission of confidential patient data. The United States and Great Britain are considering a type of key escrow, in which professional and commercial e-mail senders must reveal their keys or passwords to a secure third-party agency. When national security is involved, government officials could demand that the third party reveal the key.

E-mail developers are working on protocols that address such issues as access to e-mailed information, patient consent to transmit data by e-mail, authentication, and other aspects of confidentiality. These protocols may make it possible to identify patients and providers electronically, secure permission for records release, and track transmitted information. In the meantime, many e-mail systems are using data without patient identifiers to protect confidentiality.

What to Do

If your facility sends medical information by e-mail, find out what precautions are in place to protect patient confidentiality. The Health Insurance Portability and Accountability Act (HIPAA) requires you to remove a patient's name and social security number from medical records you send by e-mail. Typically, you must obtain the patient's written authorization before you e-mail medical information. Some exceptions apply. If you're unsure whether you need patient authorization, consult your facility's legal counsel.

When sending e-mail through the Internet, always start your message with:
- your facility's name, address, telephone number, and e-mail address
- your name

- the recipient's name (or identification number), address, telephone number, and e-mail address
- a statement emphasizing the need to maintain confidentiality

Depending on facility policy, you may also need to include instructions on verifying receipt of e-mail, such as with an e-mailed reply.

Verifying Receipt. If the intended recipient doesn't receive your e-mail, make sure you've used the correct e-mail address. Then check the e-mail system's log to determine where the message went or whether a transmission error occurred.

If your e-mail mistakenly goes to the wrong address, send an e-mail message to that address explaining that you inadvertently sent confidential information. Request that the recipient delete the first e-mail message and notify you of its deletion by e-mail. Then, e-mail the patient information to the correct address. Inform the appropriate nurse administrator, your facility's risk manager, or other appropriate staff member of the misdirected e-mail. Also, check your facility's protocol to see whether the error warrants an incident report.

What to Document

Make sure the patient or her family has authorized e-mail transmission of medical information. Include a copy of the authorization form in her medical record. If the patient expresses concerns about e-mail transmission, document them along with your response and teaching.

Also place a copy of the e-mail transmission log in the patient's medical record. If you receive a response to your e-mail, print it out and place it in the record too.

Index

A

Abbreviation use, 381-383, 382s
Abdominal examination, 20
  in gastrointestinal hemorrhage, 135
Abdominal pain, 135, 135s
Abuse suspected, 18, 308-311
  reporting requirements in, 372
  visitor restriction in, 310, 310s
Access to medical records
  in computerized systems, 388
    passwords for, 386, 388, 389s
  of law enforcement officials, 222
  media requests for, 372-373, 373s
  patient requests for, 204-208
    denial of, 207
Accidental injuries, 260-266
  smoking-related, 266-267, 268s
  in surgery, fraudulent concealment of, 185s-186s
Accuracy of documentation, 2s, 3s
  false assumptions and bias affecting, 239s
  illegal tampering affecting, 332-335
  late entries for, 377-381
  and legal alterations of mistakes, 334-335, 334s, 338s
  misleading language affecting, 283s
  patient concerns about, 207
  in surgical accident, 185s-186s
Acquired immunodeficiency syndrome, progression of HIV infection to, 155, 155s
Activity and exercise. See Exercise and activity.
Adherence
  compared to compliance, 220s
  with diet in diabetes mellitus, 144s, 219
Admission to facility of patient in custody, 222
  involuntary admission and treatment in, 222, 223s
Advance directives, 18, 363-366
  and right to refuse treatment, 215, 363, 364s, 365
Adverse events
  in drug reactions, 177-181
    gastrointestinal hemorrhage in, 134
    hypertensive crisis in, 63-64
    patient fear of, 276
  in equipment failure, 302, 303s
  incident reports on. See Incident reports.
  MedWatch program on, 180s, 303s-304s
  in transfusions, 150-154

Advice, patient requests for
  on legal issues, 317-319, 320s
  on medical issues, 360-363
Advocacy role of nurses, 360, 361s
  withholding of drug or treatment in, 369-370, 369s
Affective outcomes in patient education, 85s
Age
  of abuse victims, 308, 309
  of emancipated and mature minors, 294, 297, 298
  growth and developmental information related to, 17s
Agitation
  restraint use in, 247s-248s
  threats to harm others in, 240
AIDS, progression of HIV infection to, 155, 155s
AIR documentation format, 88s-89s
Airway assessment
  in anaphylaxis, 149
  in arrhythmias, 61
  in cardiopulmonary arrest, 54
  in cerebrovascular accident, 121, 123
  in pulmonary edema, 92-93
  in shock, 48
  in unresponsive patient, 126-127
Alcohol, as contraband possession, 269-272
Allergic reactions
  anaphylaxis in, 147-150
  to antibiotics in pneumonia, 73
  duplicate documentation on, 149-150, 149s
  history of, 13
  to transfusions, 150, 151
American Nurses Association, 4
  on advocacy role of nurses, 361s
  on collegiality, 336s
  on disclosure of patient information, 373s
  on negligence reporting, 352
Analgesia, 106
  patient-controlled, 106, 107s
Anaphylaxis, 147-150
  shock in, 46
Anesthesia, postoperative interventions in, 189-193
Antibiotic therapy
  in pneumonia, 73
  in sepsis, 175
  in wound infections, 172

Anticoagulant therapy
  in peripheral pulse loss, 26
  in pulmonary embolism, 90
Antiretroviral therapy in HIV infection,
      157-158
Anxiety of patients, 251-254
  in pulmonary edema, 94
Aphasia in cerebrovascular accident,
      122-123, 125
Arm circumference measurements in
      peripheral pulse loss, 24, 25s
Arrhythmias, 57-63
  in cardiopulmonary arrest, 55
  in heart failure, 44
  in hypertensive crisis, 67
  in myocardial infarction, 37
  in pulmonary edema, 94
Arterial blood gas analysis. *See* Gases,
      arterial blood.
Arterial catheterization
  for continuous monitoring in hypertensive
      crisis, 64, 65s
  of pulmonary artery. *See* Pulmonary artery
      catheterization.
Aspiration
  pneumonia in, 69, 131, 133
  in tube feeding, 130-133
Assessment of patient, 13, 15-23
  AIR format on, 88s-89s
  focus charting on, 6
  history-taking in. *See* History-taking.
  objectivity and specificity in, 13
  physical examination in. *See* Physical
      examination.
  problem-oriented approach in, 5, 6
  self-documentation of patient on, 202-204
    advantages and disadvantages of, 203s
    in police custody, 224
Assistive personnel, unlicensed, 353-356
  in understaffed units, 360
Asthma, 81-86
Asystole, 55
Atrial arrhythmias, 57, 58s, 59, 60, 61

B
Balloon pump, intraaortic, in shock, 51
Bar code technology in drug
      administration, 387s
Bed sores, 159-166
Behavior
  abusive, 308-311
  in adverse drug reactions, 179
  in confusion, 110, 111
  hostile, 236-239, 243s
  inappropriate comments on, 239s, 337
  in seizures, 115, 116
  of visitors, 311-312
Behavioral interventions
  as environmental restraint, 245
  in hostility, 237

Belongings of patient
  contraband items in, 269-272
  disposition on death of patient, 322, 323
  in hostile behavior, 236, 238
  inventory of, 21, 305, 305s
    preoperative, 189
  missing, 304-306
  in police custody, restrictions on, 223
  in transfer or discharge of patient, 375, 376s
  in vision impairment, 289, 291
Bias in description of patient, 239s
Bladder function
  initial assessment of, 20
  in unresponsive patient, 128, 129-130
Bleeding
  gastrointestinal, 133-140
  intracerebral, 120
Blindness, 288. *See also* Vision impairment.
Block charting, 131, 132s
Blood pressure, 18, 19
  in arrhythmias, 59
  arterial catheterization for continuous
      monitoring of, 64, 65s
  in cerebrovascular accident, 123, 124
  in gastrointestinal hemorrhage, 135, 136
  in hypertensive crisis, 63-68
  in myocardial infarction, 34, 37
  in shock, 46
Blood transfusions. *See* Transfusions.
Body mass index in obesity, 291
Bowel function
  initial assessment of, 20
  in unresponsive patient, 128, 129-130
Brain death, 324-325, 325s
Brandon HMA, Inc. v. Bradshaw, 71s-72s
Breast examination, 20
Breathing evaluation, 19
  in arrhythmias, 60, 61
  in aspiration of tube feeding, 131
  in asthma, 82
  in cardiopulmonary arrest, 54
  in heart failure, 41
  in hyperglycemia, 144
  in pneumonia, 69-70
  in pneumothorax, 77
  in pulmonary edema, 92-93
  in pulmonary embolism, 87
  in sepsis, 174
  in shock, 48-49

C
Canterbury v. Spence, 299s
Capacity, mental, 112s
  in will execution, 318s-319s
Carbohydrates in hypoglycemia, 142, 143
Cardiogenic shock, 46
Cardiopulmonary arrest, 52-56
Cardiovascular system, 23-68
  in arrhythmias, 57-63
  in cardiopulmonary arrest, 52-56

Cardiovascular system—cont'd
    in cerebrovascular accident, 123
    chest pain in disorders of, 28-34
    drug-induced disorders of, 178
    in heart failure, 39-45
    in hypertensive crisis, 63-68
    initial assessment of, 19-20
    in myocardial infarction, 28, 34-39
    in peripheral pulse loss, 23-29
    in sepsis, 174
    in shock, 46, 47-48
Care plan. *See* Plan of care.
Carotid pulse palpation, 18
Catheterization
    arterial
        for continuous monitoring in
            hypertensive crisis, 64, 65s
        of pulmonary artery. *See* Pulmonary
            artery catheterization.
    venous, for therapy. *See* Intravenous therapy.
CD4 cell count in HIV infection, 155s, 156,
        157, 158
Cerebrovascular accident, 120-125
Challenging patient situations, 199-327
Charting by exception, 7
Chemical restraints, 245, 246
Chest pain, 28-34
    in heart failure, 41
    in myocardial infarction, 28, 30, 33, 34, 37
    in pneumonia, 69
    in pulmonary edema, 91
    in pulmonary embolism, 86-87
Chest tubes
    patient removal of, 280-283
    in pneumothorax, 78, 79s-80s, 80, 280
Chest x-rays
    in pneumothorax, 77-78, 80
    in pulmonary edema, 94
Children
    abuse of, 308, 309
    as emancipated minors, 294, 297, 298
    equipment tampering by, 272, 273
    growth and developmental
        information on, 17s
    informed consent for, 296-297, 298
    as mature minors, 294, 297, 298
Cigarette smoking, 266-269
Circulation assessment
    in arrhythmias, 61
    in cardiopulmonary arrest, 54
    in pulmonary edema, 92-93
    in shock, 48-49
Code sheets in cardiopulmonary arrest, 53s
Cognitive status, 19
    in confusion, 110-111
    in consent to treatment, 112s, 297-300
    impairment of
        discovery of hidden drugs in, 275
        smoking supervision in, 267, 268
    in outcome of patient education, 85s

Collegiality, nursing standard on, 336s
Comfort measures
    in gastrointestinal hemorrhage, 139
    in pain management, 106-107
    in sepsis, 176
    in serious illness, 314, 316
Communication
    abbreviation use in, 381-383
    with anxious patients, 252
    cerebrovascular accident affecting,
        122-123, 125
    in challenging patient situations, 200
    consent to treatment in, expressed and
        implied, 295s
    e-mail use in, 392-394
    with family on quality of care, 306-308
    fax transmissions in, 206, 389-392
    with health care team, documentation of, 93s
        in anaphylaxis, 149-150, 149s
        in pressure ulcers, 166
        in seizures, 117
    in health history interview, 12-13
        patient cooperation affecting, 212-215
    with hearing impaired patient, 285-288
    with hostile patients, 236, 237
    language barriers in, 18, 283-285
    nonverbal behavior in, 20
    oral statement of dying patient in, 320
    refusal of treatment in, expressed and
        implied, 215-216
    with seriously ill patients, 313, 314
    with suicidal patient, 257
    threats to harm others in, 240
    with unresponsive patient, 314
    verbal orders from physician in,
        329, 344-347
Comparative negligence, 267, 268s
Compartment syndrome, 26
Competency issues, 112s, 295-296, 298
    in confusion, 112s
    in consent to treatment, 112s, 295-296
    in false imprisonment, 227s
    in involuntary admission of patient in
        police custody, 222
    in leaving against medical advice, 225, 226
    in patient withholding of information, 214
    in refusal of treatment, 216
    in will signing and execution, 317, 318s
Compliance issues, 218-220
    compared to adherence, 220s
    in diabetes mellitus and diet restrictions,
        144s, 219
    in discovery of hidden drugs, 275-277
    in health history interview and patient
        withholding of information, 212-215
    inappropriate medical records on, 337-338
    in leaving against medical advice, 225-228
    plan of care in, 214, 214s
    in treatment refusal, 215-218, 219.
        See also Refusal of treatment.

Computerized documentation, 7-8, 386-389
  nursing information systems in, 8
Concealment of surgical accident, 185s-186s
Confidentiality issues
  in computerized documentation, 388, 389s
    and password protection, 386, 388, 389s
  in e-mail and Internet use, 392-394
  in fax transmission of medical records, 206,
    389-392, 390s
  Health Insurance Portability and Accountability
    Act on, 22s, 206, 391, 393
  in media requests for patient information,
    372-373, 373s
  in patient requests for medical records, 205, 206, 207
  in threat for harm to others, 240, 241s
Confusion, 109-114
  equipment tampering in, 272, 273
Consciousness, level of
  in cerebrovascular accident, 121, 122s
  Glasgow Coma Scale on, 127s
  glucose blood levels affecting, 128, 141, 142
  objective documentation of, 122s
  in sepsis, 173, 174
  in serious illness, 313, 314, 316
  in unresponsive patient, 125-130
Consent to treatment or procedures, 294-300
  competency issues in, 112s, 295-296
  in confusion, 111, 112s
  expressed, 295s
  in hearing impairment, 285
  implied, 295s
  lack of understanding affecting, 299-300
  by minors, 294, 296-297
  of non-English speaking patients, 284
  in organ donation, 323, 324, 326
  photography and videotaping in, 371-372, 371s
  and refusal of treatment, 215-218
  requirements for, 112s, 295s, 299-300, 299s
  and restraint use, 247
    in false imprisonment, 226, 227s, 246
  in vision impairment, 289-290
Continuity of care, role of documentation in, 1-4
Contraband items, 269-272
Contributory negligence, 268s
  in equipment tampering, 273
  in smoking-related accidents, 267
Cornea donation, 324, 325-326
Correction of medical records
  in computerized systems, 388
  illegal tampering in, 332-335
  late entries in, 211, 379s-380s
  legal alterations in, 334-335, 334s, 338s
  patient requests for, 207
Countersignature on notes, 356-358
  with disclaimer, 357s, 358
  in late entries, 379
Court cases, 4
  Brandon HMA, Inc. v. Bradshaw, 71s-72s
  Canterbury v. Spence, 299s

Court cases—cont'd
  Curtis v. Columbia Doctors' Hospital of Opelousas,
    265s-266s
  Faison v. Hillhaven Corp. et al., 104s-105s
  Gess v. United States, 384s-385s
  Hutchins v. DCH Regional Medical Center, 167s-168s
  Kodadek v. Lieberman, 185s-186s
  Lama v. Borras, 7
  NME Properties Inc. v. Rudich, 164s-165s
  Phillips v. Covenant Clinic, 339s-340s
  Pollard v. Hastings, 318s-319s
  Pugh v. Mayeaux, 346s-347s
  Rothstein v. Orange Grove Center, Inc., 379s-380s
  Sabol v. Richmond Heights General Hospital,
    258s-259s
  State v. Bright, 241s
  Thornton v. Shah, 330s-331s
  Washington State Nurses Association v. Board of
    Medical Examiners, 32s
  White v. State of Washington, 247s-248s
Crisis, hypertensive, 63-68
Criticisms, inappropriate
  of colleagues, 335-337
  of patients, 239s, 337
Cultural and religious influences, health history
  interview on, 17
Cultures in wound infections, 171
Curtis v. Columbia Doctors' Hospital of Opelousas,
  265s-266s

D

DAR framework in focus charting, 6
Deafness, 285-288
  assessment of, 19
  confusion in, 109, 111, 113
Death and dying, 320-323
  advance directives on, 18, 215, 363-366, 364s
  brain death in, 324-325, 325s
  in do not resuscitate orders, 366-369
  fears of patient in, 315s
  late entries in medical records on, 379s-380s
  organ donation in, 323-327, 379s
  reported to organ procurement organization, 324s
  in suicidal behavior, 258s-259s
  in termination of life support, 56, 363-366
  witnessing of oral will in, 320
Decision making
  competency issues in, 112s, 295-296, 298
  in durable power of attorney, 296, 298, 363, 364s
  on organ donation, 323, 326
  on termination of life support, 363-366
Decubitus ulcers, 159-166
Defibrillation in ventricular arrhythmias, 61
Dehiscence of wound, 193-197
Delegation of tasks
  in documentation, 349-350
  in understaffed units, 360
Destruction of medical records, 330s-331s, 341s
Developmental information, 16, 17s

Diabetes mellitus
  dietary compliance in, 144s, 219
  hyperglycemia in, 143-147
  hypoglycemia in, 140
  myocardial infarction in, 35
  self-monitoring of glucose levels in, 145, 146s
  sepsis in, 173, 174
Diagnosis, nursing, PIE documentation of, 6
Dictionaries with non-English terms and phrases, 284s
Diet. *See* Nutrition.
Discharge of patient, 14, 374-377
  education and teaching in, 21, 375, 377
  in police custody, 225
Disclaimer added to countersignature on notes,
    357s, 358
Disclosure of information
  to law enforcement officials, 222
  in media requests for patient information,
    372-373, 373s
  in patient requests for medical records, 204-208
    denial of, 207
  and patient withholding of information, 212-215
Distributive shock, 46
Do not resuscitate orders, 366-369
Donation of organs, 323-327, 379s
  in brain death, 324-325, 325s
  by living donors, 326, 327
Dressings in wound infections, 171
Driver's license regulations in seizure history, 119
Drugs
  in adverse drug reaction therapy, 179
  adverse reactions to, 177-181
    gastrointestinal hemorrhage in, 134
    hypertensive crisis in, 63-64
    MedWatch program on, 180s
    patient fear of, 276
  in anaphylaxis, 149
  in arrhythmias, 61, 62
  in asthma, 83
  bar code system on, 387s
  in cardiopulmonary arrest, 55
  as chemical restraint, 245, 246
  compliance with therapy, 219
    in discovery of hidden drugs, 275-277
  in confusion, 113
  as contraband possession, 269-272
  coworker administration of, 351
  errors in administration of, 351
    in understaffed units, 359
  in gastrointestinal hemorrhage, 137
  in heart failure, 42-43
  hidden, discovery of, 275-277
  in HIV infection, 156, 157-158, 159
  in hypertensive crisis, 67-68
  medication administration records on, 73, 75s, 351
  in myocardial infarction, 38
  in pain, 106
    in chest, 31-32
    discovery of hidden drugs in, 276

Drugs—cont'd
  in pain—cont'd
    history of, 103
    legal issues in, 104s-105s
    patient-controlled analgesia in, 106, 107s
  in peripheral pulse loss, 26
  physician's assistant orders on, 32s
  in pneumonia, 73
  in pulmonary edema, 95
  in pulmonary embolism, 90
  in seizures, 118
  in sepsis, 175-176
  in shock, 49-50
  in transfusion reactions, 153-154
  in tuberculosis, 100
  withheld in questionable orders, 369-370, 369s
  in wound infections, 171, 172
Durable power of attorney, 296, 298, 363, 364s

E

E-mail, 392-394
Ear examination, 19
Edema
  in heart failure, 42
  in peripheral pulse loss, 24
    extremity circumference measurements in, 24, 25s
  pulmonary, 91-96
Education of patient and family, 14, 21-23
  in adverse drug reactions, 181
  affective outcomes in, 85s
  in anaphylaxis, 150
  in anxiety, 253-254
  in arrhythmias, 62-63
  in aspiration of tube feeding, 133
  in asthma, 84-86
  in brain death, 324-325, 325s
  in cardiopulmonary arrest, 56
  in cerebrovascular accident, 125
  in chest pain, 33-34
  cognitive outcomes in, 85s
  in confusion, 114
  in discharge preparations, 21, 375, 377
  in discovery of hidden drugs, 276
  in gastrointestinal hemorrhage, 139-140
  in heart failure, 45
  in HIV infection, 158-159
  in hyperglycemia, 145-147
  in hypertensive crisis, 68
  in hypoglycemia, 143
  for informed consent, 294-300, 299s
  in initial orientation, 21
  in intravenous infiltration, 184
  in leaving against medical advice, 226-227
  limitations on advice provided in
    in legal issues, 317-319, 320s
    in medical issues, 360-363
  in myocardial infarction, 38-39
  in obesity, 293
  in peripheral pulse loss, 27-28

Education of patient and family—cont'd
  in pneumonia, 74-75
  in pneumothorax, 80-81
  in pressure ulcers, 166
  psychomotor outcomes in, 85s
  in pulmonary edema, 96
  in pulmonary embolism, 90-91
  in refusal of treatment, 217
  in restraint use, 249
  in seizures, 118-119
  in sepsis, 177
  in severe pain, 108
  in shock, 51-52
  in smoking, 267, 269
  in surgery, 193
  in transfusion reactions, 154
  in tuberculosis, 101-102
  in unresponsive patient, 130
  in wound dehiscence or evisceration, 196-197
  in wound infections, 172
Educational level of patient, assessment and
    documentation of, 17
Elderly
  abuse of, 308, 309
  developmental information on, 17s
Electrocardiography
  in chest pain, 30, 31
  in heart failure, 43-44
  in hypertensive crisis, 66, 67
  lead placement in, 58s
  in myocardial infarction, 37
  in new arrhythmias, 57-63
  in pulmonary edema, 93-94
Electrophysiology studies in arrhythmias, 62
Elimination patterns
  in heart failure, 42
  initial assessment of, 20
  in unresponsive patient, 128
E-mail, 392-394
Emancipated minors, 294, 297, 298
Embolism
  cerebral, 120
  pulmonary, 86-91
Emotional support
  in asthma, 84
  in chest pain, 33
  in HIV infection, 158
  in organ donation, 326
  in serious illness, 315s
  in severe pain, 108, 315s
Emphysema, pneumothorax in, 76, 77
Endotracheal intubation
  in cardiopulmonary arrest, 54
  in cerebrovascular accident, 123
  patient removal of tube in, 278-280
  in sepsis, 176
  in shock, 49
Energy conservation techniques in heart
    failure, 45

Environmental factors
  in home. *See* Home environment.
  as restraint, 245, 246
  in risk for accidental injury, 262
Equipment
  failure of, 301-304
    follow-through actions in, 302, 302s
    reporting of, 303, 303s-304s
  for obese patients, 293
  patient tampering with, 272-275
    in chest tube, 280-283
    in endotracheal tube, 278-280
Esophageal hemorrhage, 137
Evisceration of wound, 193-197
Exercise and activity
  in cerebrovascular accident, 124
  in chest pain, 32
  health history interview on, 17
  in heart failure, energy conservation techniques in, 45
  in obesity, 292
  in peripheral pulse loss, 27
  in pneumonia, 74
Expressed consent to treatment, 295s
Expressed refusal of treatment, 215
Eye examination, 19
  in hypertensive crisis, 66
  visual acuity testing in, 19, 289, 289s

F

Faison v. Hillhaven Corp. et al., 104s-105s
Fall prevention, 21
False imprisonment, 226, 227s, 246
Family
  abuse suspected in, 308
  in death of patient, 320, 321, 322, 323
  in health care decisions
    in do not resuscitate orders, 368, 368s
    in durable power of attorney, 296, 298, 363, 364s
    for minors, 296-297, 298
    in termination of life support, 363-366
  health history of, 16
    genogram on, 35, 36s
    in myocardial infarction, 35
  instructions provided to, 14. *See also* Education of
    patient and family.
  as interpreter
    for hearing impaired patient, 286, 288
    for non-English speaking patient, 284, 285
  of organ donor, 323, 324, 325, 326, 327
  questions on quality of care, 306-308
    and requests for medical advice, 360-363
  requesting medical advice from nurse, 360-363
  visiting hours for, 311-312
Fax transmission of medical records, 389-392
  to patients, 206
  to wrong number, 391, 392
Fears of patients
  on adverse drug reactions, 276
  in serious illness, 315s

Fever
  in sepsis, 173, 176
  in transfusion reactions, 150, 151, 153
Fibrillation
  atrial, 57, 59, 60, 61
  ventricular, 59, 60, 61
    cardiopulmonary arrest in, 55
Flash card use
  for hearing impaired patients, 286, 288
  for non-English speaking patients, 284, 285
Floating of staff to understaffed units, 358-360
Flow sheets
  disadvantages of, 47s
  in equipment tampering, 274s, 275
  in shock, 46
Fluids
  in gastrointestinal hemorrhage, 134, 136
  in heart failure, 42, 45
  in hyperglycemia, 145
  in peripheral pulse loss, 26-27
  in pneumonia, 73
  in pressure ulcers, 163
  in pulmonary edema, 95
  in sepsis, 175
  in shock, 46, 47, 50, 51
  in tuberculosis, 100
  in unresponsive patient, 128
Focus charting, 6
Food and Drug Administration MedWatch program,
  180s, 303s-304s
Fraudulent concealment
  in late entries, 379s-380s
  in surgical accident, 185s-186s

G

Gases, arterial blood
  in asthma, 82, 83
  in chest pain, 31
  in heart failure, 43
  in pneumonia, 69, 70, 72-73, 74
  in pneumothorax, 77
  in pulmonary edema, 94
  in pulmonary embolism, 88, 89
  in shock, 48, 49, 51
  in tuberculosis, 100
Gastrointestinal system
  drug-induced disorders of, 134, 178
  hemorrhage in, 133-140
  initial evaluation of, 20
Genital examination, 20
Genogram on family history, 35, 36s
Gess v. United States, 384s-385s
Glasgow Coma Scale, 126, 127s
Glucose blood levels, 140-147
  in decreased level of consciousness, 128, 141, 142
  in hyperglycemia, 143-147
  in hypoglycemia, 118, 140-143
  measurement of, 141-142, 145
    with home meter during hospitalization, 146s

Glucose blood levels—cont'd
  in seizures, 118, 141
  in sepsis, 173, 174
Goals of documentation, 2s
Growth and development information, 16
  JCAHO requirements on, 17s
Guided imagery techniques in pain management,
  107, 314

H

Habits and lifestyle
  cerebrovascular risk factors in, 121
  health history interview on, 16-17
  tuberculosis risk factors in, 97
Hair examination, 20
Handwriting
  in late entries, analysis of, 379s-380s
  in physician orders, legibility of, 347-349
Harm
  to others, patient threats on, 239-244
    description of, 242, 243s
    protection of intended victim in, 241s, 242
  potential, protection of patient from, 4
    in negligence of colleague, 352
    in questionable physician orders, 44s, 342-344,
      369-370
    withholding of drug or treatment in,
      369-370, 369s
  to self
    in accidental injury, 260-266
    in chest tube removal, 280-283
    in endotracheal tube removal, 278-280
    restraint use in, 247s-248s
    in suicide threats, 254-259
Head examination, 18-19
Healing
  in pressure ulcers, 163-166
  wound dehiscence or evisceration in, 193-197
  in wound infections, 172
Health care power of attorney, 296, 298, 363, 364s
Health care professionals
  abbreviations used by, 381-383
  countersigning notes, 356-358, 379
  delegating documentation, 349-350
  documentation of communications with, 93s
    in anaphylaxis, 149-150, 149s
    in pressure ulcers, 166
    in seizures, 117
  drug administration by coworkers, 351
  including inappropriate information in medical
    records, 239s, 331, 335-338
  in life support decisions, 363-366
  orders from
    from physicians, 342-349. *See also* Physician
      orders.
    from physician's assistant, 32s, 345-347
  patient and family questions on abilities of, 360, 362
  removing medical records from facility, 338-342
  reporting suspected negligence, 352-353

Health care professionals—cont'd
  tampering with medical records, 332-335
  in understaffed units, 358-360
Health history interview, 12-13.
    See also History-taking.
Health Insurance Portability and Accountability Act,
    22s, 206, 391, 393
  on e-mail and Internet use, 393
  on fax transmission of medical records, 206, 391
Hearing aid use, 285, 286, 287s, 288
Hearing impairment, 285-288
  assessment of, 19
  confusion in, 109, 111, 113
Heart failure, 39-45
Heart rate, 18, 19-20
  arrhythmias of, 57-63. *See also* Arrhythmias.
  electrocardiography of. *See* Electrocardiography.
Heart sounds
  in arrhythmias, 59
  in heart failure, 42
  in hypertensive crisis, 66
Height measurement, 18
Hematemesis, 134
Hematochezia, 134
Hemiplegia in cerebrovascular accident, 121
Hemodynamic monitoring
  in myocardial infarction, 37
  in pulmonary edema, 95
  in sepsis, 174, 175
  in shock, 49, 50-51
Hemolytic transfusion reactions, 150, 151, 153
Hemorrhage
  gastrointestinal, 133-140
  intracerebral, 120
Hemothorax, 78, 280
Hidden drugs, discovery of, 275-277
History-taking, 12-13
  direct quotation of patient in, 13
  genogram in, 35, 36s
  in initial assessment, 15-18
  patient withholding of information in, 212-215
  sources of information in, 12
HIV infection, 154-159
  progression to AIDS, 155, 155s
Homans' sign, 123
Home environment
  abuse suspected in, 309
  challenging patient situations in, 201
  discharge of patient to, 375, 377
  initial assessment of, 18
  safety issues in, 18, 201
Hostile behavior, 236-239
  description of, 243s
  threats to harm others in, 239-244
  types of, 236
Human immunodeficiency virus (HIV) infections,
    154-159
  progression to AIDS, 155, 155s
Hutchins v. DCH Regional Medical Center, 167s-168s

Hygiene measures in unresponsive patient, 129
Hyperglycemia, 143-147
Hypertension
  cerebrovascular accident in, 120, 123
  crisis in, 63-68
  myocardial infarction in, 34
Hypoglycemia, 140-143
  seizures in, 118, 141
Hypotension
  in gastrointestinal hemorrhage, 135
  in shock, 46
Hypovolemia
  in gastrointestinal hemorrhage, 134, 135, 136
  shock in, 46
Hypoxemia in sepsis, 174, 176

I

Identification of patient, 21
  in surgery, 189, 190s
  in transfusions, 152s
Illegible physician orders, 347-349
Imagery techniques in pain management, 107, 314
Immunodeficiency syndrome, acquired, progression
    of HIV infection to, 155, 155s
Immunodeficiency virus infection, human,
    154-159
  progression to AIDS, 155, 155s
Implied consent to treatment, 295s
Implied refusal of treatment, 215-216
Inappropriate information in medical records,
    331, 335-338
  correction of, 338s
  criticisms of colleagues, 335-337
  criticisms of patients, 239s, 337
  false assumptions and bias, 239s
Incident reports, 201, 383-386
  on accidental injury, 264
  on colleague's actions, 336-337
    in suspected negligence, 353
  on contraband possessions, 272
  on equipment failure, 302-303
    follow-up on, 302, 302s
  follow-up on, 383, 384s-385s
    in equipment failure, 302, 302s
  on hostile behavior, 238
  on leaving against medical advice, 228
  on noncompliance, 219
  on patient withholding of information, 215
  on refusal of treatment, 218
  on sexual advance and harassment, 235
  on unavailable medical records, 211-212, 342
Infarction, myocardial, 34-39
  chest pain in, 28, 30, 33, 34, 37
Infections
  human immunodeficiency virus, 154-159
  opportunistic, in HIV infection, 155s, 158
  pneumonia in, 68-75, 155s
  reporting requirements in, 98s-99s, 372
  sepsis in, 46, 173-177

Infections—cont'd
tuberculosis in, 96-102, 155s
of wounds, 166-172
dehiscence or evisceration in, 194
Infiltration complication in intravenous therapy,
181-184
Informed consent, 294-300. *See also* Consent to
treatment or procedures.
Informed refusal of treatment, 217
in leaving against medical advice, 226
Inhaled medications in asthma, 83
Insulin therapy in hyperglycemia, 145
Insurance
health care, fax transmission of medical records for,
390-391
malpractice, 231
Intensive care in chest pain, 33
Internet use, 392-394
Interpreter use
for hearing impaired patients, 285, 286, 288
for non-English speaking patients, 284, 285
Interventions, documentation of, 13-14, 21
AIR format in, 88s-89s
focus charting in, 6
PIE approach in, 6
problem-oriented approach in, 5-6
on response to interventions, 6, 14, 88s-89s
Interview on health history, 12-13.
See also History-taking.
Intraaortic balloon pump in shock, 51
Intravenous therapy
in adverse drug reactions, 179
in arrhythmias, 61
in asthma, 83
in cardiopulmonary arrest, 55
in chest pain, 32
equipment tampering in, 274, 274s
essential components of documentation in, 183s
in gastrointestinal hemorrhage, 137-138
in heart failure, 43
in hyperglycemia, 145
in hypertensive crisis, 67-68
in hypoglycemia, 142
infiltration complication in, 181-184
in myocardial infarction, 38
in peripheral pulse loss, 26-27
in pneumonia, 73
in pulmonary edema, 95
in seizures, 118
in sepsis, 175
in shock, 50
in transfusion reactions, 153-154
in tuberculosis, 100
in unresponsive patient, 129
in wound dehiscence or evisceration, 195
Involuntary admission and treatment
in false imprisonment, 226, 227s
of patient in police custody, 222, 223s
Isolation measures in tuberculosis, 98, 99

J
Joint Commission on Accreditation of Healthcare
Organizations (JCAHO)
on abbreviation use, 381, 382s
on frequency of patient reassessment, 119s
on growth and developmental information, 17s
on incident reports, 383
on orders from physician's assistants, 32s
on pain management, 103s, 105s
on restraint use, 244, 245s
on safety goals in surgery, 190s
Journals
of nurses, 231, 232s
of patients in police custody, 224
Jugular vein distention, 18
in heart failure, 42
in pneumothorax, 77
in shock, 48

K
Ketoacidosis in hyperglycemia, 143
Kidney disorders, hypertensive crisis in, 63, 66, 67
Kodadek v. Lieberman, 185s-186s
Kussmaul's breathing in hyperglycemia, 144

L
Laboratory test results, 44s
in arrhythmias, 60
in confusion, 113
fax transmission of, 391
in gastrointestinal hemorrhage, 136
in HIV infection, 158
in hypertensive crisis, 66-67
for patient in police custody, 221-222
in sepsis, 174, 175
in shock, 48
in transfusion reactions, 154
in wound infections, 171
Lama v. Borras, 7
Language barriers
for hearing impaired patients, 285-288
for non-English speaking patients, 283-285
initial assessment of, 18
resource materials in, 284-285, 284s
Last will and testament, witnessing of, 316-320
Late entries in medical records, 211, 350, 377-381
countersignatures on, 379
explanation and format for, 378s
in telephone report from colleague, 350
in unavailable medical records, 211, 378s
Lawsuits
in accidental injury, 264, 265s-266s
communication with health care team in, 93s
in negligence. *See* Negligence.
patient threat of, 228-233
in suicide threat, 258s-259s
Leaving against medical advice, 225-228
Leg circumference measurements in peripheral pulse
loss, 24, 25s

Legal issues, 2s, 4, 11
  in abusive behavior, 308-309
  in accidental injuries, 263-264
    documentation preventing liability in, 265s-266s
    effective notes in, 261s-262s
    in smoking, 267, 268s
  in advance directives, 364s, 365
  in alteration of medical records, 332-335
  in block charting, 132s
  in caring for patient in police custody, 220-225
  in challenging patient situations, 200-201
  in charting by exception approach, 7
  claim investigation in, 230-231
  in communication with health care team, 93s
  comparative negligence in, 267, 268s
  competency and capacity in, 112s, 295-296
    in will execution, 318s-319s
  in contraband possessions, 270-271, 271s
  contributory negligence in, 267, 268s, 273
  in countersigning notes, 356
  in delegated documentation, 349-350
  in difficult professional problems, 329-330
  in disease reporting, 98s-99s
  in e-mail and Internet use, 393
  in equipment failure, 301
  in equipment tampering by patient, 272-273
    in endotracheal intubation, 278s
  in fax transmission of medical records, 206, 391, 392
  in follow-up of incident reports, 383, 384s-385s
  in fraudulent concealment of surgical accident,
    185s-186s
  in home health care, 201
  in hostile behavior, 236, 237, 238
  in illegible physician orders, 348, 348s
  in inappropriate information included in medical
    records, 239s, 331, 335-338
  in informed consent, 294-298, 299s
  in late entries, 377-379, 379s-380s
  in leaving against medical advice, 225, 226
  in life support decisions, 363, 365
  in missing belongings, 304-305
  in motor vehicle operation in seizure history, 119
  in noncompliance, 218
  in nonroutine care provided by unlicensed assistive
    personnel, 354, 355
  in objective documentation, 239s
  in Omnibus Budget Reconciliation Act of 1987, 309s
  in orders from physician's assistant, 32s
  in organ donation, 323, 324s
  in pain management, 104s-105s
  in Patient Self-Determination Act, 363, 365
  in patient withholding of information, 213
  in personal journals of nurses, 231, 232s
  in photographing or videotaping of patients,
    370-371, 371s
  in pneumonia monitoring, 70, 71s-72s
  in postmortem care, 321
  in postoperative wound infection and ambiguous
    charting, 167s-168s

Legal issues—cont'd
  in pressure ulcers, 163, 164s-165s
  in privacy of health records, 22s, 206, 372, 373s,
    391, 393
  qualified privilege in, 352, 352s
  in questionable physician orders, 343
  in refusal of treatment, 216s, 217
  in release of medical records to patients, 205, 205s,
    206, 207
  in restraint use, 245s, 246, 247s-248s, 250
  in retention of records on telephone triage,
    330s-331s
  in self-documentation by patients, 202, 204
  in sexual advance and harassment, 233-235
  in spoliation of evidence, 339s-340s
  in staffing levels, 359s
    of understaffed units, 358, 359, 360
  in suicide threats, 254, 258, 258s-259s
  in suspected negligence, 352-353
  in telephone orders, 346s-347s
  in telephone triage records, 330s-331s
  in threat for harm to others, 241s
  in threat of lawsuit, 228-233
    characteristics of patients in, 229s
  in unavailable medical records, 211-212, 341s
    court rulings on, 339s-340s
    on telephone triage, 330s-331s
  in witnessing last will and testament, 316-320
Liability
  in accidental injury, 264, 265s-266s
  in negligence. See Negligence.
  in nonroutine care provided by unlicensed assistive
    personnel, 355
  in suicide threat, 258s-259s
  and threat of patient lawsuit, 228-233
Life support measures
  in arrhythmias, 61
  in cardiopulmonary arrest, 54, 56
  and "do not resuscitate" orders, 366-369
  termination of, 56, 363-366
Lifestyle and personal habits
  cerebrovascular risk factors in, 121
  health history interview on, 16-17
  tuberculosis risk factors in, 97
Lip reading in hearing impairment,
    285, 286, 288
Living will, 363, 364s
  and right to refuse treatment, 215
Long-term care facilities
  abuse of patients in, 308, 309s
  mental capacity and will execution in,
    318s-319s
  monthly summaries of medical records in, 350s
  pain management in, 104s-105s
  pressure ulcer care in, 164s-165s
  restraint use in, 247s-248s
Lost belongings of patient, 304-306
Lost medical records. See Unavailable medical
    records.

M

Mallory-Weiss tear, 137
Malpractice cases, 4
  communication with health care team in, 93s
  notification of insurance company on, 231
  patient threat of, 228-233
Mature minors, 294, 297, 298
Mechanical ventilation. *See* Ventilatory support.
Media requests for patient information, 372-373, 373s
Medical advice
  leaving against, 225-228
  requests for, 360-363
Medical equipment. *See* Equipment.
Medical examiner, 321
Medical records
  abbreviation use in, 381-383
  alterations and corrections in
    in computerized systems, 388
    in illegal tampering, 332-335
    in late entries, 211, 379s-380s
    legal, for correction of mistake, 334-335, 334s, 338s
    patient requests for, 207
  computerized, 386-389
  destruction of, 330s-331s, 341s
  in do not resuscitate orders, 368, 368s
  e-mail transmission of, 392-394
  fax transmission of, 206, 389-392
  inappropriate information included in, 331, 335-338
    correction of, 338s
    criticisms of colleagues, 335-337
    criticisms of patients, 239s, 337
    false assumptions and bias, 239s
  late entries in, 211, 350, 377-381
  lost, 209, 211-212, 339s-340s. *See also* Unavailable
    medical records.
  monthly summaries of, 349, 350s
  on patient in police custody, 222
  patient requests for, 204-208
  relevance of information in, 331, 335-338
  retention of, 330s-331s, 341s
  self-documentation by patient included in, 204
  temporary or substitute, 208-212, 342
  unavailable, 208-212. *See also* Unavailable medical
    records.
Medication administration records, 73, 75s, 351
MedWatch program, 180s, 303s-304s
Melena, 134
Memory assessment, 19
  in confusion, 110
Mental status, 19
  in competency determination, 112
  in confusion, 109-114
Minors
  abuse of, 308, 309
  emancipated, 294, 297, 298
  equipment tampering by, 272, 273
  informed consent for, 296-297, 298
  mature, 294, 297, 298
Misleading notes, 283s

Missing belongings of patient, 304-306
Missing medical records. *See* Unavailable medical
    records.
Mistakes in medical records
  correction of, 334-335, 334s, 338s
    patient requests for, 207
  in inappropriate comments, 239s, 335-338
  in misleading notes, 283s
Monthly summaries of medical records, 349, 350s
Motor vehicle operation in seizure history, 119
Musculoskeletal system
  cerebrovascular accident affecting, 121-122, 124
  initial assessment of, 20
Myocardial infarction, 34-39
  chest pain in, 28, 30, 33, 34, 37

N

Nails, initial assessment of, 20
Narrative notes, 6
  in shock, 46, 47s
  in transfer or discharge of patient, 376-377
Nasogastric intubation
  aspiration of tube feeding in, 132
  in gastrointestinal hemorrhage, 136-137, 139
  verification of tube placement in, 137s
Nebulizer therapy in asthma, 83
Neck examination, 18
  jugular vein distention in, 18, 42, 48, 77
  throat and swallowing in, 19
Negligence
  in accidental injury, 265s-266s
    smoking-related, 267, 268s
  comparative, 267, 268s
  contributory, 267, 268s, 273
  in equipment tampering by patient, 272-273
    in endotracheal intubation, 278s
  in lost medical records, 339s-340s
  in pneumonia monitoring, 71s-72s
  in suicide threat, 258s-259s
  suspected, reporting of, 352-353
    qualified privilege in, 352, 352s
Nervous system
  in cerebrovascular accident, 120-125
  drug-induced disorders of, 178
  in hypertensive crisis, 66
  initial examination of, 19
  in seizures, 114-119
  smoking supervision in disorders of, 267, 268
  in unresponsive patient, 126
New York Heart Association classification system in
    heart failure, 40, 40s
Nicotine replacement therapy in smoking cessation,
    269
NME Properties Inc. v. Rudich, 164s-165s
Noncompliance, 218-220. *See also* Compliance issues.
Nose examination, 19
Nurse administrator alteration of medical
    records, 338s
Nursing diagnosis, PIE documentation of, 6

Nursing home care
  mental capacity and will execution in, 318s-319s
  pain management in, 104s-105s
  in pressure ulcers, 164s-165s
  restraint use in, 247s-248s
Nutrition
  aspiration of tube feeding in, 130-133
  in diabetes mellitus, compliance with, 144s, 219
  in gastrointestinal hemorrhage, 136-137, 139
  health history interview on, 17
  in heart failure, 40-41, 45
  in HIV infection, 158
  in hyperglycemia, 143, 144s
  in hypoglycemia, 142, 143
  in myocardial infarction, 38
  in obesity, 292, 293
  in pneumonia, 74
  in pressure ulcers, 163
  in unresponsive patient, 128, 129
  in vision impairment, 290
  in wound dehiscence or evisceration, 194
  in wound infections, 169, 172

O

Obesity, 291-294
Objective data, 13
  on consciousness level, 122s
  on hostile behavior, 238, 239s
  in incident report, 385
  lack of, in inappropriate in medical records,
    239s, 337-338
  in SOAP notes, 5
Occupational history, 16
Omnibus Budget Reconciliation Act of 1987, 309s
Opportunistic infections in HIV infection, 155s, 158
Orders
  from physician, 342-349. *See also* Physician orders.
  from physician's assistant, 32s, 345-347
Organ donation, 323-327, 379s
  in brain death, 324-325, 325s
  by living donors, 326, 327
Orientation of patient on facility policies, 21
Overweight, 291
Oxygen therapy
  in anaphylaxis, 149
  in asthma, 83
  in cardiopulmonary arrest, 54
  in chest pain, 31
  in chest tube removal by patient, 281, 282
  in endotracheal tube removal by patient, 279
  in heart failure, 43
  in hypertensive crisis, 67
  in myocardial infarction, 38
  in pneumonia, 70, 72-73
  in pneumothorax, 78
  in pulmonary edema, 94
  in pulmonary embolism, 89
  in sepsis, 176
  in shock, 49
  in tuberculosis, 100

Oxygenation status
  in aspiration of tube feeding, 131
  in asthma, 84
  in cerebrovascular accident, 123
  in chest tube removal by patient, 281, 282
  in endotracheal tube removal by patient, 279, 280
  in pneumonia, 70, 73
  in pneumothorax, 77
  in pulmonary edema, 94-95
  in pulmonary embolism, 87-88, 89
  in tuberculosis, 100-101
  in wound dehiscence or evisceration, 195

P

Pacing, cardiac, 62
Pain
  abdominal, 135, 135s
  in chest, 28-34. *See also* Chest pain.
  discovery of hidden drugs in, 276
  in heart failure, 41
  in myocardial infarction, 28, 30, 33, 34, 37
  in peripheral pulse loss, 27
  in pneumonia, 69
  in pulmonary edema, 91
  in pulmonary embolism, 86-87
  in serious illness, 314, 316
  severe, 102-108, 314, 315s
Parenteral nutrition in gastrointestinal hemorrhage, 139
Passwords for access to computerized documentation,
    386, 388, 389s
Patient-controlled analgesia, 106, 107s
Patient Self-Determination Act, 363, 365
Peripheral pulse loss, 23-29
Pheochromocytoma, hypertensive crisis in, 63, 67
Phillips v. Covenant Clinic, 339s-340s
Photographs of patients, 370-372
  identity disguised in, 371, 371s
Physical examination, 18-21
  in adverse drug reactions, 178
  of anxious patient, 253
  in arrhythmias, 59-60
  in cerebrovascular accident, 121-123
  in chest pain, 29-30
  in heart failure, 41-42
  in HIV infection, 157
  in hyperglycemia, 144
  in hypertensive crisis, 66
  in obesity, 292-293
  in peripheral pulse loss, 24, 25s
  in pulmonary embolism, 87
  in shock, 46-48
  in surgical patient, 188
  in transfusion reactions, 151-153
  in wound dehiscence or evisceration, 194-195
  in wound infections, 169-170, 170s
Physician assistant orders, 345-347
  legal obligations in, 32s
Physician orders, 342-349
  in computerized systems, 387s
  deviating from standard practice, 44s, 343

Physician orders—cont'd
"do not resuscitate," 366-369
illegible, 347-349
in pain management, 104s
pertinent negatives in, 44s
questionable, 44s, 342-344
withholding of drug or treatment in,
369-370, 369s
in self-documentation by patient, 202, 203
on slow code, 368s
for transfer or discharge of patient, 374, 375
verbal or telephone, 329, 344-347
PIE documentation, 6
Plan of care
evaluation of, 14
in hostile patients, 238
PIE documentation of, 6
in pressure ulcers, 159, 160s-161s
problem-oriented documentation of, 5, 6
in uncooperative patient, 214, 214s
Pleurodesis in pneumothorax, 78-80
Pneumonia, 68-75
in AIDS, 155s
aspiration, 69, 131, 133
Pneumothorax, 76-81
chest tube insertion in, 78, 79s-80s, 280
closed, 76, 78-80
open, 76, 78
tension, 76, 78
Police
notified on contraband possessions, 270-271,
271s, 272
patient in custody of, 220-225
Pollard v. Hastings, 318s-319s
Positioning of patient
in peripheral pulse loss, 27
in wound dehiscence or evisceration, 195
Postmortem care, 320-323
Postoperative documentation, 187-188, 189-193
in organ donation, 326
in wound dehiscence or evisceration repair, 196
in wound infection, ambiguous charting in,
167s-168s
Pregnancy
hypertensive crisis in, 63
telephone orders from physician in, 346s-347s
telephone triage logs in, 330s-331s
Preoperative documentation, 188, 189
in wound dehiscence or evisceration repair,
195-196
Pressure ulcers, 159-166
stages of, 162
Privacy rights, 22
in e-mail and Internet use, 392-394
in fax transmission of medical records, 206,
389-392, 390s
Health Insurance Portability and Accountability
Act on, 22s, 206, 391, 393
in media requests for patient information,
372-373, 373s

Privacy rights—cont'd
and patient withholding of information, 212-215
in photographing or videotaping of patients,
370-371, 371s
and right of public to know, 372
and search policies
in contraband items, 270
in hidden drugs, 277
Problem-oriented documentation, 5-6
Professional problems, 329-394
Prohibited items, 269-272
Psychiatric care
involuntary, for patient in police custody, 222
in suicidal behavior, 258s-259s
Psychomotor outcomes in patient education, 85s
Psychosocial status
in asthma, 84
in chest pain, 33
in confusion, 111
initial assessment of, 20-21
in pulmonary edema, 94
in severe pain, 108
in suicide threats, 255, 256s, 258s-259s
Pugh v. Mayeaux, 346s-347s
Pulmonary artery catheterization
in heart failure, 44
in myocardial infarction, 37
in pulmonary edema, 95
in shock, 50-51
Pulse
in arrhythmias, 59, 60
in cardiopulmonary arrest, 54
carotid, 18
peripheral, loss of, 23-29
in shock, 46, 47, 49
Pulseless electrical activity, 55
Purified protein derivative test in tuberculosis,
101, 101s

Q

Qualified privilege, 352s
Quality Nursing Care Act, 359s
Quality of care, 4, 11
colleague criticism of
in medical record, 335-337
nursing standards on, 336s
qualified privilege in, 352s
in suspected negligence, 352-353
family questions on, 306-308
and requests for medical advice, 360-363
and nurse questions on physician's order,
44s, 342-344
withholding of drug or treatment in,
369-370, 369s
in understaffed units, 358-360
from unlicensed assistive personnel, verification of,
353-356, 355s
Quality of documentation, assessment of, 3s
Quotation of patient, direct, 13

R

Radiography
  in pneumothorax, 77-78, 80
  in pulmonary edema, 94
Referrals, 14
Refusal of assignment
  in sexual advance and harassment, 233, 234
  in understaffed units, 358
Refusal of treatment, 199, 201, 215-217
  advance directives on, 215, 363, 364s, 365
  in "do not resuscitate" orders, 366-369
  expressed, 215
  by hostile patients, 236
  implied, 215-216
  leaving against medical advice in, 225-228
  by patient in police custody, 221-222
    involuntary admission and treatment in, 222, 223s
  reevaluation of treatment plan in, 219
Relaxation techniques
  in anxiety, 252
  in pain, 107, 314
Release of medical records
  to law enforcement officials, 222
  to media, 372-373, 373s
  to patients, 204-208
Relevance of information in medical records,
  331, 335-338
Religious and cultural influences, health history
  interview on, 17
Reproductive system, initial assessment of, 20
Requests for information
  in health history interview, patient refusal in,
    212-215
  by law enforcement officials, 222
  by media, 372-373, 373s
  by patients and family, 204-208
    deadline for response in, 206-207
    denial of, 207
    fee charged for, 206
    on legal issues, 317-319, 320s
    on medical advice, 360-363
Respiratory rate, 18
  in pneumonia, 69
Respiratory system, 68-102
  in anaphylaxis, 149
  in arrhythmias, 60, 61
  in aspiration of tube feeding, 130-133
  in asthma, 81-86
  in cardiopulmonary arrest, 52-56
  in cerebrovascular accident, 121, 123-124
  in chest tube removal by patient, 280-283
  in endotracheal tube removal by patient, 278-280
  in heart failure, 41, 43
  initial assessment of, 19
  in pneumonia, 68-75
  in pneumothorax, 76-81
  in pulmonary edema, 91-96
  in pulmonary embolism, 86-91
  in sepsis, 174, 176
  in shock, 48, 49

Respiratory system—cont'd
  in tuberculosis, 96-102
  in unresponsive patient, 126-127, 128-129
Response to interventions, documentation of, 14
  AIR format in, 88s-89s
  focus charting in, 6
Restraining orders, 308
Restraint use, 244-251
  chemical restraints in, 245, 246
  environmental restraints in, 245, 246
  in equipment tampering, 273
    with chest tube, 281-282
    with endotracheal tube, 279
  as false imprisonment, 226, 227s, 246
  in hostile behavior, 238
  JCAHO regulations on, 244, 245s
  legal issues in, 245, 246, 247s-248s, 250
  physical restraints in, 244-245, 246
  in refusal of treatment, 217
  in seizures, 117
Resuscitation, cardiopulmonary, 54
  in accidental injury, 263
  death of patient during, 322
  and "do not resuscitate" orders, 366-369
  termination of, 56
  in ventricular arrhythmias, 61
Retention of medical records
  importance of, 341s
  in physician requests for removal, 338-342
  on telephone triage, 330s-331s
Rights of patients
  in leaving against medical advice, 225-228
  in police custody, 220-225
  to privacy. *See* Privacy rights.
  in refusal of treatment, 215-218
  in request for medical records, 204-208
  in restraint use, 246
  in threats of harm to others, 241s, 242
  in withholding medical history, 212-215
Risk factors
  in accidental injuries, 260-262
  in cerebrovascular accident, 121
  health history interview on, 16-17
  in HIV infection, 156
  in pneumonia, 69
  in suicidal behavior, 255, 256s
  in tuberculosis, 97
Rothstein v. Orange Grove Center, Inc., 379s-380s

S

Sabol v. Richmond Heights General Hospital, 258s-259s
Safety issues, 4
  in abbreviation use, 381-383
  in accidental injury, 260-266
    smoking-related, 266-267, 268s
  in cerebrovascular accident, 124
  in computerized documentation, 388, 389s
  in confusion, 111-113
  in contraband items, 269-272
  in e-mail and Internet use, 392-394

Safety issues—cont'd
in equipment failure, 301-304
in equipment tampering by patient, 272-275
in chest tube, 280-283
in endotracheal tube, 278-280
fall prevention in, 21
in fax transmission of medical records,
389-392, 390s
in hidden drugs, 277
in home environment, 18, 201
in hostile patients, 236, 237-238
in identification of patient, 21
preoperative, 189, 190s
in transfusions, 152s
for patient in police custody, 221, 224
in questionable physician orders, 44s, 342-344,
369-370
restraint use in, 244-251
in seizures, 117
in sexual advance and harassment, 234
in suicide threats, 254-259
in surgery, 190s
in threat for harm to others, 239-244
protection of intended victim in, 241s, 242
in unresponsive patient, 130
in vision impairment, 290, 291
Screening for tuberculosis in close contacts, 101
Search policies
in contraband items, 270
in hidden drugs, 277
Seizures, 114-119
glucose blood levels in, 118, 141
Self-documentation
by nurses in personal journals, 231, 232s
by patients, 202-204
advantages and disadvantages of, 203s
in police custody, 224
Self-harm. See Harm, to self.
Sepsis, 173-177
shock in, 46, 173, 174, 176, 177
Sexual behavior of patient
health history interview on, 16-17
in unwanted sexual advance, 233-235
Shock, 46-52
anaphylactic, 46
cardiogenic, 46
distributive, 46
hypovolemic, 46
septic, 46, 173, 174, 176, 177
Sign language in hearing impairment, 285, 286, 288
Signatures
on late entries, 379
on notes of colleagues, 356-358
on telephone or verbal orders, 345, 347
on will, 316-320
Skin
care of
in cerebrovascular accident, 124
in unresponsive patient, 129
drug-induced disorders of, 178

Skin—cont'd
examination of
in heart failure, 42
in initial assessment, 20
in pneumonia, 70
in pneumothorax, 77
in pulmonary embolism, 87
in shock, 47
in unresponsive patient, 127-128
in intravenous infiltration, 181, 182
in pressure ulcers, 159-166
in wound dehiscence or evisceration, 193-197
in wound infections, 166-172
Skin test, tuberculin, 101, 101s
Slow code orders, 368s
Smoking, 266-269
nicotine replacement therapy for cessation of, 269
SOAP format of problem-oriented documentation, 5
Source-oriented documentation, 5
Specificity of assessment data, 13
Spoliation of evidence, 339s-340s
Sputum examination
in asthma, 84
in pneumonia, 70, 74
Staffing levels
legislation on, 358, 359s
in understaffed units, 358-360
Standards of practice
in charting by exception approach, 7
collegiality in, 336s
documentation guidelines in, 4
frequency of patient reassessment in, 119s
in pain management, 103s, 105s
physician orders deviating from, 44, 343
reporting colleague negligence in, 352-353
State v. Bright, 241s
Status epilepticus, 114-115
Stolen items
medical records, 209, 211-212
patient belongings, 304-306
Stool assessment, 20
in gastrointestinal hemorrhage, 134, 136
in unresponsive patient, 128
Street drugs as contraband possession, 269-272
Stroke, 120-125
Subjective data in SOAP notes, 5
Substitute or temporary medical records,
208-212, 342
recollection of previous entries in, 210s, 342
Suicidal behavior, 199, 254-259
discovery of hidden drugs in, 277
legal issues in, 258, 258s-259s
risk assessment in, 255, 256s
Surgery, 184-193
checklist on documentation in, 191s-192s
fraudulent concealment of accident during,
185s-186s
JCAHO safety goals concerning, 190s
for organ donation, 323-327
postoperative wound infections in, 167s-168s

Surgery—cont'd
  wound dehiscence or evisceration in, 193, 194
  in wound dehiscence or evisceration repair,
    195-196

T

Tachycardia
  ventricular, 59, 60, 61
    cardiopulmonary arrest in, 55
  wide-complex, 57, 58s
Tampering
  with medical equipment by patient, 272-275
    in chest tube, 280-283
    in endotracheal tube, 278-280
  with medical records by health care professional,
    332-335
    late entries in, 379s-380s
Teaching of patients and family, 14, 21-23.
    See also Education of patient and family.
Telephone use
  colleague reports in, 350
  orders from physician in, 329, 344-347
  triage in, retention of records on, 330, 330s-331s
Temporary or substitute medical records, 208-212, 342
  recollection of previous entries in, 210s, 342
Termination of life support, 56, 363-366
Theft
  of medical records, 209, 211-212
  of patient belongings, 304-306
Thornton v. Shah, 330s-331s
Threats from patients
  on harm to others, 239-244
  on lawsuit, 228-233
  on suicide, 254-259
Throat examination, 19
Thrombosis, cerebrovascular accident in, 120, 123
Time perception, pain affecting, 103
Tissue perfusion
  in heart failure, 42
  in shock, 47
  in wound dehiscence or evisceration, 195
Tobacco use, 266-269
Tracheal intubation. *See* Endotracheal intubation.
Transfer of patient, 374-377
  in chest pain, 33
  in suicide threat, 258s-259s
Transfusions
  in gastrointestinal hemorrhage, 138
  in peripheral pulse loss, 26-27
  reactions to, 150-154
  in shock, 50
Transplantation procedures, donation of organs for,
    323-327
Trauma
  in abuse, 308-311
  in accidental injury, 260-266
    smoking-related, 266-267, 268s
  pneumothorax in, 76, 77, 78
  in seizures, 116

Trauma—cont'd
Treatment refusal, 215-218. *See also* Refusal of
  treatment.
Triage on telephone, retention of medical records on,
  330, 330s-331s
Tube feeding aspiration, 130-133
Tuberculin skin test, 101, 101s
Tuberculosis, 96-102
  in AIDS, 155s

U

Ulcers of skin, 159-166
Unavailable medical records, 208-212
  in destruction of telephone triage logs,
    330s-331s
  incident report on, 211-212
  late entries in, 211, 378s
  in physician removal, 338-342
  as spoliation of evidence, 339s-340s
Uncooperative patient. *See also* Compliance
  issues.
  leaving against medical advice, 225-228
  plan of care for, 214, 214s
  withholding of information by, 212-215
Understaffed units, 358-360
  refusal of assignment to, 358
Uniform Anatomical Gift Act, 323
United Network for Organ Sharing, 324
Unlicensed assistive personnel, 353-356, 355s
  in understaffed units, 360
Unresponsive patient, 125-130, 314
  glucose blood levels in, 128, 141, 142
Urine evaluation
  in heart failure, 41, 42
  in hypertensive crisis, 66-67
  in initial assessment, 20
  in pulmonary edema, 95
  in shock, 48, 51
  in unresponsive patient, 128

V

Venous catheterization for therapy. *See* Intravenous
  therapy.
Ventilatory support
  in cerebrovascular accident, 123
  communication in, 313
  in sepsis, 176
  in shock, 49
  termination of, 366
Ventricular arrhythmias, 59, 60, 61
  cardiopulmonary arrest in, 55
Verbal physician orders, 329, 344-347
Vesicant solutions in intravenous therapy, infiltration
  of, 181, 182, 184
Videotaping of patients, 370-372
  identity disguised in, 371, 371s
Violent behavior
  in hostility, 236, 237
  threats of, 239-244

Vision impairment, 19, 288-291
  confusion in, 109, 111, 113
  safety issues in, 290, 291
  visual acuity testing in, 19, 289, 289s
Visitors
  refusal to leave, 311-312
  restrictions on, 310, 310s, 312
  special arrangements for, 312
Vital signs, 18
  in adverse drug reactions, 179
  in arrhythmias, 59
  in aspiration of tube feeding, 131
  in cerebrovascular accident, 124
  in gastrointestinal hemorrhage,
      135, 136
  in heart failure, 41, 43
  in hypertensive crisis, 64, 67
  in myocardial infarction, 37
  in pneumonia, 69, 70, 72, 73
    legal issues in monitoring of, 71s-72s
  in pneumothorax, 77
  postoperative, 189
  in sepsis, 173, 175
  in shock, 46, 49
  in transfusion reactions, 153
  in wound dehiscence or evisceration, 195
  in wound infections, 171

W
*Washington State Nurses Association v. Board of Medical
    Examiners,* 32s
Weapon possession, 269-272
Weight measurements, 18
  in heart failure, 41
  in obesity, 291, 293
White v. State of Washington, 247s-248s
Wills
  last will and testament, 316-320
    mental capacity in execution of, 318s-319s
    oral statement of dying patient, 320
    patient requests for advice on, 317-319, 320s
  living will, 215, 363, 364s
Wireless networks, 387s
Withholding of information by patients, 212-215
Withholding of treatment
  in do not resuscitate orders, 366-369
  nurse decisions on, 369-370, 369s
  in patient refusal, 215-218
Witness of will signing, 316-320
Wolff-Parkinson-White syndrome, 57
Wounds
  dehiscence and evisceration of, 193-197
  infection of, 166-172, 194
  in pressure ulcers, 159-166
  stages of, 162, 169, 170s

Printed in the United States
By Bookmasters